3rd edition

pharmacology

The National Medical Series for Independent Study

3rd edition

pharmacology

Leonard S. Jacob, M.D., Ph.D.

*Research Associate Professor
of Pharmacology
Medical College of Pennsylvania
Adjunct Associate Professor
of Pharmacology and Medicine
Temple University School
of Medicine
Philadelphia, Pennsylvania
Executive Vice President
Magainin Pharmaceuticals, Inc.
Plymouth Meeting, Pennsylvania*

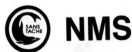 **NMS**

National Medical Series from Williams & Wilkins
Baltimore, Hong Kong, London, Sydney

Harwal Publishing Company, Malvern, Pennsylvania

Williams & Wilkins

Efforts have been made to ensure accuracy and immediacy in drug dosage schedules; however, this book is not intended as a guide to drug therapy. The reader is urged to consult the manufacturer's package insert to ascertain the recommended drug dosage, administration, and contraindications, especially relative to new and seldom-used drugs.

Library of Congress Cataloging-in-Publication Data

Jacob, Leonard S.
    Pharmacology / Leonard S. Jacob. — 3rd ed.
      p.   cm. — (The National medical series for independent study)
    Rev. ed. of: Pharmacology / editor, Leonard S. Jacob. 2nd ed.
  c 1987.
    Includes index.
    ISBN 0-683-06250-6 (alk. paper)
    1. Pharmacology—Examinations, questions, etc.   I. Pharmacology.
  II. Title. III. Series.
    [DNLM: 1. Pharmacology—examination questions. 2. Pharmacology—
  outlines. QV 18 J15p]
  RM105.J33   1992
  615'.1076—dc20
  DNLM/DLC
  for Library of Congress   91-21585
                                                   CIP

ISBN 0-683-06250-6

10 9 8 7 6 5 4 3

To Terri, Stefanie, and Ellen

Contents

Preface

The success of *Pharmacology* continues to exceed my most optimistic expectations. Continuous telephone calls and letters praising its content and presentation are most gratifying. To help students prepare for the National Board examinations has been a stated purpose of the *National Medical Series*. In reality, it serves a far greater role; namely, it allows medical students to learn in a concise but comprehensive fashion about how to treat illness.

Many physicians believe that the "pen" is as important as the scalpel. It is estimated that 80% of recommended treatment is by prescription. This book, if used judiciously, will aid in ensuring that the practitioner "will do no harm" and hopefully will help the patient.

The third edition, as the previous two, updates the dynamic discipline of pharmacology. *Pharmacology,* third edition, has been extensively revised to reflect the up-to-date treatment of new diseases, such as AIDS and Lyme disease, as well as new treatment of old diseases, such as fungal infections and congestive heart failure. Again, my hope is that *Pharmacology* will play an important role in helping to educate all those students who are committed to healing sick individuals.

Leonard S. Jacob

Acknowledgments

The writing and editing of this third edition have been made much easier with the help of my academic colleagues, from whom I continuously learn, and my students and residents who continuously challenge me. Additionally, my secretary Sandra Hitner ensures that the many journals I read each week are appropriately catalogued, creating a ready reference to the latest therapeutic information.

A special thanks is extended to Bob Zeid, who contributed to the reorganization of the endocrine and cancer chemotherapy chapters.

Finally, Jane Edwards provided superb editorial guidance. Her diligence in ensuring an outstanding text and my contribution to that in a timely fashion is both remembered and appreciated.

Leonard S. Jacob

We wish to acknowledge the significant contribution of Dr. John Lazo and Dr. Edward Hawrot as associate editors on the first edition of *Pharmacology*.

The Publisher

To the Reader

Since 1984, the *National Medical Series for Independent Study* has been helping medical students meet the challenge of education and clinical training. In today's climate of burgeoning information and complex clinical issues, a medical career is more demanding than ever. Increasingly, medical training must prepare physicians to seek and synthesize necessary information and to apply that information successfully.

The *National Medical Series* is designed to provide a logical framework for organizing, learning, reviewing, and applying the conceptual and factual information covered in basic and clinical sciences. Each book includes a comprehensive outline of the essential content of a discipline, with up to 500 study questions. The combination of an outlined text and tools for self-evaluation allows easy retrieval of salient information.

All study questions are accompanied by the correct answer, a paragraph-length explanation, and specific reference to the text where the topic is discussed. Study questions that follow each chapter use the current National Board format to reinforce the chapter content. Study questions appearing at the end of the text in the Comprehensive Exam vary in format depending on the book. Wherever possible, Comprehensive Exam questions are presented as clinical cases or scenarios intended to simulate real-life application of medical knowledge. The goal of this exam is to challenge the student to draw from information presented throughout the book.

All of the books in the *National Medical Series* are constantly being updated and revised. The authors and editors devote considerable time and effort to ensure that the information required by all medical school curricula is included. Strict editorial attention is given to accuracy, organization, and consistency. Further shaping of the series occurs in response to biannual discussions held with a panel of medical student advisors drawn from schools throughout the United States. At these meetings, the editorial staff considers the needs of medical students to learn how the *National Medical Series* can better serve them. In this regard, the Harwal staff welcomes all comments and suggestions.

General Pharmacologic Principles

I. INTRODUCTION. Pharmacology is the study of the biochemical and physiologic aspects of drug effects, including absorption, distribution, metabolism, elimination, toxicity, and specific mechanisms of drug action. The two main areas of pharmacology are pharmacokinetics and pharmacodynamics.

A. Pharmacokinetics refers to the way the body handles drug absorption, distribution, biotransformation, and excretion. Once the pharmacokinetics of a drug is determined, rational dosage regimens can be instituted.

B. Pharmacodynamics is the study of the biochemical and physiologic effects of drugs and their mechanisms of action.

II. PHARMACOKINETICS

A. General principles

1. **Drug transport.** The movement of drug molecules in the body affects absorption, distribution, and excretion. Drugs can cross cellular membranes by simple diffusion, carrier-mediated diffusion, filtration, active transport, or endocytosis. The cell membrane, being a bimolecular lipid layer, can also act as a barrier to some drugs.

   a. **Passive diffusion.** Most foreign compounds penetrate cells by diffusing as the **un-ionized moiety** through the lipid membrane. Factors affecting the passage of a molecule through a membrane are the molecule's size and charge, the lipid–water partition coefficient, and the concentration gradient. The two types of passive drug transport are **simple diffusion** and **filtration**.

      (1) **Simple diffusion**

         (a) Simple diffusion is based on **Fick's law**:

         $$dQ/dt = (- D)(A)(dc/dx)$$

         where dQ/dt is the rate of drug flux (i.e., the change in concentration of a drug within a given time); D is a temperature-dependent diffusion constant of the molecule; A is the area of the absorbing surface; and dc/dx is the concentration gradient.

         (i) The greater the concentration gradient, the greater the rate of absorption.

         (ii) The larger the absorbing surface, the greater the drug flux.

         (iii) The diffusion constant, D, is directly proportional to the temperature and is inversely related to the molecular size.

         (iv) The greater the lipid–water partition coefficient, the greater the drug flux.

         (b) In simple diffusion, molecules cross the lipid membrane in an **uncharged form**. The distribution of the uncharged form is a function of the pK_a of the compound and the pH of the medium and is expressed by the **Henderson-Hasselbalch equation:**

         (i) If the drug is a weak acid:

         $$pK_a = pH + \log \frac{\text{concentration of un-ionized acid}}{\text{concentration of ionized acid}}$$

         (ii) If the drug is a weak base:

         $$pK_a = pH + \log \frac{\text{concentration of ionized base}}{\text{concentration of un-ionized base}}$$

         (c) The pH of the medium, therefore, affects the absorption and excretion of a passively diffused drug.

(i) Aspirin and other weak acids are best absorbed in the stomach because of its acidic environment.

(ii) Alkalinic drugs are best absorbed in the small intestine, which has a higher pH.

(iii) Since the pH of urine is acidic, a weakly acidic drug can be extensively re-absorbed into the body from the urine. If the pH of the urine is increased, excretion of the drug can be increased.

(2) **Filtration**

(a) Water, ions, and some polar and nonpolar molecules of low molecular weight can diffuse through membranes, suggesting that **pores** or **channels** may exist.

(b) The capillaries of some vascular beds (e.g., in the kidney) have large pores, which permit the passage of molecules as large as proteins.

b. **Carrier-mediated facilitated diffusion**

(1) In this type of transport, movement across the membrane is facilitated by a macro-molecule.

(2) The properties of carrier-mediated diffusion are as follows:

(a) It is a saturable process; that is, external concentrations can be achieved in which increasing the external/internal concentration gradient will not increase the rate of influx.

(b) It is selective for the chemical structure of a drug; that is, the carrier mechanism transports only those drugs having a specific molecular configuration.

(c) It requires no energy.

(d) It cannot move against a concentration gradient and, therefore, is still a diffusion process.

c. **Active transport**

(1) Active transport is similar to carrier-mediated diffusion in several ways:

(a) Movement across the membrane is mediated by a macromolecule.

(b) It is a saturable process.

(c) It is selective for chemical structure.

(2) Several important features, however, distinguish active transport from diffusion processes:

(a) Active transport requires metabolic energy; this is often generated by the enzyme known as Na^+-K^+-ATPase.

(b) It transports molecules against a concentration gradient.

d. **Endocytosis** is a minor method by which some drugs are transported into cells.

(1) A vacuolar apparatus in some cells is responsible for this process.

(2) There exist both **fluid-phase endocytosis** for substances such as sucrose and **adsorptive-phase endocytosis** for substances such as insulin.

2. **Bioavailability** is the relative rate and extent to which an administered drug reaches the general circulation; this is especially important when a drug is administered orally. Factors that influence bioavailability are:

a. Solubility of the drug in the contents of the stomach

b. Dietary patterns

c. Tablet size

d. Quality control in manufacturing and formulation

B. **Absorption** is the rate at which a drug leaves the site of administration and the extent to which this occurs. The absorption of a drug through the mucosal lining of the gastrointestinal tract or through capillary walls depends on the physical and chemical properties of the drug.

1. **Route of administration** is an important determinant of the rate and efficiency of absorption.

a. **Alimentary routes** are the most common routes of administration.

(1) **Examples of alimentary routes**

(a) Oral

(b) Rectal

(c) Sublingual

(d) Buccal

(2) **Advantages of alimentary administration**

(a) An alimentary route is generally the safest route of administration. The delivery of the drug into the circulation is slow after oral administration, so that rapid, high blood levels are avoided and adverse effects are less likely.

(b) The dosage forms available for alimentary administration are convenient and do not require sterile technique.

(3) Disadvantages of alimentary administration
  (a) The rate of absorption varies. This becomes a problem if a small range in blood levels separates a drug's desired therapeutic effect from its toxic effects.
  (b) Irritation of mucosal surfaces can occur.
  (c) Patient compliance is not ensured.
  (d) With oral administration of some drugs, extensive hepatic metabolism may occur before the drug reaches its site of action. This is known as the **first-pass effect**. Passage through the liver and the resulting initial hepatic metabolism are avoided by administering the drug sublingually.
b. Parenteral routes bypass the alimentary tract.
  (1) Examples of parenteral routes
    (a) Intravenous
    (b) Intramuscular
    (c) Subcutaneous
    (d) Intraperitoneal
    (e) Intra-arterial
    (f) Intrathecal
    (g) Transdermal
  (2) Advantages of parenteral administration
    (a) The drug gets to the site of action more quickly, providing a rapid response, which may be required in an emergency.
    (b) The dose can often be more accurately delivered.
    (c) Parenteral administration can be used when the alimentary route is not feasible (e.g., when the patient is unconscious).
    (d) Large volumes can be delivered intravenously.
  (3) Disadvantages of parenteral administration
    (a) More rapid absorption can lead to increased adverse effects.
    (b) A sterile formulation and an aseptic technique are required.
    (c) Local irritation may occur at the site of injection.
    (d) Parenteral administration is not suitable for insoluble substances.
c. Miscellaneous routes
  (1) Topical administration is useful in the treatment of patients with local conditions; with topical administration, there is usually little systemic absorption. Drugs can be applied to various mucous membranes and skin.
  (2) Inhalation provides a rapid access to circulation; it is the common route of administration for gaseous and volatile drugs.

2. Factors affecting drug absorption
  a. Solubility of the drug affects absorption.
  b. Dosage affects the drug's concentration at its site of action and, thus, greatly influences the biologic response to the drug. The larger the dose, the greater the effect, until a maximum effect is achieved. This is called the **dose–response relationship**.
  c. Route of administration. The route of administration affects the area of absorbing surface available to the drug. Drugs are absorbed more quickly from large surface areas.
    (1) After any route of administration except intravenous administration, the absorption of most drugs follows **first-order (exponential) kinetics;** thus, a constant *fraction* of drug is absorbed.
    (2) After intravenous administration, the absorption of a drug follows **zero-order kinetics;** thus, a constant *amount* (i.e., 100%) of drug is absorbed.

C. Distribution. After absorption or injection, drugs may be distributed into interstitial or cellular fluids.

1. Drug distribution
  a. Once in the circulatory system, some drugs can **bind** nonspecifically and reversibly to various **plasma proteins;** that is, to albumin or globulins.
    (1) In this case, the bound and free drug reach an equilibrium.
    (2) Only the **free drug** exerts a biologic effect; the bound drug stays in the vascular space, and is not metabolized or eliminated.
  b. Some areas of the body (e.g., the brain) are not readily accessible to drugs due to **anatomic barriers**. The placenta also provides a barrier to some drugs.

    c. Some drugs may be **sequestered** in storage depots; for example, lipid-soluble drugs in fatty tissue. The drug stored in these depots is in equilibrium with free circulating drug.

    d. Eventually, the drug achieves a free state and is excreted either directly or after it has been metabolized.

    e. Factors modifying the **distribution** of a drug to a particular region of the body:

      (1) Physical and chemical characteristics of the drug (lipid to water partition coefficient)

      (2) Cardiac output

      (3) Capillary permeability in various tissues

      (4) Lipid content of the tissue

      (5) Binding to plasma proteins and tissues

2. Clinical distribution

    a. One-compartment model. This is the simplest and most commonly used pharmacokinetic model system.

      (1) Distribution of the drug within the compartment is assumed to be **uniform** and is assumed to occur **rapidly** in comparison to absorption and elimination.

      (2) The **apparent volume of distribution (V_d)** is a quantitative estimate of the tissue localization of the drug.

        (a) It can be determined by measuring the plasma level of the drug:

$$V_d = \frac{\text{total amount of drug in body}}{\text{concentration of drug in plasma}}$$

        (b) In general, a high V_d indicates high lipophilicity or many receptors for the drug.

      (3) The **total body clearance** is the volume of blood or plasma that is effectively cleared of drug in a specified unit of time.

        (a) Clearance is related to V_d and to the time required for the plasma drug concentration or the amount in the body to decrease by 50%, which is called **half-life ($t_{1/2}$)**. Clearance is, therefore, related to the **elimination rate constant (k)**:

$$\begin{aligned} \text{Clearance} &= V_d(k) \\ &= \frac{V_d(0.693)}{t_{1/2}} \end{aligned}$$

        (b) This formula assumes a specific V_d, but the V_d changes over time.

    b. Two-compartment model

      (1) This model is generally used for drugs that are not administered intravenously because it can better describe both distribution and elimination.

      (2) The distribution rate constant in this model is known as the **alpha half-life,** or $t_{1/2\alpha}$.

      (3) The elimination rate constant in this model, known as the **beta half-life,** or $t_{1/2\beta}$, is therapeutically more important than the $t_{1/2\alpha}$.

    c. The multicompartment model is used for drugs that are stored in body depots and for drugs with extensive metabolism or elimination mechanisms.

D. Drug metabolism/biotransformation is the process of chemical alteration of drugs in the body.

1. Principles

    a. The liver is the major site of metabolism for many drugs or other xenobiotics, but other organs, such as the lungs, kidneys, and adrenal glands, can also metabolize drugs.

    b. Many lipid-soluble, weak organic acids or bases are not readily eliminated from the body and must be conjugated or metabolized to compounds that are more polar and less lipid-soluble before being excreted.

    c. Metabolism often, but not always, results in **inactivation** of the compound.

    d. Some drugs are **activated** by metabolism. These substances are called **prodrugs.**

2. Biochemical reactions involved in drug metabolism occur in two phases: Phase 1 reactions (e.g., oxidation, reduction, hydrolysis) alter chemical reactivity and increase aqueous solubility; phase 2 reactions (e.g., conjugation) further increase the solubility, promoting elimination.

    a. Oxidation, the most common metabolic reaction, involves the addition of oxygen or the removal of hydrogen from the drug.

      (1) Microsomal oxidation

        (a) The smooth endoplasmic reticulum of cells in many organs, especially the liver, contain **membrane-associated enzymes,** which are responsible for drug oxidation.

(b) The subcellular components of the endoplasmic reticulum, called **microsomes,** can be isolated by centrifugation of organ homogenates.

(c) The primary components of this enzyme system are **cytochrome P-450 reductase** and **cytochrome P-450**. Several distinct isozymes of cytochrome P-450 exist within the microsomal membrane.

(d) This enzyme system has been termed a **mixed-function oxygenase** because one oxygen atom in molecular oxygen is incorporated into a drug in the form of a hydroxyl (−OH) moiety, and the other is incorporated into water. Reduced nicotinamide adenine dinucleotide phosphate (NADPH) provides the reducing equivalents.

(e) Types of microsomal oxidation reactions are:

   (i) Carbon oxidation–hydroxylation of aliphatic or aromatic groups (e.g., pentobarbital and phenytoin)

   (ii) *N*- or *O*-dealkylation (e.g., diazepam and codeine)

   (iii) *N*-oxidation or *N*-hydroxylation (e.g., 2-acetylaminofluorene)

   (iv) Sulfoxide formulation (e.g., chlorpromazine)

   (v) Deamination (e.g., amphetamine)

   (vi) Desulfuration (e.g., thiobarbital)

(f) The microsomal oxidative system also metabolizes endogenous fatty acids and steroids.

(g) A number of drugs and environmental substances can induce (increase) or inhibit the microsomal enzyme system (see Chapter 13 II D 5).

(2) Nonmicrosomal oxidation

(a) Soluble enzymes found in the cytosol or mitochondria of cells are responsible for the metabolism of relatively few compounds. These enzyme activities are, however, important.

(b) Examples include:

   (i) **Alcohol dehydrogenase** and **aldehyde dehydrogenase,** which oxidize ethanol to acetaldehyde and acetate, respectively, in reactions requiring oxidized nicotinamide adenine dinucleotide (NAD$^+$)

   (ii) **Xanthine oxidase,** which converts hypoxanthine to xanthine and xanthine to uric acid

   (iii) **Tyrosine hydroxylase,** which is important in the synthesis of adrenergic neurotransmitters because it hydroxylates tyrosine to dopa (L-β-3,4-dihydroxyphenylalanine)

   (iv) **Monoamine oxidase,** which is important to the metabolism of catecholamines and serotonin

b. Reduction occurs in both the microsomal and nonmicrosomal metabolizing systems; it is less common than oxidation.

(1) Examples of microsomal reduction include nitro (chloramphenicol) and azo (prontosil).

(2) Examples of nonmicrosomal reduction include aldehyde (chloral hydrate), ketone (naloxone), and quinone (menadione).

c. Hydrolysis

(1) Nonmicrosomal hydrolases exist in a variety of body systems, including the plasma. Examples of **nonmicrosomal hydrolases** are:

   (a) Nonspecific **esterases** for drugs, such as acetylcholine, succinylcholine, and procaine

   (b) **Peptidases** (e.g., proinsulin)

   (c) **Amidases** for drugs, such as procainamide and indomethacin

(2) Microsomal hydrolases have also been identified.

d. Conjugation involves the coupling of a drug or its metabolite with an endogenous substrate, usually inorganic sulfate, a methyl group, acetic acid, an amino acid, or a carbohydrate. Usually, a conjugate is a readily excreted polar substance.

(1) Glucuronide conjugation is the most common conjugation reaction. It occurs frequently with phenols, alcohols, and carboxylic acids.

   (a) Activated glucuronic acid (uridine diphosphoglucuronic acid; UDP-glucuronide) is formed from glucose 1-phosphate, which then reacts as follows:

$$\text{UDP-glucuronide} + \text{ROH} \rightarrow \text{RO-glucuronide} + \text{UDP}$$

where ROH is the drug or its metabolite.

(b) Glucuronides are generally inactive and are rapidly excreted in urine or bile by anionic transport systems.

(c) Glucuronides eliminated in the bile can be hydrolyzed by intestinal or bacterial β-glucuronidases, and free drug can be reabsorbed. This **enterohepatic recirculation** can greatly extend the action of a drug.

(2) Other conjugation reactions. All conjugations except glucuronide formation are catalyzed by nonmicrosomal enzymes. These reactions include:

(a) Sulfate formation, in which phenols, alcohols, and aromatic amines are converted to sulfates and sulfanilates; 3'-phosphoadenosine 5'-phosphosulfate (PAPS) is the sulfate donor (e.g., steroids)

(b) *O-, S-,* and *N*-methylation; *S*-adenosylmethionine is the methyl donor (e.g., norepinephrine)

(c) *N*-acetylation; acetyl coenzyme A is the acetyl donor (e.g., isoniazid)

(d) Glycine and glutamine conjugation with acids (e.g., salicylic acid)

(e) Glutathione conjugation (e.g., ethacrynic acid)

3. Factors affecting drug metabolism

a. Genetics. The most important factor is genetically determined polymorphisms. The acetylation of isoniazid and the hydrolysis of succinylcholine are genetically controlled.

b. Chemical properties of the drug. Certain drugs may stimulate or inhibit the metabolism of the other drugs (e.g., phenobarbital stimulates the metabolism of diphenylhydantoin).

c. Route of administration. The oral route, for example, can result in extensive hepatic metabolism of some drugs (the **first-pass effect**).

d. Diet. Starvation can deplete glycine stores and alter glycine conjugation.

e. Dosage. Toxic doses can deplete enzymes needed for detoxification reactions.

f. Age. The liver cannot detoxify drugs, such as chloramphenicol, as well in neonates as it can in adults.

g. Gender. Young males are more prone to sedation from barbiturates than females.

h. Disease. Liver disease decreases the ability to metabolize drugs, while kidney disease hampers the excretion of drugs.

i. Species differences. Experimental findings in animals do not necessarily translate to humans.

j. Circadian rhythm. In rats and mice, the rate of hepatic metabolism of some drugs follows a diurnal rhythm. This may be true in humans as well.

E. Drug excretion is the process by which a drug or metabolite is eliminated from the body.

1. Rate of elimination

a. For most drugs, **elimination from the blood** follows exponential (first-order) kinetics.

b. The elimination process can be saturated after high doses of some drugs, and elimination will then follow zero-order kinetics. Ethanol is a prototypic example.

c. For drugs that are eliminated by first-order kinetics, the fractional change in the amount of drug in the plasma or blood per unit of time is expressed by the **half-life ($t_{1/2}$)**—or by the **elimination rate constant (k)**, which is equal to $0.693/t_{1/2}$.

2. Routes of elimination

a. The **kidney** is the most important organ for excretion of drugs. Excretion of drugs and their metabolites into the urine involves three processes:

(1) Glomerular filtration. Water-soluble and polar compounds are unable to diffuse back into circulation and are excreted unless a specific transport exists for their reabsorption.

(2) Active tubular secretion. Mechanisms for active tubular secretion exist in the proximal tubule. Drugs such as organic acids (e.g., penicillin, bases, quinine) are transported by these systems.

(3) Passive tubular reabsorption

b. The **biliary tract and the feces** are important routes of excretion for some drugs that are metabolized in the liver.

c. Other routes. Drugs and their metabolites can also be eliminated in expired air, sweat, saliva, tears, and breast milk. Drugs eliminated through these routes tend to be lipid-soluble and nonionized.

F. Effect of repeated doses

1. A drug accumulates in the body if the time interval between doses is less than four of its half-lives, in which case the total body stores of the drug increase exponentially to a plateau. This plateau is known as the **steady-state concentration**.

2. The **average total body store** of a drug at the plateau is a function of the dose, the interval between doses, and the elimination half-life of the drug.
   a. When the drug is administered in intervals that equal its half-life of elimination, the average total body store of the drug is approximately equal to 1.5 times the amount administered.
   b. When the drug is given by constant infusion, the plasma concentration will be within 10% of the desired steady-state concentration after four elimination half-lives.

III. PHARMACODYNAMICS

A. Mechanisms of drug action

1. It is currently believed that most drugs interact with macromolecular components (called **receptors**) of a cell or an organism to begin biochemical and physiologic changes that produce the drug's observed effects or **response**.
   a. Receptors bind ligands and transduce signals.
   b. Drug receptors are identified primarily by the effect or lack of effect of antagonists and the relative strength of agonists.
      (1) A drug is called an **agonist** if it produces some of the effects of endogenous compounds when it interacts with the receptor. The agonist, acetylcholine, has intrinsic activity.
      (2) An **antagonist** is a drug that has no intrinsic activity yet can reduce or abolish the effect of an agonist.
         (a) Examples of pure antagonists are atropine and curare, which inhibit the effect of acetylcholine.
         (b) Atropine and curare occupy cholinergic receptor sites (curare in nicotinic skeletal muscle, atropine in muscarinic smooth muscle; see Chapter 2 I D), preventing the further binding of acetylcholine to these receptors.
      (3) Some drugs (e.g., nalorphine) are **partial antagonists;** that is, they possess some intrinsic activity.
   c. In general, the effect (E) is a function of the quantity of the drug–receptor complex (DR), and can be expressed as:

$$E = \alpha\,[DR]$$

      (1) The magnitude of E depends on the amount of DR, which, in turn, depends on the amount of drug given. Once all receptors are saturated, the maximum effect is achieved.
      (2) Alpha (α) is a constant for a given drug and is a partial determinant of whether an effect occurs.
      (3) Alpha (α) is determined experimentally and is considered to be a measure of a drug's **intrinsic activity;** that is, its inherent ability to produce an effect. If α is a zero, the drug has no intrinsic pharmacologic activity, and, therefore, if the drug binds to the receptor, it must be an effective antagonist.

2. Other drugs may not cause a response by interacting with receptors. These drugs may combine with small molecules or ions found in the body (e.g., chelating agents).

B. Receptors are specific drug-binding sites in a cell or on its surface, which mediate the action of the drug. Some drugs (e.g., mannitol) are believed not to have specific receptors.

1. **Ion channel**
   a. Hormones and neurotransmitters enhance the movement of ions across membranes.
   b. The hormone or neurotransmitter receptor may be an ion channel.
   c. Ion receptors are confined to excitable tissue (e.g., central nervous system, neuromuscular junction, autonomic ganglia).
   d. Agonists that activate ion channel receptors produce depolarization or hyperpolarization.
   e. Examples of ion channel receptors include the nicotinic acetylcholine receptor, the gamma-aminobutyric acid (GABA) receptor, the glutamine receptor, and the glycine receptor.

2. **G proteins**
   a. Receptors on the inner face of the plasma membrane regulate or facilitate effector proteins through a group of guanosine triphosphate (GTP) proteins known as G proteins.
   b. Some hormone peptide receptors and neurotransmitter receptors (e.g., α and β adrenergic and muscarinic receptors) depend on G proteins to mediate their actions on cells.
   c. Each G protein can respond to several different receptors and regulate several effectors.

d. Effectors include adenylyl cyclase and phospholipases C and A_2 and channels specific for Na^+, K^+, and Ca^{2+}.

e. Each cell can express several G proteins. Each G protein consists of α, β, and γ subunits. Specificity for receptor–effector coupling lies within the α portion.

f. Termination of signal transmission results from hydrolysis of GTP to guanosine diphosphate (GDP) by GTPase that is intrinsic to the α subunit.

3. Hormones

a. Steroid hormones bind to intracellular receptors. These receptors are proteins associated with the nuclear matrix.

b. The steroid receptor complex ultimately increases binding of RNA polymerase and the expression of regulated genes.

c. Examples of such receptors include those for estrogen, progesterone, glucocorticoid, triiodothyronine (T_3), thyroxine (T_4), and vitamin D.

4. Tyrosine kinases

a. A variety of growth factors and growth-promoting hormones [e.g., colony-stimulating factor (CSF), epidermal growth factor (EGF), insulin-life growth factor (IGF-1)] and certain oncogenes interact with receptors that have tyrosine-specific protein kinase activity.

b. These receptors are located on the plasma membrane and are critical proteins in cell growth and differentiation.

C. Receptor regulation

1. Certain receptors when exposed to an agonist repeatedly can become desensitized or down-regulated. For example, β-adrenergic bronchodilators used in the treatment of patients with asthma can become less effective over time when administered at the same concentration. The signal from the stimulated receptor can become depressed, or the receptor itself can be altered.

2. Supersensitivity of receptors to agonists can occur with chronic administration of an antagonist. For instance, the abrupt discontinuation of propranolol in a patient who had been taking it chronically, could precipitate dysrhythmias. Supersensitivity may result from the synthesis of additional receptors (up-regulation).

D. Dose–response relationships

1. Quantal dose–response curve

a. A **quantal response** is an all-or-none response to a drug and relates to the frequency with which a specified dose of a drug produces a specific response in a population (e.g., death among the mice in a preclinical study or a 20% decrease in blood pressure among the patients in a clinical trial).

b. The smallest amount of a drug that will produce a quantal response is not the same for all members of a population. If the frequency of response is plotted against the minimum dose necessary to produce the response, the result is often a gaussian distribution. A graphic representation of this gaussian **frequency distribution curve** is shown in Figure 1-1.

c. The **quantal dose–response curve** is a cumulative graph of the frequency distribution curve (Figure 1-2).

2. Graded dose–response curve (Figure 1-3)

a. As the dosage administered to a single subject or isolated tissue is increased, the pharmacologic effect will also increase (**graded dose–response**).

b. At a certain dose, the resulting effect will reach a maximum level (**ceiling effect**).

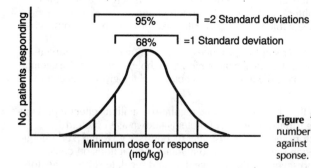

Figure 1-1. Frequency distribution curve, plotting the number of patients showing a quantal response to a drug against the minimum dose needed to produce the response.

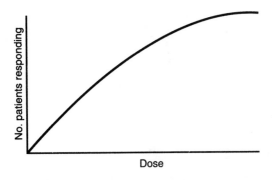

Figure 1-2. Quantal dose–response curve, cumulating the data used in plotting Figure 1-1.

  c. Efficacy versus potency
    (1) Efficacy is the maximum effect of a drug, E_{max} (see Figure 1-3).
      (a) Efficacy is independent of the slope or position of the dose–response curve. In Figure 1-3, drugs A and B have equal efficacies (i.e., the same E_{max}).
      (b) Drugs such as aspirin and morphine produce the same pharmacologic effect (analgesia) but have very different levels of efficacy.
    (2) Potency, a comparative measure, refers to the different doses of two drugs that are needed to produce the same effect.
      (a) In Figure 1-3, drug A is more potent than drug B, since the dose of drug B (D_B) must be larger than the dose of drug A (D_A) to produce a given effect (E_1).
      (b) Meaningful comparisons of potency can be made only when the drugs being compared have log dose–response curves (see III D 3) of the same slope.
      (c) K_D (the dissociation constant for the drug–receptor complex) and the ED_{50} [see III D 3 a (1)] are measures of drug **potency**.
    (3) Potency is independent of efficacy, and efficacy is usually more important than potency in selecting drugs for clinical use.

  3. Log dose–response curve
    a. To construct the log–dose response curve, the log of the dose is plotted on the abscissa and the drug effect on the ordinate. This causes the hyperbolic graded dose–response curve to become sigmoidal. Log dose–response curves for two drugs, A and B, are shown in Figure 1-4.
    (1) The **ED_{50},** the smallest dose showing an effect that is 50% of the maximum, is a measure of drug **potency:** The smaller the ED_{50}, the greater the potency. Thus, in Figure 1-4, drug A is more potent than drug B.
    (2) Efficacy is indicated by the **height** of the log dose–response curve. Drug B in Figure 1-4 is less efficacious than drug A; the E_{max} of the two drugs is, therefore, different.
    b. One advantage of plotting on a logarithmic scale is that drugs with the same action at a receptor, but with different potencies, usually will show dose–response curves that are parallel.

  4. Antagonism between drugs
    a. Pharmacologic antagonism occurs when an antagonist prevents an agonist from interacting with its receptors to produce an effect. This type of antagonism can be either competitive or noncompetitive.

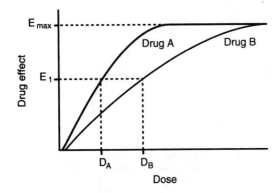

Figure 1-3. Graded dose–response curves for two drugs, A and B. E_{max} = maximum effect; D_A and D_B = amount (dose) of drug A and drug B, respectively, needed to produce the drug effect, E_1.

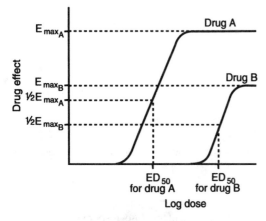

Figure 1-4. Log dose–response curves for two drugs, A and B. E_{max} = maximum effect; ED_{50} = smallest dose showing an effect that is 50% of the E_{max}.

   (1) Competitive antagonism
       (a) Competitive antagonists compete with agonists in a reversible fashion for the same receptor site.
       (b) When the antagonist is present, the log dose–response curve is shifted to the right, indicating that a higher concentration of agonist is necessary to achieve the same response as when the antagonist is absent.
       (c) In the presence of the antagonist, if enough agonist is given, the E_{max} can be achieved, indicating that the action of the antagonist has been overcome. This results in a **parallel shift** of the dose–response curve, as shown in Figure 1-5.
   (2) Noncompetitive antagonism
       (a) The noncompetitive antagonist binds irreversibly to the receptor site or to another site that inhibits the response to the agonist.
       (b) No matter how much agonist is given, the action of the antagonist cannot be overcome.
       (c) This results in a **nonparallel shift** of the log dose–response curve with a lower E_{max} (Figure 1-6).
b. Physiologic antagonism. With pharmacologic antagonism, the agonist and antagonist compete for the *same* receptor site. In contrast, with physiologic antagonism, the drugs act independently on two *different* receptors.
   (1) Physiologic antagonism is exemplified by one drug acting on the sympathetic nervous system causing the heart rate to increase and causing vasoconstriction; while another drug acting on the parasympathetic nervous system decreases the heart rate and causes vasodilation.
   (2) Using physiologic antagonists is generally less preferable than using a receptor-specific antagonist. Since physiologic antagonists work on different receptors, they produce effects that are harder to control than the effects of a receptor-specific antagonist.
c. Antagonism by neutralization (also called **chemical antagonism**) occurs when two drugs combine with one another to form an inactive compound. For example, drugs containing sulfhydryl (—SH) groups, when combined with mercury or arsenic, no longer show agonistic actions.

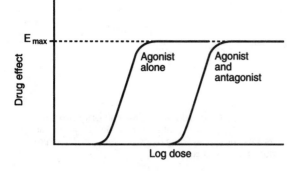

Figure 1-5. Shift in the log dose–response curve that occurs when an agonist is administered in the presence of a competitive antagonist.

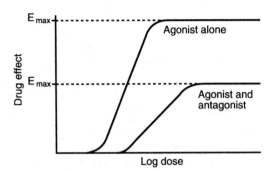

Figure 1-6. Shift in the log dose–response curve and lowering of the maximum effect (E_{max}) that occur when an agonist is given in the presence of a noncompetitive antagonist.

5. Enhancement of drug effects

a. Additive drug effects occur if two drugs with the same effect, when given together, produce an effect that is **equal in magnitude** to the sum of the effects when the drugs are given individually:

$$E_{AB} = E_A + E_B \qquad 1 + 1 = 2$$

b. Synergism occurs if two drugs with the same effect, when given together, produce an effect that is **greater in magnitude** than the sum of the effects when the drugs are given individually:

$$E_{AB} > E_A + E_B \qquad 1 + 1 > 2$$

c. Potentiation occurs if a drug lacking an effect of its own increases the effect of a second, active drug:

$$E_{AB} > E_A + E_B \qquad 0 + 1 > 1$$

6. Therapeutic index (TI) and margin of safety

a. The **therapeutic index** is a ratio used to evaluate the safety and usefulness of a drug for an indication. It is a measurement that describes the relationship between doses of a drug required to produce undesired and desired effects.

(1) The formula for the therapeutic index is:

$$TI = \frac{LD_{50}}{ED_{50}}$$

where LD_{50} is the mimimum dose that is *lethal* or toxic for 50% of the population, and ED_{50} is the minimum dose that is *effective* for 50% of the population.*

(2) Ideally, the LD_{50} should be a much higher dose than the ED_{50}, so that the therapeutic index would be large.

b. Standard margin of safety. The therapeutic index may be misleading if the log dose–response curves for effectiveness and toxicity have different slopes (i.e., are not parallel). Therefore, the standard margin of safety may be more useful.

(1) The formula for the standard margin of safety is:

$$\frac{(LD_1)}{(ED_{99})} - 1 \times 100$$

(2) The standard margin of safety shows the percentage by which the ED_{99} (the dose effective in 99% of the population) must be increased to cause toxic effects in 1% of the population.

(3) For example, if 100 mg of a drug causes toxicity in 1% of the population and 10 mg is effective in 99%, then the drug's standard margin of safety is $(100/10) - 1 \times 100$, or 900. Therefore, the dose that is effective in 99% must be increased 900% to be toxic to 1% of the population.

---

*Note that the definition for ED_{50} here is for a population rather than a single individual or tissue, and thus it differs from the ED_{50} in III D 3 a (1).

STUDY QUESTIONS

Directions: Each of the numbered items or incomplete statements in this section is followed by answers or by completions of the statement. Select the **one** lettered answer or completion that is **best** in each case.

1. All of the following statements about Fick's law as it pertains to simple diffusion are true EXCEPT

(A) the greater the concentration gradient, the greater the rate of absorption
(B) the smaller the surface area, the greater the drug flux
(C) the greater the lipid–water partition coefficient, the greater the drug flux
(D) diffusion constant is directly proportional to the temperature
(E) diffusion constant is inversely related to the molecular size

2. Correct statements concerning characteristics of a particular route of drug administration include all of the following EXCEPT

(A) intravenous administration provides a rapid response
(B) oral administration requires that the patient be alert
(C) intramuscular administration requires sterile technique
(D) subcutaneous administration may cause local irritation
(E) inhalation administration provides slow access to the general circulation

3. The first-pass effect occurs most often after which route of drug administration?

(A) Oral
(B) Sublingual
(C) Intravenous
(D) Subcutaneous
(E) Intramuscular

4. Properties of drug absorption include all of the following EXCEPT

(A) the route of administration is an important factor affecting drug absorption
(B) the rate of absorption varies after oral administration
(C) after rectal administration, drug absorption follows first-order kinetics
(D) after intramuscular administration, drug absorption follows first-order kinetics
(E) with intravenous administration, drug absorption follows first-order kinetics

5. All of the following statements about efficacy and potency are true EXCEPT that

(A) efficacy is usually a more important clinical consideration than potency
(B) efficacy is indicated by the height of the log dose–response curve
(C) the ED_{50} is a measure of a drug's efficacy
(D) drugs that produce a similar pharmacologic effect can have very different levels of efficacy
(E) on a log dose–response curve, two drugs with the same action but with different potencies will usually have parallel curves

6. A patient with a systemic infection is being treated with an antibiotic whose elimination half-life ($t_{1/2\beta}$) is 8 hours. To maintain the patient's total body store at 300 mg of the antibiotic, what should the dosage be?

(A) 100 mg every 8 hours
(B) 200 mg every 8 hours
(C) 300 mg every 8 hours
(D) 400 mg every 8 hours
(E) 500 mg every 8 hours

7. Which of the following statements best describes a drug receptor?

(A) Gamma globulin can bind to a drug and serve as a drug receptor
(B) A drug cannot act unless it is first bound to a receptor
(C) A drug cannot act unless it is first released from a receptor
(D) Drug receptors play a role in the bioavailability of a drug
(E) A drug can act as an antagonist even if it is bound to a drug receptor

8. All of the following statements regarding receptor classes are true EXCEPT

(A) ion channels are confined to excitable tissue
(B) each cell is capable of producing only one G protein
(C) steroids bind to intracellular receptors
(D) a hormone or neurotransmitter receptor may be an ion channel
(E) certain growth factors interact with receptors that have tyrosine-specific protein kinase activity

9. The maximum effect (E_{max}) achieved by a drug is a measure of

(A) potency
(B) efficacy
(C) the quantal response
(D) antagonist magnitude
(E) the therapeutic index (TI)

Directions: Each item below contains four suggested answers of which **one or more** is correct. Choose the answer

A if **1, 2, and 3** are correct
B if **1 and 3** are correct
C if **2 and 4** are correct
D if **4** is correct
E if **1, 2, 3, and 4** are correct

10. Correct statements about drug transport include which of the following?

(1) Little, if any, of an ionized drug passively diffuses into cells
(2) Bioavailability refers to the percentage of drug that is not bound to plasma protein
(3) Simple diffusion depends upon the area of the absorbing surface
(4) Simple diffusion is a saturable process

11. Absorption of a drug from the gastrointestinal tract is influenced by

(1) the patient's dietary patterns
(2) the plasma half-life of the drug
(3) the pH of the stomach
(4) stress

7-E   10-B
8-B   11-B
9-B

12. Which of the following properties would characterize a drug when it is bound to plasma albumin?

(1) It is biologically inactive
(2) It can pass through the glomerulus
(3) It usually can become unbound
(4) It is promptly metabolized

13. Tissues that often are not readily accessible to drugs include which of the following?

(1) Fetus
(2) Kidneys
(3) Brain
(4) Testes

14. A high volume of distribution for a molecule indicates which of the following effects?

(1) High total body water
(2) Many receptors for the molecule
(3) Low rate of excretion
(4) High lipophilicity

15. Correct statements concerning drug metabolism include which of the following?

(1) Oxidation is the most common type of metabolic reaction
(2) Glucuronides eliminated in the bile can be hydrolyzed and the free drug reabsorbed
(3) Most drug metabolism takes place in the microsomal system of the liver
(4) Conjugation reactions involve linking two or more exogenously administered drug molecules together

16. True statements concerning the hepatic microsomal metabolizing enzyme system include which of the following?

(1) It requires NADPH and molecular oxygen
(2) It is concerned only with exogenous substances
(3) Its oxidation reactions include hydrocarbon chain hydroxylations and *N*- and *O*-dealkylations
(4) It includes alcohol dehydrogenase activity

17. Propranolol is a competitive antagonist of norepinephrine. When the log dose–response curve seen with both norepinephrine and propranolol is compared to that seen with norepinephrine alone, the norepinephrine–propranolol curve would

(1) have the same E_{max} as the norepinephrine curve
(2) be shifted to the right of the norepinephrine curve
(3) be parallel to the norepinephrine curve
(4) have the same ED_{50} as the norepinephrine curve

18. True statements about potency and efficacy include which of the following?

(1) The slope of the dose–response curve gives a good idea of a drug's efficacy
(2) Potency refers to the different amounts of two or more drugs that are needed to produce the same effect
(3) The log dose–response curve allows comparison of the relative potency of two drugs but not a comparison of their efficacy
(4) Potency and efficacy are unrelated properties

ANSWERS AND EXPLANATIONS

1. The answer is B *[II A 1 a]*
Fick's law is expressed as:

$$dQ/dt = (-D)(A)(dc/dx)$$

where dQ/dt is the rate of drug flux, D is the temperature-dependent diffusion constant of the molecule, A is the area of the absorbing surface, and dc/dx is the concentration gradient. Thus, the larger the surface area, the greater the drug flux. All of the other statements in the question are true.

2. The answer is E *[II B 1]*
The more rapid response after intravenous administration can be critical in an emergency. All forms of parenteral administration (i.e., administration by injection) require the use of sterile technique, and all can cause local irritation, depending on the drug being given. For a drug to be administered orally, the patient must be conscious and alert to avoid the risk of aspiration. Inhalation provides rapid access to the general circulation (e.g., gaseous anesthetics).

3. The answer is A *[II B 1 a (3) (d)]*
After oral administration, a drug is absorbed through the gastrointestinal mucosa and then passes through the liver. Some drugs (e.g., propranolol) can undergo extensive hepatic metabolism (first-pass effect) before reaching the site of action. With most other routes of administration, the first-pass effect does not occur because extensive hepatic passage immediately after drug absorption is avoided.

4. The answer is E *[II B 1, 2]*
The route of administration is an important determinant of the rate and efficiency of absorption of a drug. Delivery of the drug into the circulation is relatively slow after oral administration, and the rate of absorption is variable. Parenteral routes of administration bypass the alimentary tract and usually result in rapid, direct drug absorption. After intravenous administration, the absorption of a drug follows zero-order kinetics; thus, a constant **amount** (i.e., 100%) of the drug is absorbed. After any other route of administration, the absorption of most drugs follows first-order (exponential) kinetics; thus, a constant **fraction** of the drug is absorbed.

5. The answer is C *[III D 2 c, 3]*
The ED_{50} is a measure of a drug's potency, not its efficacy. The smaller the ED_{50}, the greater the potency of the drug. All of the other statements in the question are true.

6. The answer is B *[II F]*
A drug accumulates in the body if the time interval between doses is less than four half-lives, in which case the total body store of the drug increases exponentially to a plateau. The average total body store of a drug at the plateau is a function of the dose, the interval between doses, and the elimination half-life of the drug. When the drug is administered at the half-life of elimination, the average total body store of the drug is approximately equal to 1.5 times the amount administered.

7. The answer is E *[III A 1, B]*
A drug receptor is a specific drug-binding site in a cell or on its surface that mediates the action of the drug. Some drugs bind to various plasma proteins, such as gamma globulin, but these molecules do not serve as drug receptors. Most drugs combine reversibly with their receptors to form a drug–receptor complex, and it is this complex that exerts a biologic effect (e.g., a decrease in blood pressure). However, some drugs are believed not to have specific receptors and act by some other mechanism. If a drug has no inherent pharmacologic activity but binds to a receptor, it acts as an antagonist.

8. The answer is B *[III B 1–3]*
All of the statements listed in the question are true except that each cell can express several G proteins, and each G protein can respond to several different receptors and regulate several effectors.

9. The answer is B *[III D 2 c, 6]*
E_{max} reflects the efficacy of a drug and is indicated by the height of the dose–response curve. Potency refers to the different doses of two drugs that are needed to produce the same effect. Potency is independent of efficacy, and efficacy is more important than potency in selecting drugs for a particular clinical situation. The quantal response of a drug relates to the all-or-none relationship seen in a population with a given dose of a drug. The therapeutic index (TI) is defined as the LD_{50}/ED_{50} and is independent of the E_{max}.

10. The answer is B (1, 3)   *[II A 1, 2]*

Ionized drugs will not passively diffuse across cell membranes. Simple diffusion is not saturable, requires no energy, and is governed by Fick's law; thus, it is a function of the area of the absorbing surface, the diffusion constant of the drug, and the concentration gradient. Bioavailability is a measure of the relative rate at which an administered drug reaches the general circulation.

11. The answer is B (1, 3)   *[II A 2, B]*

Tablet size, solubility of the drug in the contents of the stomach, quality control of the manufacturer, the patient's dietary patterns, and the pH of the surrounding environment influence the absorption of a drug from the gastrointestinal tract. In general, the plasma half-life of a drug is independent of the absorption process, and stress has not been shown to be an important factor.

12. The answer is B (1, 3)   *[II C 1 a]*

Only the free drug is biologically active; while a drug is bound to plasma proteins, it does not produce its desired pharmacologic effects. Moreover, the bound drug cannot leave the vascular space and is not metabolized or eliminated. Binding to albumin is a reversible process.

13. The answer is B (1, 3)   *[II C 1 b]*

Drugs frequently cannot enter the brain readily because of the blood–brain barrier. This is due primarily to the continuous layer of endothelial cells with tight gap junctions that line the cerebral capillaries. The fetus is also protected from many drugs because the fetal circulation is separated from the maternal circulation by several placental layers. Both the kidneys and the testes are exposed to circulating drugs.

14. The answer is C (2, 4)   *[II C 2 a (2)]*

In a one-compartment model, a high volume of distribution indicates that a drug is very lipophilic or that it interacts with many receptors.

15. The answer is A (1, 2, 3)   *[II D 1 a, 2 a, d (1)]*

Glucuronides that are eliminated in the bile can be hydrolyzed by β-glucuronidases, and the free drug will then be reabsorbed into the blood. This "enterohepatic recirculation" can be very important in increasing the half-life of a drug. Most drug metabolism occurs by oxidation in the hepatic microsomal metabolizing system. In conjugation reactions, exogenous compounds react with endogenous functional groups to produce a more polar compound.

16. The answer is B (1, 3)   *[II D 2 a (1)]*

In the hepatic microsomal metabolizing system, molecular oxygen is incorporated into the substrate, and NADPH is required as a reducing equivalent to reduce oxygen. This enzyme system oxidizes both exogenous and endogenous substrates. Oxidation reactions include hydrocarbon chain hydroxylations as well as N- and O-dealkylations. Alcohol dehydrogenase activity is a nonmicrosomal oxidation reaction.

17. The answer is A (1, 2, 3)   *[III D 4 a]*

With competitive antagonism, the log dose–response curve will be parallel and shifted to the right and will have the same E_{max}. The shift to the right indicates that a higher dose of agonist is necessary to achieve the same response as when the antagonist is absent. Therefore, the ED_{50} for the combination would be higher than the ED_{50} for the agonist alone, even though the E_{max} remains the same. With noncompetitive antagonism, there is a nonparallel shift of the log dose–response curve with a lower E_{max}.

18. The answer is C (2, 4)   *[III D 2 c, 3]*

The maximum effect of a drug (E_{max}) is a measure of the drug's efficacy. Potency is a comparative measure that refers to the different doses of two or more drugs that are needed to produce the same effect. The log dose–response curve allows both the efficacy and the potency of two or more drugs to be compared. The height (not the slope) of the log dose–response curve indicates a drug's efficacy, while drugs with the same action but with different potencies will usually have parallel curves. Potency is independent of efficacy, and efficacy is usually more important than potency in selecting drugs for use in a clinical situation.

Drugs Affecting Peripheral Neurohumoral Transmission

I. PERIPHERAL EFFERENT NERVOUS SYSTEM. The peripheral efferent nervous system consists of the **somatic** and the **autonomic nervous systems**.

A. The somatic nervous system innervates and controls the motor function of the body. Axons from the spinal cord innervate skeletal muscle; the neurotransmitter (see I C) is acetylcholine.

B. Autonomic nervous system. Axons from preganglionic neurons within the spinal cord connect to neurons in ganglia outside the spinal cord. Postganglionic axons from the ganglia innervate smooth and cardiac muscle and exocrine glands. The autonomic nervous system has two parts: the **parasympathetic** and **sympathetic nervous systems**. These two divisions control homeostatic functions that are primarily involuntary.

   1. Parasympathetic nervous system
      a. Location of preganglionic neurons. In the parasympathetic (craniosacral) nervous system, preganglionic neurons are located in cranial and sacral portions of the spinal cord.
      b. Location of ganglia. In the parasympathetic nervous system, the ganglia are close to the innervated organ, so that the preganglionic axons are long and the postganglionic axons are short.
      c. Innervation of organs
         (1) The parasympathetic nervous system innervates the heart, bronchial smooth muscle, iris, salivary glands, and urinary bladder.
         (2) Under normal conditions, the heart, eye, gastrointestinal tract, urinary bladder, bronchi, and salivary glands are under parasympathetic control.

   2. Sympathetic nervous system
      a. Location of preganglionic neurons. In the sympathetic (thoracolumbar) nervous system, the neurons are located in lumbar and thoracic portions of the spinal cord.
      b. Location of the ganglia. In the sympathetic nervous system, the ganglia are close to the spinal cord, so that the preganglionic axons are short and the postganglionic axons are long.

C. Neurotransmitters. These are chemical mediators that transmit nerve impulses across junctions such as synapses (see Chapter 3 I A).

   1. At the **ganglionic synapse** in both the sympathetic and the parasympathetic nervous systems, the neurotransmitter is **acetylcholine** (see IV A).

   2. At the **postganglionic synapse,** the two systems differ.
      a. The **parasympathetic** neurotransmitter is **acetylcholine**.
      b. The **sympathetic** transmitter is usually **norepinephrine** (see II A), but at sweat glands and at some blood vessels, it is **acetylcholine**.

D. Receptors of the nervous system. More than one type of receptor exists for each neurotransmitter. The receptors are distinguished in part on the basis of their affinity for various agonists and antagonists.

   1. Cholinergic receptors (for acetylcholine) are broadly subdivided into **muscarinic** and **nicotinic receptors**.
      a. Muscarinic receptors

(1) Muscarinic receptors are further subdivided into M_1 and M_2 receptors. Muscarinic receptors of both types are found in the central nervous system (CNS). In addition, M_1 receptors are also found at autonomic ganglia; M_2 receptors at end-organ effector sites.

(2) Muscarine is the classic agonist for muscarinic receptors, and atropine is an antagonist.

b. Nicotinic receptors are found in the CNS, in autonomic ganglia, and in striated muscle.

(1) Nicotine, the classic agonist, first stimulates and then blocks autonomic ganglia and skeletal muscle end-plates.

(2) *d*-Tubocurarine blocks nicotinic receptors in striated muscle and in autonomic ganglia, especially the former, while hexamethonium preferentially blocks ganglionic nicotinic receptors.

c. The various cholinergic receptors and their sites are summarized in Table 2-1.

2. Adrenergic receptors [for norepinephrine (noradrenalin) and epinephrine (adrenalin)] are also of several types.

a. α-Adrenergic receptors. Agonists, in decreasing order of potency, are epinephrine > norepinephrine > isoproterenol. Antagonists are phentolamine and phenoxybenzamine. Some α-adrenergic receptors precede the synapse between nerve terminal and effector organ; others are postsynaptic.

(1) $α_1$-Adrenergic receptors are **postsynaptic** receptors. They are found on blood vessels, on the radial muscle of the eye, in the gastrointestinal tract, and on the splenic capsule.

(2) $α_2$-Adrenergic receptors are **presynaptic** or **postsynaptic;** all seem to serve an inhibitory function. Isoproterenol is ineffective on $α_2$ receptors.

(a) Presynaptic $α_2$ receptors are found at adrenergic and cholinergic nerve terminals. Presynaptic $α_2$ receptors, when activated, inhibit the release of further neurotransmitter.

(b) Postsynaptic $α_2$ receptors are found in blood vessels and in the CNS.

b. β-Adrenergic receptors. Agonists for β receptors are isoproterenol, epinephrine, and norepinephrine. Propranolol is an antagonist. The β receptors also subdivided on the basis of their relative response to agonists and antagonists.

(1) $β_1$-Adrenergic receptors are found predominantly on cells in the heart and intestine. The relative potency of agonists is isoproterenol > epinephrine and norepinephrine.

(2) $β_2$-Adrenergic receptors are found at other sites, most importantly, on bronchial and vascular smooth muscle. The relative potency of agonists is isoproterenol > epinephrine >> norepinephrine.

E. Direct effects of autonomic stimulation on various organs. Stimulation of effector organs may be either direct or indirect. A **direct** effect occurs when the nerve innervating an organ is stimulated. **Indirect** responses are mediated by changes caused in other organs.

1. Direct effects of parasympathetic and sympathetic stimulation on various organs

a. Heart

(1) Sympathetic stimulation increases the heart rate (**chronotropic effect**) and the contractile force (**inotropic effect**).

(2) Parasympathetic stimulation decreases the heart rate but has little effect on contractile force because there is no parasympathetic innervation of the ventricles.

b. Blood vessels

(1) Sympathetic stimulation

(a) Stimulation of α receptors causes constriction of the arteries, arterioles, and veins.

(b) Stimulation of β receptors causes dilation of skeletal muscle arteries.

(2) Parasympathetic stimulation has no effect on blood vessels because most have no parasympathetic innervation.

Table 2-1. Sites of Cholinergic Receptors

| | Receptors | | |
| | Muscarinic | | |
Site	M_1	M_2	Nicotinic
Skeletal muscle	−	−	+
Autonomic ganglia	+	−	+
Central nervous system	+	+	+
End organ innervation	−	+	−

    c. Gastrointestinal tract. Sympathetic stimulation decreases the activity of the gastrointestinal tract, while **parasympathetic stimulation** increases it.

    d. Eye
      (1) Sympathetic stimulation contracts the radial muscle, causing dilation of the pupil.
      (2) Parasympathetic stimulation produces contraction of the circular and ciliary muscles, causing pupillary constriction and changes in accommodation.

    e. Bronchial smooth muscle is relaxed by sympathetic stimulation and contracted by parasympathetic stimulation.

    f. Glycogenolysis is increased in liver and muscle by sympathetic stimulation.

2. Table 2-2 summarizes the effects of autonomic stimulation on various end organs, depending on the type of receptor stimulated.

F. Drug effects on neurohumoral transmission

1. Drugs can affect neurohumoral transmission at various steps. They can affect the:
    a. Synthesis, storage, or release of a neurotransmitter
    b. Interaction between transmitter and receptor
    c. Enzymatic destruction of a neurotransmitter
    d. Transport of a transmitter into cells
    e. Recovery of a cell membrane after the transmitter–receptor interaction

2. Figure 2-1 and Table 2-3 show the mechanisms and sites of drug effects on the sympathetic nervous system.

II. SYMPATHOMIMETIC (ADRENERGIC) AGENTS. These are drugs that mimic the actions of the sympathetic nervous system.

A. Catecholamines: norepinephrine and epinephrine (Figure 2-2)

1. Chemistry
    a. Tyrosine is hydroxylated on the aromatic ring by tyrosine hydroxylase, yielding **dopa** (dihydroxyphenylalanine); this step is the rate-limiting step in the biosynthesis of adrenergic transmitters.

Table 2-2. Receptor–End Organ Response

Organ	Receptor Type	End Organ Effect
Heart	β_1	Increased inotropism and chronotropism
	M_2	Decreased inotropism and chronotropism
Coronary and pulmonary arterioles, blood vessels to skeletal muscle	β_2 (predominant type)	Dilation
	α	Constriction
	M_2	Dilation
Other arterioles	α	Constriction
	β	Dilation
	M_2	Dilation
Veins	α	Constriction
	β_2	Dilation
Bronchi	β_2	Relaxation
	M_2	Constriction
Gastrointestinal tract	α,β	Decreased motility and secretion
	M_2	Increased motility and secretion
Bladder	α,β	Retention
	M_2	Evacuation
Eye	α_1	Mydriasis
	β	Relaxation of ciliary muscle
	M_2	Miosis, constriction of ciliary muscle

Adapted from Lefkowitz RJ, Hoffman BB, Taylor P: Drugs acting at synaptic and neuroeffector junctional sites. In *Goodman and Gilman's The Pharmacological Basis of Therapeutics*, 8th ed. Edited by Gilman AG, et al. New York, Pergamon Press, 1990, p 89.

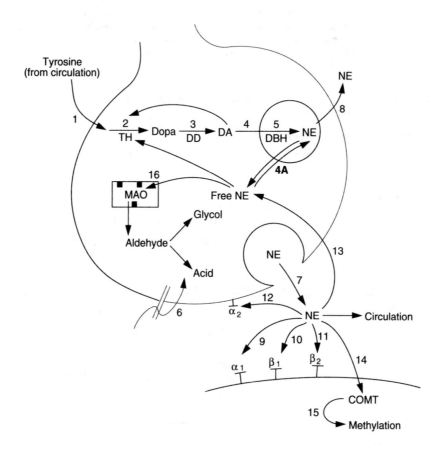

Figure 2-1. Site of action of drugs affecting the sympathetic nervous system. The figure depicts the events taking place at the junction of a sympathetic nerve terminal and an end-organ cell.

Tyrosine from the circulation enters the nerve terminal (**1**) and is converted, first (**2**) via tyrosine hydroxylase (*TH*) into dopa and then (**3**) via dopa decarboxylase (*DD*) into dopamine (*DA*). Dopamine enters the vesicles of the nerve terminal (**4**), where it is converted (**5**), via dopamine β-hydroxylase (*DBH*), into norepinephrine (*NE*), which is stored in the vesicles. Free NE in the axoplasm also enters and leaves the vesicles (**4A**).

In the process of nerve impulse transmission across the neuroeffector junction, the nerve terminal is depolarized (**6**) by an action potential. The storage vesicle fuses with the plasma membrane, and the neurotransmitter NE is released into the junction (**7**) by exocytosis. Indirect-acting sympathomimetics can also cause NE to leave the vesicles and enter the neuroeffector junction (**8**).

Once released from the nerve cell, NE activates the postsynaptic α_1, β_1, and β_2 receptors (**9, 10, 11**) on the effector cell, thereby producing the effector response. NE also activates the presynaptic α_2 receptors (**12**) on the nerve terminal itself.

Several mechanisms terminate the action of NE. Most important is the reentry of NE into the nerve terminal (a process known as uptake-1) [**13**]. Some of the NE enters the effector cell (uptake-2) [**14**], and some enters the circulation.

Two enzymes play a role in the metabolism of NE. The NE that enters the effector cell is methylated (**15**) by catechol-O-methyltransferase (*COMT*) to normetanephrine. The NE in the axoplasm of the nerve terminal is converted (**16**) by monoamine oxidase (*MAO*) in the nerve cell's mitochondria, first to the aldehyde, and then to the glycol or to 3-methoxy-4-hydroxymandelic acid (vanillylmandelic acid, or VMA). The glycol and the acid are the major metabolites excreted in the urine.

Drugs that affect the sympathetic nervous system act at specific steps in the above process. Such drugs, and the processes they inhibit, are listed in Table 2-3. (Adapted from Molinoff PB: The regulation of the noradrenergic neuron. *J Psychiatr Res* 11:339–345, 1974.)

Table 2-3. Sites of Action of Drugs Affecting the Sympathetic Nervous System*

Site*	Process*	Inhibitor
1	Tyrosine uptake	None
2	Tyrosine hydroxylase (TH)	α-Methyl-p-tyrosine, dopamine (DA), norepinephrine (NE)
3	Dopa decarboxylase (DD)	α-Methyldopa
4	Movement of DA into vesicles	Reserpine
4A	Movement of NE back into vesicles	
5	Dopamine β-hydroxylase (DBH)	Disulfiram
6	Depolarization of adrenergic terminals	Bretylium, guanethidine
7	Exocytotic release of NE	See site 6
8	Release by indirect-acting sympathomimetics	Cocaine (blocks uptake), reserpine (eliminates stores)
9	α$_1$-Adrenergic receptors (postsynaptic)	Phentolamine, tolazoline, phenoxybenzamine, ergotamine, prazosin
10	β$_1$-Adrenergic receptors	Propranolol (also β$_2$), atenolol, metoprolol
11	β$_2$-Adrenergic receptors	Propranolol (also β$_1$)
12	α$_2$-Adrenergic receptors (presynaptic)	See site 9 (not prazosin)
13	Norepinephrine uptake (U-1)	Cocaine, imipramine, ouabain, bretylium, guanethidine, phenoxybenzamine
14	Extraneuronal uptake (U-2)	Phenoxybenzamine, corticosterone, normetanephrine
15	Catechol-O-methyltransferase	Pyrogallol
16	Monoamine oxidase	Phenelzine (a hydrazine), tranylcypromine (derivative of amphetamine)

*Site numbers and processes are as in Figure 2-1.
Adapted from Molinoff PB: Drugs affecting the sympathetic nervous system. In lecture notes for course in medical pharmacology. University of Pennsylvania School of Medicine, August, 1985.

    b. Dopa is decarboxylated to give **dopamine**.
    c. Dopamine is hydroxylated on the β-carbon to give **norepinephrine**.
    d. **Epinephrine** is formed in the adrenal medulla by the methylation of norepinephrine. The medulla releases 85% epinephrine and 15% norepinephrine.

2. Pharmacokinetics of epinephrine and norepinephrine
    a. Absorption is poor with oral administration because the drugs are rapidly conjugated and oxidized.
    b. Absorption is slow with subcutaneous administration because the drugs cause local vasoconstriction.
    c. Nebulized and inhaled solutions are usually used for their actions on the respiratory tract.
    d. The drugs can be given intravenously, but this route must be used with caution so that the heart does not fibrillate.

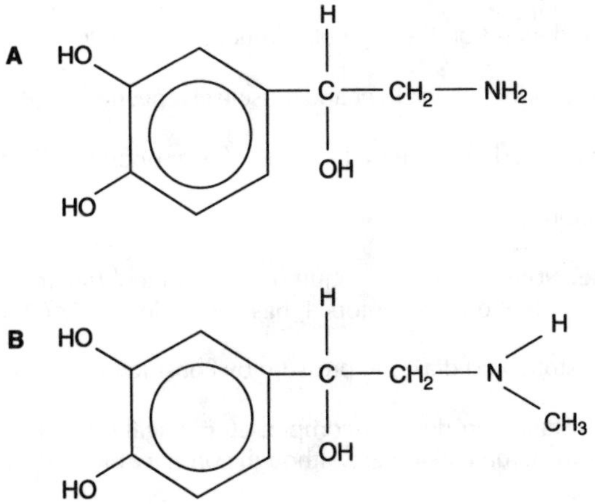

Figure 2-2. Structures of norepinephrine (*A*) and epinephrine (*B*).

    e. The liver is important in the degradation of epinephrine and norepinephrine. The majority of the dose is metabolized by catechol-O-methyltransferase (COMT) and monoamine oxidase (MAO), and the metabolites are excreted in the urine.

3. Pharmacologic effects of epinephrine. Epinephrine interacts strongly with both β and α receptors. Its effects on some body systems depend on the concentration of epinephrine as well as the type of receptor. At low concentrations, β effects predominate, and at high concentrations, α effects predominate.

    a. Effects on blood pressure

        (1) A large dose of epinephrine, administered intravenously, causes an increase in blood pressure, the systolic pressure increasing more than the diastolic. Subsequently, the mean pressure falls below normal before returning to the control value. The rise in pressure is due to:

            (a) Vasoconstriction through activation of α receptors

            (b) Increased ventricular contraction through activation of β receptors

            (c) An initial increase in heart rate, which, at the height of the vasopressor response, will be slowed by a compensatory vagal discharge

        (2) Low doses cause a fall in blood pressure because the β_2 (vasodilator) receptors are more sensitive to epinephrine than are the α (vasoconstrictor) receptors.

    b. Vascular effects. Epinephrine exerts its action on small arterioles and precapillary sphincters. Its vascular effects include:

        (1) Decreased cutaneous blood flow

        (2) Increased blood flow to skeletal muscle at low concentrations and decreased flow at higher concentrations

        (3) Increased hepatic blood flow with increased splanchnic vascular resistance

        (4) Increased renal vascular resistance, producing decreased renal blood flow

        (5) Increased arterial and venous pulmonary pressure

        (6) Increased coronary blood flow, caused indirectly by an increase in the work of the heart, and mediated by local effectors

    c. Effects on the heart produced by epinephrine include:

        (1) A direct effect on β_1 receptors, producing a slight initial increase in heart rate, which is slowed by a compensatory vagal discharge

        (2) Increased stroke volume

        (3) Increased cardiac output

        (4) A propensity toward arrhythmias

    d. Effects on smooth muscle depend on the predominant type of adrenergic receptor in the muscle.

        (1) Epinephrine relaxes gastrointestinal smooth muscle (α_2- and β-receptor stimulation), while it usually increases sphincter contraction (α stimulation).

        (2) Uterine contractions may be inhibited (β) or stimulated (α), depending on menstrual phase or state of gestation.

        (3) In the bladder, the detrusor muscle relaxes (β), while the trigone and sphincter contract (α).

        (4) Bronchiolar smooth muscle relaxes (β_2).

    e. Metabolic effects of epinephrine also depend on the type of adrenergic receptor. These effects include:

        (1) An increase in glucose and lactate production via liver and muscle glycogenolysis (β_2)

        (2) Inhibition of insulin secretion (α)

        (3) An increase in free fatty acids, mediated by cyclic adenosine 3',5'-monophosphate [cyclic AMP] (β_1)

        (4) An increase in oxygen consumption

4. Pharmacologic effects of norepinephrine. Norepinephrine is equipotent to epinephrine in its reaction on β_1 receptors, and slightly less potent on α receptors. It has very little effect on β_2 receptors.

    a. An intravenous infusion raises both systolic and diastolic pressure by constriction of vascular smooth muscle (α receptors).

    b. The increased peripheral vascular resistance produces a compensatory vagal reflex that slows the heart rate. Cardiac output may actually decrease although coronary blood flow is increased.

5. Termination of action

    a. Transport, or uptake into the cells, is an important mechanism for terminating the action of many neurotransmitters. There are two active **amine transport systems:**

        (1) A system in the plasma membrane transports amines from the extracellular fluid to the cytosol.

        (2) A system in the secretory granular membrane transports amines into granules.

    b. Deactivation by conversion to inactive metabolites is also a way of terminating action. Two enzymes are involved:

        (1) COMT adds a methyl group to the hydroxyl of the catechol ring.

        (2) MAO removes the amine group. When metabolic breakdown or transport is prevented (as in patients taking MAO inhibitors or tricyclic antidepressants), then the dosage of sympathomimetic agents must be reduced.

6. Therapeutic uses

    a. Epinephrine is used:

        (1) To treat bronchospasm

        (2) For relief of hypersensitivity reactions; it is the primary treatment for anaphylactic shock

        (3) To prolong the duration of infiltrative anesthesia

        (4) To restore cardiac activity in cardiac arrest

        (5) To facilitate aqueous drainage in chronic open-angle glaucoma

    b. Norepinephrine is used for treating hypotension during anesthesia when tissue perfusion is good.

7. Adverse effects. Both epinephrine and norepinephrine can cause:

    a. Anxiety

    b. Headache

    c. Cerebral hemorrhage from the vasopressor effects

    d. Cardiac arrhythmias, especially in the presence of digitalis and certain anesthetic agents

    e. Pulmonary edema from pulmonary hypertension

B. Isoproterenol

1. Pharmacokinetics

    a. Absorption of orally administered isoproterenol is unreliable.

    b. It is readily absorbed when given parenterally or as an inhaled aerosol.

    c. It is principally metabolized by COMT; MAO plays a much smaller role than in epinephrine or norepinephrine metabolism.

2. Pharmacologic effects

    a. Isoproterenol has an N-alkyl substitution, which makes it act almost entirely on β receptors and have very little effect on α receptors.

    b. Intravenous infusion produces a reduction of peripheral vascular resistance in skeletal muscles and in renal and mesenteric vascular beds.

    c. Diastolic blood pressure falls, but owing to increased venous return and positive inotropic and chronotropic effects, cardiac output is increased.

    d. Systolic blood pressure may increase, but mean pressure decreases.

    e. Renal blood flow decreases in normotensive individuals, but it increases in patients with nonhemorrhagic shock.

    f. Relaxation of both bronchial and gastrointestinal smooth muscle occurs.

    g. A release of free fatty acids occurs; hyperglycemia is less than with epinephrine.

    h. Pancreatic islet cells are activated, stimulating insulin secretion.

3. Therapeutic uses. Isoproterenol is used as a bronchodilator and as a cardiac stimulant.

4. Adverse effects

    a. These are similar to the adverse effects of epinephrine.

    b. Overdosage by inhalation can induce fatal ventricular arrhythmias.

    c. Tolerance to the desired effects occurs with overuse in the asthmatic.

C. Dopamine

1. Chemistry. Dopamine is an intermediate in the synthesis of norepinephrine (see II A 1).

2. Pharmacokinetics. Dopamine resembles epinephrine and norepinephrine in its pharmacokinetics.

3. **Central dopamine receptors (D_1, D_2, D_3)**
   a. The central D_1 receptor site is excitatory and directly activates the adenylate cyclase system.
   b. The D_2 receptor site is inhibitory in some brain tissues and uses cAMP as its intracellular messenger. Pituitary-related side effects of neuroleptics are thought to be mediated through D_2 receptors in the pituitary.
   c. The D_3 receptor is localized in the limbic system and is not found in the pituitary. It is principally associated with emotional and cognitive behavior.

4. **Pharmacologic effects**
   a. Dopamine is an important neurotransmitter in the CNS. It is a direct agonist, acting on β_1 receptors and also releases norepinephrine from nerve terminals. The result is a positive inotropic effect on the myocardium.
   b. Low or intermediate doses of dopamine reduce arterial resistance in the mesentery and kidney; this raises the glomerular filtration rate. The effect is mediated by a receptor for dopamine.
   c. Dopamine increases systolic pressure but has little effect on diastolic pressure.
   d. At higher doses, it acts on α receptors and causes vasoconstriction with a consequent reduction in renal function.

5. **Therapeutic uses.** Dopamine is used in the treatment of cardiogenic and septic shock and in chronic refractory congestive heart failure.

6. **Adverse effects**
   a. Overdosage results in excessive sympathomimetic activity.
   b. Anginal pain, arrhythmias, nausea, and hypertension can occur, but these effects are short-lived because of dopamine's rapid metabolism.

D. Dobutamine

1. **Pharmacokinetics**
   a. Dobutamine is not absorbed when given orally.
   b. It has a half-life of 2 minutes when given by intravenous injection.

2. **Pharmacologic effects**
   a. Though dobutamine resembles dopamine chemically, it is a direct β_1-receptor agonist. It has a greater inotropic than chronotropic effect.
   b. Dobutamine does not act on dopaminergic receptors.

3. **Therapeutic uses.** Dobutamine is used to improve myocardial function in congestive heart failure. Oxygen demands are less than with other sympathetic agonists because dobutamine causes minimal changes in heart rate and systolic pressure.

4. **Adverse effects**
   a. Dobutamine increases atrioventricular conduction and must, therefore, be used with caution in atrial fibrillation.
   b. Other adverse effects are similar to those of other catecholamines.

E. Phenylephrine

1. **Pharmacologic effects**
   a. Phenylephrine is a direct-acting sympathomimetic agent. Its effects are similar to those of norepinephrine, but it is less potent and has a longer duration of action.
   b. Vasoconstriction, increased atrial pressure, and reflex bradycardia occur with parenteral administration.

2. **Therapeutic uses.** Phenylephrine is used:
   a. As a nasal decongestant
   b. As a pressor agent
   c. To provide local vasoconstriction as:
      (1) A 10% ophthalmic solution
      (2) An adjunct for use with local anesthetics
   d. For relief of paroxysmal atrial tachycardia

3. **Adverse effects**
   a. Large doses cause cardiac irregularities.

   b. Ophthalmic solutions, like intranasal solutions, can be systemically absorbed. Their use in patients taking β blockers increases the risk of cardiac irregularities, myocardial infarction, and intracranial hemorrhage.
   c. Rebound nasal congestion can occur with chronic use as a nasal decongestant.

F. Ephedrine

1. Pharmacokinetics
   a. Ephedrine is absorbed when taken orally.
   b. It is resistant to COMT and MAO, so that its action is prolonged.

2. Pharmacologic effects
   a. Ephedrine is a **mixed-acting** sympathomimetic agent; that is, it has both direct and indirect actions.
   - **(1)** Its **primary action** is **indirect:** It causes the release of norepinephrine from storage in nerve terminals, apparently by competing with norepinephrine for transport into the granules.
   - **(2)** It also produces direct stimulation of adrenergic receptors.
   b. When administered intravenously its action is similar to that of epinephrine. However,
   - **(1)** Its pressor response occurs more slowly and lasts 10 times longer.
   - **(2)** Its potency is 1/250 that of epinephrine in producing an equivalent pressor response.
   c. Ephedrine increases arterial pressure by causing peripheral vasoconstriction and cardiac stimulation.
   d. Its effects on the bronchi and other smooth muscle are qualitatively similar to those of epinephrine.
   e. It causes CNS stimulation, which can result in effects such as insomnia, nervousness, nausea, and agitation.
   f. Tachyphylaxis occurs with repeated administration.

3. Therapeutic uses. Ephedrine is used:
   a. In the treatment of bronchial asthma
   b. As a nasal decongestant
   c. As a pressor agent in spinal anesthesia
   d. As a mydriatic

4. Adverse effects
   a. These are similar to the adverse effects seen with epinephrine.
   b. In addition, CNS effects may occur.
   c. Ephedrine must be used with caution in patients with cardiovascular disease or hyperthyroidism because it is a powerful heart stimulator.

G. Amphetamine

1. Pharmacologic effects
   a. Amphetamine acts indirectly by releasing norepinephrine.
   b. Amphetamine is also a CNS stimulant (see Chapter 3 VIII A).
   c. The dextrorotatory (*d*-) form is more active in the CNS than the levorotatory (*l*-) form.
   d. Amphetamine depresses the appetite, decreasing food intake, by affecting the feeding center in the lateral hypothalamus.
   e. It increases metabolism to a small extent.

2. Therapeutic uses
   a. Amphetamine is used in the treatment of narcolepsy and the hyperkinetic syndrome in children (see Chapter 3 VIII A 2).
   b. The control of obesity is not a recommended use because abuse of amphetamine is not rare and because tolerance to the anorexic effects develops within a few weeks.

3. Adverse effects
   a. Tolerance to amphetamine can occur within several weeks.
   b. Psychic and physical dependence can occur.
   c. Toxic psychosis can result from large doses.
   d. Prolonged use can lead to mental depression and fatigue.
   e. Reactions attributable to CNS stimulation occur, such as restlessness or insomnia.
   f. Cardiovascular stimulation can result in tachycardia and hypertension.
   g. Mydriasis and dry mouth can occur.

h. Amphetamine is contraindicated in patients with cardiovascular disease, because it stimulates the heart, and also in those receiving MAO inhibitors or guanethidine, since these compounds increase norepinephrine concentrations outside the cells, as amphetamine does.

i. Treatment of acute intoxication should include:

(1) Acidification of the urine by ammonium chloride administration

(2) Administering chlorpromazine, which is effective for treating both the CNS symptoms and the elevated blood pressure because of its α-blocking activity

H. Methamphetamine and hydroxyamphetamine

1. Methamphetamine is related chemically to both amphetamine and ephedrine.

a. A mixed-acting sympathomimetic agent, it is equal to amphetamine in central stimulant activity and is more potent than ephedrine in pressor activity.

b. Therapeutic indications are limited to those that make use of its CNS effects, such as narcolepsy.

2. Hydroxyamphetamine has an action resembling that of ephedrine but without CNS effects. It is used as a mydriatic, decongestant, and pressor agent.

I. Mephentermine

1. Mephentermine is a mixed-acting sympathomimetic. Its peripheral vasopressor actions are similar to those of methamphetamine; it lacks significant central actions.

2. Its major therapeutic use is in the treatment of hypotension.

J. Methoxamine

1. Methoxamine is a direct-acting stimulator of α-adrenergic receptors with pharmacologic properties similar to those of phenylephrine.

2. It produces little CNS stimulation.

3. Its large pressor effect is due to an increase in total peripheral resistance.

4. It causes a reflex bradycardia.

5. Methoxamine is used therapeutically in hypotensive states and to end attacks of paroxysmal atrial tachycardia.

K. Metaraminol

1. Metaraminol is a mixed-acting sympathomimetic that is similar to norepinephrine in its actions, although it is less potent.

2. Metaraminol increases systolic and diastolic blood pressure via vasoconstriction, and produces a marked reflex bradycardia.

3. It has little stimulant effect on the CNS.

4. Its major therapeutic use is in the treatment of hypotensive states.

L. β_2-Stimulating bronchodilators

1. Pharmacologic effects. The adrenergic agents that are primarily β_2 agonists have a relaxing effect on bronchial smooth muscle and show little effect on cardiac β_1 receptors.

2. Therapeutic uses. These agents are used therapeutically for the treatment of bronchial asthma or bronchospasm where their lack of cardiac stimulation is a decided advantage. They are used chiefly as aerosol inhalants; oral and injectable forms are also available.

3. Adverse effects of the β_2 agonists are similar to those seen with the sympathomimetic drugs listed above. Even though their effects are primarily bronchial, they should be used with caution in patients with cardiovascular disease or hyperthyroidism because they can still stimulate (though minimally) β_1 receptors of the heart.

4. Specific agents

a. Metaproterenol has a more rapid onset of bronchodilating action in asthma than either albuterol or terbutaline.

b. Albuterol is somewhat more bronchoselective than isoproterenol when given as an inhalant. In asthma, the effects of albuterol are apparent within 15 minutes, are maximal at about 60–90 minutes, and last about 3–4 hours.

c. Terbutaline, when used in the treatment of bronchial asthma, has a longer duration of action than metaproterenol. It may have more side effects than other sympathomimetic agents.

d. Bitolterol is a prodrug that is converted in the lung to **colterol,** an active catecholamine. It may have a longer duration of action than terbutaline, metaproterenol, or albuterol. It may cause tremor due to stimulation of skeletal muscle, in addition to the adverse effects seen with all sympathomimetic agents.

III. SYMPATHETIC ANTAGONISTS. Synonyms for this class of drugs are numerous: They are also called **sympatholytics, antiadrenergic agents,** and **adrenergic blocking agents.**

A. α-Adrenergic blocking agents (α blockers)

1. Phenoxybenzamine

a. Mechanism of action

(1) Phenoxybenzamine is a haloalkylamine and is closely related to the nitrogen mustards.

(2) It binds covalently to the α receptor, producing an irreversible blockade.

(3) Phenoxybenzamine is somewhat more potent in blocking α_1 (postsynaptic) receptors than in blocking α_2 (presynaptic) receptors.

b. Pharmacologic effects. Phenoxybenzamine antagonizes sympathetic responses mediated by α-adrenergic receptors.

(1) **Cardiovascular effects.** Phenoxybenzamine induces postural hypotension due to a lack of compensatory sympathetic vasoconstriction. In addition, it increases cardiac output and decreases total peripheral resistance.

(2) Most **metabolic effects** produced by catecholamines are the result of their effects on β receptors, and thus, α-adrenergic blocking agents do not have significant metabolic actions.

(3) **CNS effects.** Phenoxybenzamine stimulates the CNS, producing nausea, hyperventilation, and loss of time perception.

c. Therapeutic uses. Phenoxybenzamine is used:

(1) For acute hypertensive episodes due to sympathomimetics, MAO inhibitors, or pheochromocytomas

(2) To reverse vasoconstriction in shock (if use is attempted in shock, the patient must have an elevated central venous pressure)

(3) To relieve vasospasm in Raynaud's phenomenon

(4) For control of autonomic hyperreflexia due to spinal cord transection

d. Adverse effects

(1) Postural hypotension and reflex tachycardia may occur, especially in patients who are hypovolemic.

(2) Ejaculation may be inhibited.

(3) Miosis and nasal stuffiness may occur.

(4) Nausea and vomiting may occur with oral administration.

(5) Injections cause local tissue irritation.

2. Phentolamine and tolazoline act by a reversible α-adrenergic blockade.

a. Pharmacologic effects

(1) These agents produce vasodilation and reflex cardiac stimulation.

(2) They decrease peripheral resistance and increase venous capacity.

(3) Both stimulate salivary, lacrimal, pancreatic, and respiratory tract secretions.

(4) They cause a gastric secretion that resembles the effect of histamine.

(5) Phentolamine is more potent than tolazoline.

(6) Tolazoline is absorbed when given orally and is rapidly excreted by the kidneys; phentolamine is excreted more slowly. Both can be given parenterally.

b. Therapeutic uses

(1) Phentolamine has been used to control acute hypertensive episodes due to sympathomimetics.

      (2) In the past, phentolamine was used as a diagnostic test for pheochromocytoma, but it has been replaced by assays for urinary catecholamines.

      (3) Tolazoline can be used in the treatment of neonates with persistent pulmonary hypertension despite oxygen therapy and mechanical ventilation.

      (4) Tolazoline has been used experimentally to relieve vasospasm and in the treatment of Raynaud's phenomenon.

  c. Adverse effects

      (1) Both drugs can cause cardiac stimulation, leading to arrhythmias and anginal pain, especially after parenteral administration; they must be used with caution in patients with coronary artery disease.

      (2) Tolazoline can produce a paradoxical hypertension.

      (3) Because they induce gastrointestinal stimulation, both drugs must be used with caution in patients with peptic ulcer disease.

3. Prazosin is a selective blocker of postsynaptic α_1 receptors, producing vasodilation.

  a. Pharmacologic effects

      (1) Prazosin reduces vascular tone in both resistance and capacitance vessels.

      (2) Because prazosin has no effect on α_2 receptors, neurotransmitter feedback inhibition is maintained, so that prazosin causes only a small degree of tachycardia.

      (3) It decreases arterial pressure with little change in cardiac output, heart rate, and right atrial pressure.

  b. Further information about prazosin can be found in Chapter 5 IV F 2.

4. Ergot alkaloids

  a. Mechanism of action

      (1) These agents are weak α-adrenergic blockers as well as being serotonin antagonists (see Chapter 8 V B).

      (2) They are also partial agonists at α-adrenergic receptors, and agonists at tryptaminergic and dopaminergic receptors.

  b. Pharmacologic effects

      (1) Ergot alkaloids are CNS stimulants and, therefore, may cause effects such as confusion, irregular respiration, and anxiety.

      (2) They directly stimulate smooth muscle.

      (3) They cause a significant elevation of blood pressure via peripheral vasoconstriction.

  c. Therapeutic uses

      (1) Ergotamine tartrate, by virtue of its vasoconstricting effects, is used in the treatment of migraine headaches.

      (2) Ergonovine maleate is a powerful oxytocic but lacks the adrenergic blocking activity of ergotamine. It causes direct contraction of uterine smooth muscle and is used to decrease postpartum bleeding.

      (3) Methylergonovine maleate is also used to decrease postpartum uterine bleeding.

      (4) Methysergide (see also Chapter 8 V B 1) is used for prophylaxis of migraine attacks.

  d. Adverse effects

      (1) Ergot preparations often cause nausea and vomiting.

      (2) Their vasoconstricting effects can cause vascular insufficiency, leading to gangrene.

B. β-Adrenergic blocking agents (β blockers) [Table 2-4]

1. Propranolol is a nonselective β antagonist: It competes for both β_1 and β_2 receptors.

  a. Pharmacokinetics

      (1) Although propranolol is completely absorbed from the gastrointestinal tract, a large portion of the drug is extracted by the liver before it enters the systemic circulation.

      (2) Wide variation in the hepatic metabolism of the drug among individuals causes significant differences in the plasma concentrations attained.

      (3) Propranolol is approximately 90% bound to plasma proteins.

      (4) The elimination half-time is approximately 3 hours for a small dose, but it is prolonged with larger doses and is significantly prolonged in the presence of cirrhosis.

      (5) A metabolic product, 4-hydroxypropranolol, is active but has a short half-life.

  b. Pharmacologic effects

      (1) Propranolol decreases the heart rate and cardiac output and prolongs systole.

      (2) It decreases total coronary blood flow and oxygen consumption.

      (3) It reduces blood flow to most tissues except the brain.

Table 2-4. β-Blockers for Hypertension

Drug	β-Blocking Selectivity
Carteolol	Nonselective, intrinsic sympathomimetic
Labetolol	Nonselective β- and selective α_1-blocking activity
Nadolol	Nonselective
Penbutolol	Nonselective, intrinsic sympathomimetic
Pindolol	Nonselective, intrinsic sympathomimetic
Propranolol	Nonselective
Timolol	Nonselective
Acebutolol	β_1-selective, intrinsic sympathomimetic
Atenolol	β_1-selective
Betaxolol	B_1-selective
Metoprolol	B_1-selective

    (4) Propranolol's antihypertensive effect is slow to develop, and the mechanisms that cause the effect are not clear. However, propranolol inhibits the renal secretion of renin, which may play a part.

    (5) It depresses sodium (Na^+) excretion because it alters renal hemodynamics, an effect that is secondary to the decrease in cardiac output.

    (6) Propranolol increases airway resistance by β_2 blockade.

    (7) Since most of the effects of catecholamines on carbohydrate and fat metabolism are mediated by β receptors, propranolol will interfere with these events.

  c. Therapeutic uses. Propranolol is used for:

    (1) Treatment of hypertension, often in combination with a diuretic

    (2) Prophylaxis of angina pectoris (see Chapter 5 III B)

    (3) Prophylaxis of supraventricular and ventricular arrhythmias (see Chapter 5 II E 1)

    (4) Long-term prophylaxis in patients who have had a myocardial infarction and are at high risk for infarction or sudden death

    (5) Management of hypertrophic obstructive cardiomyopathies to reduce the force of myocardial contractions

    (6) Management of hyperthyroidism and anxiety states to decrease the heart rate

    (7) Prophylaxis of migraine headaches

  d. Adverse effects and precautions

    (1) Propranolol can induce heart failure, especially in patients with compromised myocardial function.

    (2) Rapid withdrawal can lead to "supersensitivity" of β-adrenergic receptors, which can provoke anginal attacks, arrhythmias, or myocardial infarction.

    (3) Because propranolol increases airway resistance, it must be used with caution in asthmatics.

    (4) Because of its effects on carbohydrate metabolism, the hypoglycemic action of insulin may be augmented. Therefore, diabetics being treated with insulin and persons prone to hypoglycemia must use propranolol with caution.

    (5) Rash, fever, and purpura are characteristic of an allergic response and require discontinuation of the drug.

    (6) Prolonged use may cause fatigue, depression, nightmares, sexual dysfunction, and peripheral arterial insufficiency.

    (7) Because of its effects on peripheral blood flow, propranolol is contraindicated in patients with Raynaud's phenomenon.

2. Timolol is a nonselective β-adrenergic antagonist that is 5–10 times more potent than propranolol.

  a. Timolol lowers intraocular pressure by reducing the production of aqueous humor; the mechanism is not clear.

  b. It does not change the size of the pupil, and vision is not affected.

  c. Timolol, in the form of eyedrops, is, therefore, useful in the treatment of glaucoma.

  d. Other uses are the same as for propranolol.

  e. Timolol decreases the frequency of migraine attacks but not their duration or severity.

  f. Systemic absorption can occur with ocular use, but the amount absorbed is usually not enough to affect patients with asthma or heart failure.

3. **Nadolol** is a nonselective β-adrenergic blocking agent that is not metabolized and is excreted unchanged in the urine. Its effect and adverse reactions are similar to those of propranolol.

4. **Labetalol** is a nonselective β blocker, which also has α_1-blocking activity. It is used in the treatment of mild to severe hypertension.
    a. Labetalol reduces peripheral vascular resistance while preventing reflex tachycardia.
    b. When combined with either prazosin or hydralazine, labetalol is faster-acting than other β blockers.
    c. It can be given intravenously in hypertensive emergencies.
    d. Labetalol may cause postural hypotension and jaundice in addition to the adverse effects seen with other β blockers.

5. **Pindolol** is a nonselective β blocker, which also has some degree of intrinsic sympathomimetic (α-adrenergic) activity. Unlike the case with propranolol, no rebound tachycardia occurs upon abrupt withdrawal of pindolol.

6. **Acebutolol** is a β blocker with mild intrinsic sympathomimetic activity (ISA).
    a. Its β_1-blocking effects exceed its β_2-blocking effects.
    b. Because of its ISA, it may not cause as slow a bradycardia as propranolol does.
    c. **Adverse effects,** in addition to those seen with other β blockers, include arthritis, myalgia and arthralgia, and the presence of antinuclear antibodies.

7. **Metoprolol** is a selective β_1-adrenergic antagonist.
    a. **Pharmacologic effects**
        (1) Metoprolol inhibits the inotropic and chronotropic cardiac responses to isoproterenol.
        (2) It is 1/50 as potent as propranolol in inhibiting the vasodilator response to isoproterenol; however, it is long-acting.
        (3) It is absorbed well when given orally.
    b. **Therapeutic uses.** Metoprolol is used chiefly in the treatment of hypertension.
    c. **Adverse effects**
        (1) Metoprolol produces fewer deleterious effects in asthmatic patients because of its selective β_1-adrenergic antagonism, but its use in asthmatics still requires caution.
        (2) Other adverse effects are similar to those of propranolol.

8. **Atenolol** is a selective β_1-adrenergic antagonist, which is administered once a day.

9. **Betaxolol** is a selective β_1-adrenergic antagonist, which is administered once a day. It is more lipophilic than atenolol. It is also available as a topical formulation for the treatment of glaucoma.

C. **Agents that inhibit the action of adrenergic nerves**

1. **Reserpine**
    a. **Mechanism of action.** Reserpine, a rauwolfia alkaloid, acts via catecholamine depletion. It inhibits the uptake of norepinephrine into vesicles, and intraneuronal degradation of norepinephrine by MAO then occurs. This action takes place both centrally and peripherally.
    b. **Pharmacologic effects**
        (1) Large doses given parenterally may cause a transient sympathomimetic effect as stored catecholamines are released from the cell, because uptake into vesicles is inhibited.
        (2) Blood pressure decreases, which usually triggers reflex tachycardia in normal people through sympathetic stimulation. However, because sympathetic stores are depleted, bradycardia may ensue in people taking reserpine.
        (3) Sedation often results, owing to the depleted stores of catecholamines and serotonin (5-hydroxytryptamine, 5-HT) in the brain.
    c. **Therapeutic uses.** The major therapeutic use of reserpine is in the treatment of hypertension (see Chapter 5 IV H 1).
    d. **Adverse effects**
        (1) Sedation
        (2) Psychic depression that may result in suicide
        (3) Abdominal cramps and diarrhea
        (4) Gastrointestinal ulceration
        (5) Possible increased incidence of breast carcinoma

2. **Guanethidine**
    a. **Mechanism of action**
        (1) Guanethidine acts presynaptically. It impairs the response to sympathetic stimulation by inhibiting the release of neurotransmitters from peripheral adrenergic neurons.

(2) Guanethidine is taken up by adrenergic nerves and displaces norepinephrine from intraneuronal storage granules. This action does not inhibit the release of granule contents; that occurs through another, unknown, mechanism.

(3) Much of the norepinephrine released from the adrenergic nerve terminals is deaminated by intraneuronal MAO. Some norepinephrine will still leak from the cell.

b. Pharmacokinetics

(1) With oral administration, absorption varies and the onset of action is slow.

(2) The drug is rapidly cleared by the kidney.

c. Pharmacologic effects

(1) A large intravenous dose causes a transient increase in blood pressure.

(2) This is followed by a fall in systemic and pulmonary arterial pressures that is much more intense in the erect than in the supine individual.

d. Therapeutic uses. The major therapeutic indication is a potent, long-acting antihypertensive agent (see Chapter 5 IV H 2).

e. Adverse effects include:

(1) Postural hypotension

(2) Syncope, especially with strenuous exercise

(3) Diarrhea

(4) Edema

f. Guanethidine is contraindicated in patients taking MAO inhibitors.

g. The antihypertensive effects of guanethidine may be reversed by tricyclic antidepressants or indirect-acting sympathomimetic amines, such as ephedrine or phenylpropanolamine.

3. Guanadrel is similar to guanethidine in its mode of action and indications, but it has a shorter duration of action.

a. Guanadrel causes less morning hypotension and less diarrhea than guanethidine does.

b. Like guanethidine, guanadrel is contraindicated in patients taking MAO inhibitors, and its effects may be reversed by the same types of drugs as for guanethidine.

c. Guanadrel causes water retention and should, therefore, be given in combination with a diuretic.

4. Bretylium

a. Pharmacologic effects

(1) Bretylium is taken up by adrenergic nerve terminals and produces a block in the release of norepinephrine.

(2) It also inhibits the re-uptake of norepinephrine into nerve terminals.

(3) Initially, bretylium produces a sympathomimetic effect, before it blocks the action of the nerves.

b. Therapeutic uses. Bretylium is no longer used for hypertension but is used mainly as an antiarrhythmic agent (see Chapter 5 II F 1). It is poorly absorbed when given orally.

c. Adverse effects include cardiac stimulation due to the sympathomimetic effects of bretylium, and strong hypotension.

IV. PARASYMPATHETIC (CHOLINERGIC) AGONISTS

A. Acetylcholine

1. Chemistry. Acetylcholine is a quaternary ammonium ester (Figure 2-3) that is rapidly hydrolyzed by acetylcholinesterase and plasma cholinesterase.

2. Pharmacologic effects

a. Cardiovascular effects

(1) Acetylcholine produces:

(a) A negative inotropic effect

(b) A negative chronotropic effect

(c) Vasodilation

(2) Its actions on the heart are the same as the effects of vagal stimulation.

(3) Large intravenous doses cause an increase in blood pressure, owing to the release of catecholamines from the adrenal medulla and activation of sympathetic ganglia.

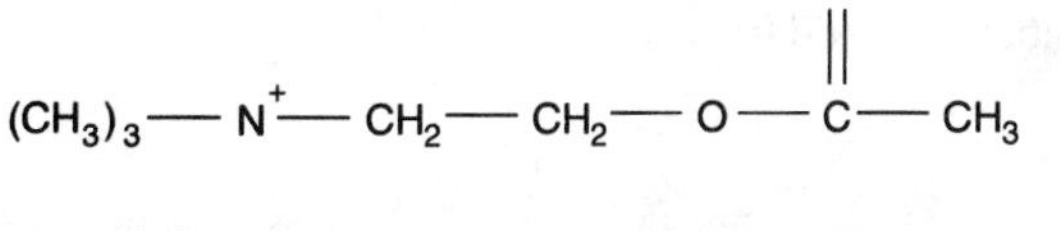

$$(CH_3)_3 - N^+ - CH_2 - CH_2 - O - \overset{\overset{\displaystyle O}{\|}}{C} - CH_3$$

Figure 2-3. Acetylcholine.

b. Effects on other systems
   (1) Acetylcholine increases gastrointestinal motility and secretory activity.
   (2) It contracts smooth muscle in the uterus, ureters, bladder, and bronchioles, and the constrictor muscles of the iris.
   (3) It stimulates the salivary, sweat, and lacrimal glands.

3. Therapeutic uses. Acetylcholine is used as a miotic in cataract surgery.

B. Methacholine (acetyl-β-methylcholine)

1. Chemistry. Methacholine differs chemically from acetylcholine by the addition of a methyl group to the β position of choline. As a result:
   a. Methacholine is hydrolyzed only by acetylcholinesterase and, therefore, has a longer duration of action than acetylcholine.
   b. It becomes virtually a pure muscarinic-acting agent.

2. Pharmacologic effects. The effects of methacholine on the cardiovascular system and other systems are similar to those of acetylcholine.

C. Carbachol (carbamylcholine)

1. Carbachol has a carbamic acid–ester link, which is not readily susceptible to hydrolysis by cholinesterases.

2. Carbachol has all the pharmacologic properties of acetylcholine. It exerts both nicotinic and muscarinic effects.

3. Carbachol is used ophthalmically as a miotic agent.

D. Bethanechol

1. Chemically, bethanechol has the structural features of both methacholine and carbachol. It is resistant to hydrolysis by cholinesterases and is mainly muscarinic in action.

2. Bethanechol shows no negative inotropic or chronotropic cardiovascular effects.

3. It is used therapeutically for abdominal distention, esophageal reflux, and urinary bladder distention.

E. Pilocarpine

1. Pilocarpine is a tertiary amine alkaloid.

2. Its actions are similar to those of methacholine. When applied locally to the eye, it causes miosis and an eventual fall in intraocular pressure.

3. Its major therapeutic indication is in the treatment of glaucoma.

F. Metoclopramide

1. Metoclopramide stimulates the motility of the upper gastrointestinal tract.

2. It is useful for the treatment of diabetic gastroparesis (delayed gastric emptying) and gastroesophageal reflux disease.

3. It is also an antiemetic and is used for this purpose during cancer chemotherapy.

4. Adverse effects include possibly irreversible tardive dyskinesia [see Chapter 3 V B 5 a (3)]; acute dystonia; and prolactin secretion, which can cause loss of libido, galactorrhea, and menstrual disorders.

G. Adverse effects and precautions for parasympathetic agonists

1. Atropine will often block serious adverse effects, such as the increase in gastrointestinal motility, muscle paralysis, and stimulation of glandular secretion, that can occur with these drugs.

2. Use of these drugs is contraindicated in patients with coronary insufficiency, hyperthyroidism, peptic ulcer, or asthma. In addition, **metoclopramide** is contraindicated in patients taking phenothiazines, butyrophenones, or thioxanthenes, and in patients with pheochromocytoma or acute porphyria.

V. ANTICHOLINESTERASE AGENTS

A. Physostigmine

1. **Mechanism of action.** This alkaloid forms a reversible complex at the site of acetylcholinesterase where acetylcholine is broken down.

2. **Pharmacokinetics**
   a. Physostigmine is well absorbed from the gastrointestinal tract, subcutaneous tissues, and mucous membranes.
   b. Its metabolism is at the ester linkage by hydrolytic cleavage.

3. **Pharmacologic effects.** The pharmacologic properties of physostigmine mimic those of acetylcholine.
   a. It produces miosis and, thus, can antagonize the mydriasis induced by atropine.
   b. When given in large doses, it causes fasciculation, then paralysis, of skeletal muscle because of the accumulation of acetylcholine at the neuromuscular junction that results when acetylcholine is not broken down.

4. **Therapeutic uses**
   a. Treatment of atropine, phenothiazine, and tricyclic antidepressant intoxication
   b. Treatment of glaucoma, especially simple and secondary glaucoma
   c. Treatment of early stages of Alzheimer's disease, since degeneration of cortical cholinergic axons has been seen at autopsy in some patients with this disorder

B. Neostigmine

1. **Chemistry.** Neostigmine is a synthetic reversible anticholinesterase that contains a quaternary nitrogen.

2. **Pharmacokinetics**
   a. Neostigmine is not well absorbed orally.
   b. It does not penetrate the blood–brain barrier, which minimizes the toxicity due to inhibition of acetylcholinesterase that is in the brain.
   c. It is destroyed by plasma esterases and is excreted in the urine.

3. **Pharmacologic effects**
   a. The pharmacologic properties of neostigmine mimic those of acetylcholine.
   b. It also has a direct action on nicotinic receptors, in addition to blocking acetylcholinesterase.
   c. It reverses the neuromuscular blockade produced by curare and its derivatives; the mechanism of action involves the release of increased amounts of acetylcholine from nerve endings, cholinesterase inhibition, and a direct action on skeletal muscle cholinergic receptors.

4. **Therapeutic uses**
   a. Neostigmine is used to reverse the effects of competitive neuromuscular blocking agents (see VIII).
   b. It is used in the management of paralytic ileus and atony of the urinary bladder.
   c. It is also used in the symptomatic treatment of myasthenia gravis.

C. Endrophonium

1. **Pharmacokinetics.** Endrophonium is more rapidly absorbed and has a shorter duration of action than neostigmine. It is administered parenterally.

2. **Pharmacologic effects.** In its actions, edrophonium is similar to neostigmine, except that with high doses it can stimulate the neuromuscular junction without affecting muscarinic effector organs.

3. **Therapeutic uses**
   a. Diagnosis of myasthenia gravis
   b. Antagonism of curare-like agents

D. Other physostigmine-like anticholinesterases

1. **Pyridostigmine** and **ambenonium** are used in the symptomatic treatment of myasthenia gravis.

2. **Demecarium** is used as an ophthalmic solution for the treatment of chronic glaucoma.

E. Organophosphate cholinesterase inhibitors

1. Preparations
a. **Diisopropyl fluorophosphate (DFP)** is an organophosphate compound, which forms a co-valent bond between its phosphorus atom and the esteratic site of cholinesterase. The enzyme-inhibitor complex thus formed is irreversible. Its use is limited to the treatment of certain types of glaucoma.
b. **Echothiophate** is a long-acting organophosphate cholinesterase inhibitor with pharmacologic properties similar to those of DFP. Spontaneous regeneration of the phosphorylated enzyme can occur. Its major use is in the treatment of glaucoma.
c. **Parathion** is an organophosphate anticholinesterase agent used as an insecticide. Its active form is **paraoxon,** a metabolite. Pharmacologic and adverse effects are similar to those of DFP.

2. Adverse effects of DFP and other organophosphate cholinesterase inhibitors include:
a. Miosis
b. Increased bronchial secretions, profuse sweating, and increased lacrimation
c. Anorexia, vomiting, and involuntary diarrhea
d. Bradycardia
e. Weakness of all skeletal muscles, but especially those of respiration, after twitching and fasciculations
f. Anxiety, confusion, and convulsions, followed by vasomotor depression

3. Reversal of cholinesterase inhibition. Pyridine-2-aldoxime methyl chloride (PAM, pralidoxime) reverses the effects of the organophosphate anticholinesterase agents.
a. It combines with and splits off the phosphorus from the esteratic site on cholinesterase in such a way that the enzyme is restored.
b. With reactivation of the enzyme, the effects of acetylcholine begin to disappear.
c. Treatment must be within hours, because the phosphorylated enzyme slowly changes to a form that cannot be reversed.

VI. PARASYMPATHETIC ANTAGONISTS

A. Atropine is an alkaloid derived from the plant *Atropa belladona* (deadly nightshade). The active component is the racemic mixture *dl*-hyoscyamine, an ester compound of tropic acid and the organic base tropine.

1. Mechanism of action
a. Atropine competes reversibly with acetylcholine at muscarinic receptors.
b. At very high concentrations, it blocks acetylcholine at ganglionic synapses and motor nerve endings.
c. Atropine antagonizes the action of acetylcholine in the CNS.

2. Pharmacokinetics
a. Atropine is rapidly but poorly absorbed when given orally.
b. It disappears rapidly from the blood and is excreted in the urine.

3. Pharmacologic effects
a. **Effects on the heart**
(1) The heart rate slows initially, owing to medullary stimulation of the cardioinhibitory center.
(2) Tachycardia then follows with increased cardiac output and shortening of the P–R interval. Higher doses cause only tachycardia.
b. **Effects on blood pressure**
(1) Oral or intramuscular doses have little effect on blood pressure.
(2) With intravenous injection, total peripheral resistance increases.
(3) Owing to the rise in heart rate and cardiac output, arterial pressure increases.
(4) Atropine has a direct vasodilating effect on small blood vessels.
c. **Effects on the CNS**
(1) Large doses can produce hallucinations and, ultimately, coma, but therapeutic doses exert little effect.
(2) Atropine possesses antitremor activity via a central antimuscarinic mechanism.

    d. Effects on involuntary muscles

      (1) Atropine decreases the amplitude and frequency of peristaltic contractions and reduces the tone of the stomach, small intestine, and colon.

      (2) It also relaxes the smooth muscle of the biliary tract.

      (3) Bladder and ureter tone are decreased, while vesical sphincter tone is increased.

    e. Effects on the eye. Atropine blocks the acetylcholine response of the ciliary muscle of the lens and of the circular smooth muscles of the iris, producing cycloplegia and mydriasis.

    f. Effects on secretions

      (1) Sweat gland secretions are greatly reduced.

      (2) Bronchial and salivary secretions are decreased.

      (3) There is a reduction in gastric secretion during both the psychic and gastric phases, and a reduction in total acid content, especially at doses greater than 1 mg.

    g. Effects on the bronchi. Atropine produces slight bronchodilation.

  4. Therapeutic uses

    a. Ophthalmic administration is used for producing cycloplegia and mydriasis.

    b. Its ability to reduce secretions in the upper and lower respiratory tract makes it useful as a preanesthetic agent.

    c. It is used in myocardial infarction to treat sinus node bradycardia or a high-grade A-V block.

    d. It is effective for prophylaxis of motion sickness.

    e. Combined with an opioid, it is used for the treatment of renal and biliary colic.

    f. It may be used in large doses for the treatment of poisoning by anticholinesterase agents and for the rapid type of mushroom poisoning, because it antagonizes the actions of acetylcholine.

  5. Adverse effects

    a. Rapid pulse

    b. Dilated pupils, resulting in photophobia

    c. Dry mouth

    d. Flushed skin

    e. A rise in body temperature, especially in children

    f. Restlessness, confusion, and disorientation

  6. The **antidote** in atropine poisoning is physostigmine.

B. Scopolamine (hyoscine), like atropine, is an alkaloid and is an ester of tropic acid but with the organic base scopine.

  1. Pharmacologic effects. Like atropine, scopolamine has antimuscarinic actions.

    a. It is more potent than atropine in producing mydriasis and cycloplegia, in decreasing bronchial, salivary, and sweat gland secretions, and in its sedative effect.

    b. It is less potent than atropine in its effects on the heart, bronchial muscles, and intestines.

    c. Atropine has a longer duration of action, and in therapeutic doses, it does not depress the CNS.

  2. Therapeutic uses and adverse effects are generally similar to those of atropine. Scopolamine is excellent for motion sickness.

C. Propantheline is a synthetic antimuscarinic agent. High doses produce skeletal neuromuscular blockade. It is useful in the treatment of bladder spasm and enuresis.

D. Dicyclomine is another synthetic antimuscarinic drug.

  1. At normal therapeutic doses, it decreases spasm in most smooth muscles without producing atropine-like effects on the heart, eye, or salivary and sweat glands.

  2. It is thought to act by direct relaxation of muscle rather than by competitive antagonism of acetylcholine at muscarinic receptors.

E. Homatropine and eucatropine are used in ophthalmology.

  1. Homatropine is a rapidly acting muscarinic blocking agent used to produce cycloplegia and mydriasis for ophthalmic refractions.

  2. Eucatropine is used as a mydriatic.

VII. GANGLIONIC STIMULATORS AND BLOCKERS

A. Nicotine

1. Mechanism of action
   a. Nicotine interacts with the acetylcholine receptor on the postsynaptic membrane of autonomic ganglia.
   b. It causes an initial stimulation of the ganglion similar to the effect of acetylcholine.
   c. Large amounts produce a prolonged blockade following the initial stimulation.
   d. In small doses, it causes the release of catecholamines from the adrenal medulla, while larger doses prevent their release.
   e. Nicotine affects chemoreceptors in the carotid and aortic bodies and centers in the medulla oblongata.

2. Pharmacokinetics
   a. Nicotine is readily absorbed through the skin, respiratory tract, and buccal membranes.
   b. It is metabolized in the liver, kidney, and lung, and is eliminated via the kidney.
   c. It is excreted in the breast milk of lactating women who are heavy smokers.

3. Pharmacologic effects
   a. Nicotine is a CNS stimulant.
      (1) Via motor cortex excitation, it produces tremors which, with larger doses, can be followed by convulsions.
      (2) Small doses stimulate respiration while toxic doses depress it.
      (3) Nicotine stimulates the release of antidiuretic hormone.
   b. Tachycardia, increased blood pressure, and increased total peripheral resistance result from stimulation of sympathetic ganglia and the adrenal medulla.
   c. Increased bowel motility results predominantly from parasympathetic ganglionic stimulation.
   d. Salivary and bronchial secretions are first stimulated, then blocked.

4. No therapeutic uses for nicotine exist. Its inherent toxicity has been applied in the control of insects. Its presence in tobacco is, of course, of major medical importance.

B. Hexamethonium

1. Chemistry. Hexamethonium $[(CH_3)_3—N^+—(CH_2)_6—^+N—(CH_3)_3]$ has a bridge of six methylene groups between two quaternary nitrogen atoms. The addition of more intervening carbon groups decreases the activity at the ganglionic receptor and increases activity at the skeletal muscle receptor. Ten carbons (as in **decamethonium**) will produce maximal activity at the skeletal muscle receptor.

2. Mechanism of action. Hexamethonium produces competitive ganglionic blockade by occupying ganglionic cholinergic receptors.

3. Pharmacologic effects
   a. Hexamethonium reduces systemic vascular resistance, venous return, and cardiac output.
   b. Gastric secretions are reduced in volume and acidity, and gastric motility is reduced.
   c. Salivary secretions are decreased, and some bronchodilation occurs.
   d. The glomerular filtration rate is decreased and renal vascular resistance is increased.
   e. Urinary excretion may be impaired because of reduced bladder contractions.
   f. Partial mydriasis and loss of accommodation may occur.
   g. Dryness of the skin and flushing occur.

4. Therapeutic uses. Hexamethonium is not used therapeutically.

C. Trimethaphan is a sulfonium ganglionic blocking agent with a very short duration of action.

1. It is used therapeutically in treating hypertensive crises, in the management of autonomic hyperreflexia, and to provide controlled hypotension to reduce bleeding in the operative field during surgery.

2. It may reduce pulmonary edema associated with congestive heart failure by decreasing the return of blood to the right heart.

D. Mecamylamine, a ganglionic blocking agent, can be taken orally for the treatment of hypertension.

VIII. NEUROMUSCULAR BLOCKING AGENTS. These agents, which act by blocking transmission at the neuromuscular junction, can be divided into two classes on the basis of their mechanism of action: **depolarizing agents** and **competitive,** or **stabilizing, blocking agents**.

A. Mechanism of action

1. **Depolarizing agents** (succinylcholine, decamethonium)
   a. Like acetylcholine, depolarizing agents react with receptors at the muscle end-plate leading to depolarization of the excitable membrane. This **phase I block** is seen clinically as fasciculation.
   b. With prolonged exposure, a reduction in receptor sensitivity occurs, leading to a **phase II,** or **desensitization, block** manifested by flaccid paralysis. This phase II block is not competitive in nature.

2. **Competitive blocking agents** (tubocurarine, gallamine, pancuronium, atracurium, vecuronium, metocurine, pipercuronium)
   a. Competitive blocking agents combine with acetylcholine receptors at the muscle end-plate but do not activate them.
   b. By decreasing the number of available acetylcholine receptors, these agents reduce the height of the end-plate potential; thus, the threshold for excitation is not reached.

B. Pharmacokinetics

1. After injection of a neuromuscular blocking agent, it is found in high concentration in venous blood flowing to the heart and ultimately in the extracellular space around the muscle end-plate.

2. Succinylcholine has a rapid onset of action, which facilitates rapid endotracheal intubation.

3. Atracurium has a longer onset of action than succinylcholine, and spontaneous recovery occurs after 30–60 minutes.

4. **Metabolism**
   a. Metabolism of gallamine, tubocurarine, and decamethonium is negligible.
   b. Pancuronium is deacetylated, and its metabolites show some activity.
   c. Succinylcholine is rapidly metabolized to succinylmonocholine and choline, which accounts for its brief duration of action.
   d. Atracurium is inactivated in the plasma by enzymatic ester hydrolysis and by a nonenzymatic process known as Hofmann elimination.

C. Therapeutic uses

1. Neuromuscular blocking agents are used:
   a. As surgical adjuvants to anesthesia
      (1) For promoting skeletal muscle relaxation
      (2) For facilitating endotracheal intubation
   b. With electroconvulsant shock therapy to prevent trauma
   c. In the diagnosis of myasthenia gravis (tubocurarine), although provocative tests of this sort are potentially hazardous procedures

2. Atracurium may be useful in patients with renal failure, since it does not rely on the kidney for excretion.

3. **Pipercuronium** does not have vagolytic activity nor does it cause histamine release.

D. Adverse effects

1. **All neuromuscular blocking agents**
   a. These agents do not affect the sensorium, so that despite the paralysis, individuals remain conscious and are able to feel pain.
   b. Prolonged apnea may occur.

2. **Depolarizing agents**
   a. The fasciculations can cause muscle pain; this occurs most frequently in young patients.
   b. Fasciculation of the abdominal muscles can result in increased intragastric pressure. This is important in patients at risk of aspirating gastric contents.
   c. Contraction of extraocular muscles can lead to an increase in intraocular pressure.

    d. The muscle fasciculations and the increased intraocular and intragastric pressure may be diminished by the prior administration of a small dose of a competitive blocking agent.

    e. Succinylcholine may exert some action at other acetylcholine receptors, such as stimulation of autonomic ganglia and muscarinic receptors.

    f. The resulting effects, such as bradycardia and increased bronchial secretions, are seen more commonly with repeated intravenous administration in children; cardiac arrest has occurred.

    g. In some genetically predisposed individuals, the combination of succinylcholine and halothane results in a rapid and potentially fatal rise in temperature (malignant hyperthermia).

  3. Tubocurarine

    a. A dose-related fall in arterial pressure, the most common side effect, is the result of both ganglionic blockade and histamine release.

    b. Histamine release can also result in bronchospasm.

  4. Metocurine causes histamine release less often than tubocurarine does, and **atracurium** is a less potent histamine releaser than either tubocurarine or metocurine.

  5. Vecuronium causes no histamine release; thus, the risk of histamine-induced hypotension or bronchoconstriction is reduced.

  6. Gallamine causes tachycardia and increased arterial pressure, the results of both vagolytic and tyramine-like effects.

  7. Pancuronium also causes an increase in the heart rate and in arterial pressure, but to a lesser extent than gallamine does; the mechanism is not understood.

  8. Pipercuronium can have a prolonged duration of action in patients with renal failure.

E. Factors influencing the action of neuromuscular blocking agents

  1. Serum cholinesterase is determined genetically; the normally transient effects of succinylcholine will be greatly prolonged in an individual with deficient serum cholinesterase.

  2. Because serum cholinesterase is synthesized in the liver, hepatic disease can double the duration of action of succinylcholine.

  3. Echothiophate, an irreversible cholinesterase inhibitor used in the treatment of glaucoma, can significantly decrease cholinesterase activity and thereby increase the duration of action of succinylcholine.

  4. Patients with myasthenia gravis are highly sensitive to competitive neuromuscular blocking agents, and phase II block occurs sooner than in normal individuals when depolarizing blockers are given.

  5. Patients with Eaton-Lambert syndrome (small cell, or oat cell, carcinoma of the lung) have increased sensitivity to both competitive and depolarizing neuromuscular blockers.

  6. Depolarizing neuromuscular blockers increase serum potassium; this is exacerbated in conditions that are associated with hyperkalemia, such as burns.

  7. Aminoglycoside antibiotics and lincomycin exert a synergistic neuromuscular blockade when given with either competitive or depolarizing neuromuscular blocking agents; the mechanism is presynaptic.

  8. All inhalation anesthetics increase the effects of neuromuscular blocking agents.

F. Reversal of neuromuscular blockade

  1. Competitive neuromuscular blockers can be antagonized by cholinesterase inhibitors, such as edrophonium, neostigmine, or pyridostigmine.

  2. No antagonists currently exist for depolarizing blockers.

    a. Controlled ventilation is used until spontaneous recovery occurs.

    b. If an anticholinesterase is given, phase I block increases, but an anticholinesterase may reverse phase II block.

STUDY QUESTIONS

Directions: Each of the numbered items or incomplete statements in this section is followed by answers or by completions of the statement. Select the **one** lettered answer or completion that is **best** in each case.

1. A patient who is using a direct-acting sympath-omimetic agent as a decongestant is most likely to be taking

(A) ephedrine
(B) amphetamine
(C) phenylephrine
(D) metaraminol
(E) mephentermine

2. A patient is taking a mixed-acting sympathomi-metic as a nasal decongestant. This agent, which exhibits tachyphylaxis and qualitatively resembles epinephrine in its cardiovascular effects, most likely is

(A) ephedrine
(B) phenylephrine
(C) metaproterenol
(D) terbutaline
(E) amphetamine

3. Which of the following agents would bring a rapid heart rate (120 beats/minute) back to normal?

(A) Isoproterenol
(B) Phentolamine
(C) Propranolol
(D) Phenoxybenzamine
(E) Edrophonium

4. A 29-year-old woman says that her eyes will not stay open despite the fact that she is not tired. On physical examination, her facial musculature weakens as she continues to talk. Which of the following drugs would be most useful in helping to make a diagnosis in this patient?

(A) Physostigmine
(B) Neostigmine
(C) Pyridostigmine
(D) Edrophonium
(E) Demecarium

5. Atropine is useful in treating poisoning pro-duced by organophosphate insecticides because it

(A) reactivates inhibited acetylcholinesterase
(B) stimulates α receptors directly
(C) stimulates β receptors directly
(D) inhibits normal ganglionic transmission
(E) blocks the action of acetylcholine at both cen-tral and peripheral sites

1-C   4-D
2-A   5-E
3-C

Directions: Each item below contains four suggested answers of which **one or more** is correct. Choose the answer

A if **1, 2, and 3** are correct
B if **1 and 3** are correct
C if **2 and 4** are correct
D if **4** is correct
E if **1, 2, 3, and 4** are correct

6. β-Adrenergic agonists include which of the following substances?

(1) Epinephrine
(2) Isoproterenol
(3) Norepinephrine
(4) Phentolamine

7. A 15-year-old girl presents with complaints of frequent migraine headaches. Which of the following drugs might help to prevent them?

(1) Aspirin
(2) Propranolol
(3) Ibuprofen
(4) Methysergide

8. Dopamine can be used to treat which of the following?

(1) Parkinson's disease
(2) Cardiogenic shock
(3) Side effects of phenothiazines
(4) Congestive heart failure

9. Characteristics of amphetamine include which of the following?

(1) It is a sympatholytic agent
(2) It causes mood elevation
(3) It stimulates MAO
(4) It depresses hunger centers in the hypothalamus

10. Selective β₁-adrenergic blocking agents include which of the following?

(1) Atenolol
(2) Timolol
(3) Metoprolol
(4) Propranolol

11. Mechanisms by which labetalol produces a reduction in blood pressure when administered to hypertensive patients include which of the following?

(1) Nonselective β-receptor blocking activity
(2) Ganglionic blocking activity
(3) α₁-Receptor blocking activity
(4) Adrenergic neural blocking activity

12. Characteristics of carbachol include which of the following?

(1) It is a parasympathetic agent
(2) It is purely muscarinic in action
(3) It is resistant to acetylcholinesterase
(4) It causes mydriasis

13. True statements concerning the effects of drugs on gastrointestinal motility include which of the following?

(1) Atropine delays gastric emptying
(2) Opiates stimulate gastric emptying
(3) Metoclopramide stimulates gastrointestinal motility
(4) Scopolamine stimulates gastrointestinal motility

14. Characteristics of pancuronium include which of the following?

(1) Its effects on the heart are similar to the effects of succinylcholine
(2) It acts by the same mechanism as tubocurarine
(3) It produces analgesia
(4) It can increase arterial pressure

Directions: The group of items in this section consists of lettered options followed by a set of numbered items. For each item, select the **one** lettered option that is most closely associated with it. Each lettered option may be selected once, more than once, or not at all.

Questions 15–19

Match each characteristic to the β-adrenergic blocking agent with which it is most likely to be associated.

(A) Acebutolol
(B) Labetalol
(C) Metoprolol
(D) Pindolol
(E) Timolol

15. This nonselective β blocker is used to treat glaucoma

16. This nonselective β blocker also has α_1-blocking activity

17. This nonselective β blocker has some α-adrenergic activity

18. This β blocker has a stronger β_1-blocking effect than β_2-blocking effect

19. This β blocker is a selective β_1-adrenergic antagonist

15-E   18-A
16-B   19-C
17-D

ANSWERS AND EXPLANATIONS

1. The answer is C *[II E 1 a, 2 a]*
All of the substances listed in the question are sympathomimetic agents. Ephedrine, amphetamine, me-phentermine, and metaraminol are all mixed-acting agents. Phenylephrine is direct-acting and is used clinically as a decongestant.

2. The answer is A *[II F 2, 3 b]*
Phenylephrine, metaproterenol, and terbutaline are all direct-acting sympathomimetic agents, while am-phetamine is indirect-acting. Ephedrine is mixed-acting and is used as a nasal decongestant. While its primary action is indirect, causing release of norepinephrine from storage in nerve terminals, it also di-rectly stimulates sympathetic receptors.

3. The answer is C *[III B 1]*
Propranolol is an effective agent for treating an abnormal tachycardia. Its mechanism of action is β-adrenergic blockade. Propranolol decreases the heart rate, reduces cardiac output, and prolongs sys-tole. It reduces total coronary blood flow to most tissues (except the brain) and lowers oxygen consump-tion.

4. The answer is D *[V C 3 a]*
If the patient's symptoms are due to myasthenia gravis, they will be reversed by a cholinesterase inhibitor. Although neostigmine and pyridostigmine are used for the symptomatic treatment of myasthenia gravis, edrophonium is more useful for the diagnosis of this disorder because it is more rapidly absorbed and has a shorter duration of action. Demecarium and physostigmine are used in the treatment of glaucoma; the latter drug is also useful for reversing the anticholinergic effects of various drugs.

5. The answer is E *[VI A 1, 4 f]*
Atropine is both a central and a peripheral muscarinic blocker. Atropine competes reversibly with ace-tylcholine at muscarinic receptors, antagonizes the action of acetylcholine in the CNS, and, at high con-centrations, blocks acetylcholine action at ganglionic synapses and motor nerve endings.

6. The answer is A (1, 2, 3) *[I D 2 b]*
Isoproterenol, epinephrine, and norepinephrine are agonists for all adrenergic receptors, α and β. The relative potency at β_1 receptors is isoproterenol > epinephrine and norepinephrine. The relative potency of these agonists at β_2 receptors is isoproterenol > epinephrine >> norepinephrine. Phentolamine is an α-adrenergic antagonist.

7. The answer is C (2, 4) *[III A 4 c, B 1 c (7); Ch 8 V B 1 b; Ch 9 II A 4 b, G 3 b]*
Aspirin and ibuprofen are both analgesics and can be used for the treatment of migraine headaches but not for the prevention of acute attacks. Propranolol, a β-adrenergic receptor blocker, and methysergide, a semisynthetic ergot alkaloid, are both effective for the prophylaxis of migraine headaches.

8. The answer is C (2, 4) *[II C 4; Ch 3 IV A]*
Dopamine, an intermediate in the biosynthesis of norepinephrine, is an important neurotransmitter in the CNS. Dopamine is a β_1-adrenergic agonist with positive inotropic effects on the myocardium and is, therefore, used in the treatment of cardiogenic and septic shock and in chronic refractory congestive heart failure. In Parkinson's disease, a dopamine deficiency in the stratum appears to cause the neurologic symptoms. However, the drug dopamine does not cross the blood–brain barrier, and, therefore, levodopa (l-dopa), the precursor of dopamine, is given instead. The neurologic side effects of antipsychotic agents, such as the phenothiazines, resemble the symptoms of Parkinson's disease, but again dopamine would be ineffective as therapy.

9. The answer is C (2, 4) *[II G]*
Amphetamine is a mixed-acting sympathomimetic agent that causes mood elevation. It does not stimulate MAO but blocks it. Amphetamine has been used in the treatment of obesity because of its effects on the lateral hypothalamic feeding center.

10. The answer is B (1, 3) *[III B 1, 2, 7, 8]*
Atenolol and metoprolol are selective β_1 blockers, whereas timolol and propranolol are nonselective: They compete for both β_1 and β_2 receptors. Nonselective β blockers are more likely to cause broncho-spasm than selective β_1 blockers. Nevertheless, all β-adrenergic blocking agents must be used with cau-tion in patients with asthma or chronic obstructive pulmonary disease.

11. The answer is B (1, 3) *[III B 4]*
Labetalol is a nonselective β blocker that also has α_1-receptor blocking activity, properties that make it useful in the treatment of mild to severe hypertension. Labetalol does not possess adrenergic neural or ganglionic blocking activity.

12. The answer is B (1, 3) *[IV C]*
Carbachol (carbamylcholine) is a parasympathetic agent that is resistant to cholinesterase because of its carbamic acid–ester link. It exerts both muscarinic and nicotinic effects. Because it is a parasympathetic agonist, it causes miosis, not mydriasis.

13. The answer is B (1, 3) *[IV F 1; VI A 3 d; Ch 3 IX B 1 b (3); Ch 13 II B 2 b (2)]*
Both atropine and scopolamine delay gastric emptying and inhibit gastrointestinal activity because of their anticholinergic properties. Opiates delay gastric emptying, while metoclopramide stimulates gastrointestinal motility. Drugs that alter gastric emptying and intestinal motility can affect the absorption of other drugs.

14. The answer is C (2, 4) *[VIII A, D]*
Pancuronium is, like tubocurarine, a competitive muscular blocker. Unlike tubocurarine, it can cause an increase in arterial pressure, whereas tubocurarine causes histamine-induced hypotension. Unlike succinylcholine, pancuronium can increase the heart rate. None of the neuromuscular blocking agents affect awareness of pain.

15–19. The answers are: 15-E *[III B 2]*, **16-B** *[III B 4]*, **17-D** *[III B 5]*, **18-A** *[III B 6]*, **19-C** *[III B 7]*
Timolol is a nonselective β-adrenergic blocking agent (i.e., it competes for both β_1 and β_2 receptors); it lowers intraocular pressure by reducing the production of aqueous humor. Timolol eyedrops are used for the treatment of glaucoma.

Labetalol is another nonselective β blocker; it also has α_1-blocking activity. Labetalol is a potent antihypertensive agent.

Pindolol is a nonselective β blocker that also has some degree of intrinsic sympathomimetic (α-adrenergic) activity.

Acebutolol is primarily a β_1-blocking agent but has some β_2-blocking activity. It can cause arthralgia and myalgia as well as the usual untoward effects seen with β blockers.

Metoprolol is a selective β_1-adrenergic antagonist that is used to treat hypertension. It is less likely to cause problems in asthmatic patients than nonselective β blockers, but must still be used with caution in such patients.

3
Agents Acting on the Central Nervous System

I. INTRODUCTION

A. Transmission of nerve impulses (see Chapter 2 Figure 2-1).

1. **Information transfer.** The brain and spinal cord are involved in information transfer via electrical signals passing along axons (**action potentials**).

2. **Synaptic transmission**
   a. The **locus of communication** between neurons is the **synapse**.
      (1) In general, a chemical **neurotransmitter** is released from a presynaptic neuron, diffuses across the synaptic cleft, and interacts with a special cell-surface receptor located on a second, postsynaptic, neuron.
      (2) The neurotransmitter–receptor complex initiates a sequence of events (e.g., the opening of channels for particular ions), which can either excite, inhibit, or otherwise modulate the electrical activity of the postsynaptic neuron.
   b. Synaptic transmission between neurons can be affected by altering the levels of neurotransmitter in the presynaptic neuron. This can be accomplished by various agents, which:
      (1) Block or enhance the biosynthesis of the neurotransmitter
      (2) Block or enhance the metabolic degradation of the neurotransmitter
      (3) Alter the reuptake and reutilization of the neurotransmitter in presynaptic terminals
   c. It is possible to alter the amount of neurotransmitter that is released by activating **presynaptic receptors (autoreceptors)** that are located at some synapses.
   d. Many drugs are believed to bind to receptors and, bypassing the normal neurotransmitter, either to activate or block the response of the postsynaptic neuron, serving, respectively, as agonists or antagonists.
   e. Some drugs may act directly on ion channels, bypassing the neurotransmitter–receptor interaction entirely.

3. **Mechanism of action.** Although the basic mechanisms underlying many of these agents that act on the central nervous system (CNS) are only partially understood, most are believed to alter either the basic cellular functioning of neurons or the communication between neurons.
   a. Any agent that slows or blocks the axonal electrical conduction (e.g., a local anesthetic) will have an effect on behavior.
   b. At therapeutic doses, most of the pharmacologically useful agents that affect the CNS are believed to act at various specific synaptic sites.

B. Blood–brain barrier. The ability of an agent to affect CNS function is dependent on its ability to cross or mediate an effect across the **blood–brain barrier**.

1. The blood–brain barrier restricts the passage of polar compounds and macromolecules from the blood into the brain interstitium.
   a. Agents that are lipid-soluble, are un-ionized to physiologic pH, and bind poorly to plasma proteins are better able to diffuse across the blood–brain barrier.
   b. Some metabolically important compounds (e.g., nutrients) apparently are actively transported across this barrier.

2. The morphologic basis for the blood–brain barrier appears to be the structure of the endothelial cell layer lining the brain capillaries. Transendothelial vesicular transport (pinocytosis) is a primary cellular mechanism by which plasma protein constituents and macromolecules pass through the cerebrovascular endothelium.

II. SEDATIVE–HYPNOTICS

A. Barbiturates

1. Chemistry

   a. The parent compound, **barbituric acid** (Figure 3-1), is derived from a dehydration of urea and malonic acid. Barbituric acid itself has no depressant effect on the CNS.

   b. The common barbiturates are listed in Table 3-1; the radicals given in the table are those shown in Figure 3-1 (R_1 and R_2).

   c. Changes in structure that favor increased lipid solubility will speed up the onset of action, shorten the duration of action, and increase the hypnotic potency.

   d. When the oxygen at C-2 of oxybarbiturates is replaced with a sulfur, it becomes a thiobarbiturate, a compound with enhanced lipid solubility.

2. Classification. Barbiturates are classified on the basis of their onset and duration of action.

   a. Ultra–short-acting barbiturates (e.g., **thiopental**) act within seconds, and their duration of action is 30 minutes. Their principal use is as intravenous adjuvants to anesthesia.

   b. Short-acting barbiturates (e.g., **pentobarbital**) have a duration of action of about 2 hours; their principal use is as sleep-inducing hypnotics.

   c. Intermediate-acting barbiturates (e.g., **amobarbital**) have an effect lasting 3–5 hours. Their principal use is as hypnotics; however, they have a "hangover" liability, the result of residual depression of the CNS.

   d. Long-acting barbiturates (e.g., **phenobarbital**) have a duration of action greater than 6 hours. They are effective hypnotics and sedatives and at low doses are used as antiepileptic agents, but they are likely to cause hangover.

3. Mechanism of action

   a. At low doses, barbiturates either have a γ-aminobutyric acid (GABA)-like action or enhance the effects of GABA, an inhibitory neurotransmitter.

   b. When GABA receptors are activated, chloride channels open. Chloride enters the cell, hyperpolarizes it, and produces decreased excitation.

   c. There is also a picrotoxin site associated with the GABA receptor to which barbiturates bind. The greater the affinity of a barbiturate for the picrotoxin binding site, the greater will be its potency.

   d. Barbiturates are less selective than benzodiazepines, which also have GABA-like actions, because elevating the dose of barbiturates produces a generalized CNS depression in addition to selective depression at synaptic sites.

4. Pharmacokinetics

   a. The duration of action of a barbiturate depends on:

   (1) Its rate of metabolic (hepatic) degradation

   (2) Its degree of lipid solubility

   (3) The extent to which it binds to serum proteins, which reduces renal excretion

   b. Long-acting barbiturates are metabolized principally in the liver by a slow oxidation of the radicals at C-5, which produces more polar derivatives with low lipid solubility.

   c. Ultra–short-acting barbiturates are highly lipid-soluble and, thus, have a short onset and duration of action.

   (1) High lipid solubility allows rapid transport across the blood–brain barrier.

   (2) Removal of the ultra–short-acting barbiturates from the brain occurs via redistribution to other tissues (e.g., muscle).

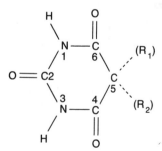

Figure 3-1. Structure of barbituric acid. The radicals (R_1 and R_2) of the common barbiturates are given in Table 3-1.

Table 3-1. Common Barbiturates: Radicals and Duration of Action

Drug	Radical 1 $(R_1)^*$	Radical 2 $(R_2)^*$	Duration of Action
Thiopental	Ethyl	1-Methylbutyl	Ultra-short
Hexobarbital	Methyl	1-Cyclohexen-1-yl	Short
Pentobarbital	Ethyl	1-Methylbutyl	Short
Secobarbital	Allyl	1-Methylbutyl	Short
Amobarbital	Ethyl	Isopentyl	Intermediate
Butabarbital	Ethyl	*sec*-Butyl	Intermediate
Barbital	Ethyl	Ethyl	Long
Phenobarbital	Ethyl	Phenyl	Long

*See Figure 3-1.

  d. Barbiturates are absorbed from the stomach, small intestine, rectum, and intramuscular sites.
  e. They readily cross the placental barrier, and concentrations in the fetal blood approach those in maternal blood.
  f. Barbiturates and their metabolites are principally excreted via the renal route.
   (1) If renal function is impaired, barbiturates can cause severe CNS and cardiovascular depression.
   (2) Alkalinization of the urine profoundly expedites the excretion of barbiturates with lower lipid solubility, such as phenobarbital. These drugs are only partially bound to plasma protein and are weak organic acids.

 5. Pharmacologic effects
  a. Barbiturates depress the CNS at all levels in a dose-dependent fashion. A barbiturate plus another CNS depressant (e.g., a phenothiazine, ethanol, or an antihistamine) can result in marked depression.
  b. As hypnotics, they decrease the amount of time spent in REM sleep.
  c. Barbiturates are not analgesic and, at low doses, are thought to be hyperalgesic.
  d. All barbiturates will suppress convulsant activity if given in sufficient doses.
  e. Respiration is depressed at multiple levels. As CNS depression develops and the neurogenic respiratory drive is eliminated, the respiratory drive shifts to the carotid and aortic bodies. The hypoxic drive is affected at lower doses than the chemoreceptor drive, but it persists beyond complete blockade of the response to carbon dioxide. Eventually, at high doses, the hypoxic drive also fails.
  f. At sedative doses, barbiturates have little effect on the cardiovascular system.
   (1) As the dose of barbiturate is increased, depressed ganglionic transmission results in decreased blood pressure and heart rate.
   (2) Toxic dose levels can cause circulatory collapse, which is due, in part, to medullary vasomotor depression.
  g. Most barbiturates, but especially phenobarbital, are capable of inducing the hepatic microsomal drug-metabolizing enzyme system.
   (1) This results in increased degradation of the barbiturate, ultimately leading to barbiturate tolerance.
   (2) It also causes increased inactivation of other compounds, such as the anticoagulants, phenytoin, digitoxin, theophylline, and glucocorticoids, leading to potentially serious problems with drug interactions.
  h. Anesthetic doses of barbiturates may suppress renal tubular transport.
  i. Barbiturate-induced porphyria can occur as a result of more rapid hemoglobin degradation.

 6. Therapeutic uses
  a. Although still used as sedative–hypnotic agents, barbiturates are being replaced for this purpose by the benzodiazepines (see II B 6; VI C) because of the following disadvantages:
   (1) They have a narrow therapeutic-to-toxic dosage range.
   (2) They suppress REM sleep.
   (3) Tolerance develops relatively quickly.
   (4) They have a high potential for physical dependence and abuse.
   (5) Drug interactions secondary to microsomal enzyme induction are frequent.

b. Due to their rapid onset of action, barbiturates (i.e., phenobarbital, pentobarbital, amobarbital, thiopental) are used in the emergency treatment of convulsions as in status epilepticus (see III A), but in adults, the benzodiazepines are the drugs of choice.

c. The ultra–short-acting thiobarbiturates are useful as intravenous adjuncts to surgical anesthetics.

d. Barbiturates, especially in anesthetic doses, significantly decrease oxygen utilization by the brain, which may be of value in lessening cerebral edema caused by surgery or trauma and in protecting against cerebral infarction during cerebral ischemia.

e. The ability of barbiturates to stimulate liver glucuronyl transferase has been applied successfully in the treatment of hyperbilirubinemia and kernicterus in the neonate.

7. Adverse effects

a. Depressant effects include oversedation and a decrease in REM sleep.

b. Skin eruptions and porphyria can occur.

c. Barbiturate dependence

(1) Physiologic as well as psychological dependence can occur.

(2) Withdrawal of a barbiturate may result in grand mal seizures, severe tremors, vivid hallucinations, and psychoses. Abrupt withdrawal should, therefore, be avoided.

d. Acute barbiturate overdosage

(1) An overdose can result in coma, diminished reflexes (although deep tendon reflexes are usually intact), severe respiratory depression, hypotension leading to cardiovascular collapse, and renal failure.

(2) **Treatment of acute overdosage**

(a) Primary treatment consists of supporting respiration and circulation.

(b) Excretion of the drug is fostered by alkalinizing the urine and promoting diuresis. These measures are most effective with the long-acting barbiturates.

(c) Hemodialysis or peritoneal dialysis is useful and often needed.

B. Nonbarbiturate sedative–hypnotics

1. Chloral hydrate

a. Pharmacokinetics

(1) Chloral hydrate is metabolized in the liver by alcohol dehydrogenase to trichloroethanol, which is thought to be the active metabolite producing the CNS effects. In addition, it enhances the ability of hepatic microsomes to metabolize drugs.

(2) Trichloroethanol and, to a lesser extent, chloral hydrate are oxidized to trichloroacetic acid, which is excreted in the kidney as the glucuronide conjugate.

b. Therapeutic uses

(1) Chloral hydrate is a relatively safe hypnotic drug, inducing sleep in a half hour, which lasts about 6 hours. It causes a relatively small reduction in REM sleep.

(2) It is used mainly in children and the elderly and is most effective when used for 1–3 nights to treat transient insomnia.

(3) Chloral hydrate should not be used in patients with significant liver or kidney disease.

c. Adverse effects

(1) Chloral hydrate is quite bad-tasting and is irritating to the gastrointestinal tract.

(2) The CNS depressant effects are potentiated by alcohol (the combination being dubbed a "Mickey Finn").

(3) Addiction can occur, and when it does, the patient often presents with chronic gastritis and skin eruptions. Dependent individuals may lose the mechanisms that detoxify the drug.

2. Paraldehyde

a. Chemistry. Paraldehyde is a trimer of acetaldehyde; its structure is shown in Figure 3-2.

b. Mechanism of action

(1) Paraldehyde produces hypnosis in about 15 minutes, and its effects last 4–8 hours.

(2) Its CNS depressant activity resembles that of alcohol, chloral hydrate, and the barbiturates.

c. Route of administration. Paraldehyde can be administered orally, parenterally, or rectally. When used rectally, it is combined with two volumes of olive oil.

d. Therapeutic uses

(1) It is used exclusively for patients undergoing withdrawal from alcohol.

(2) It is used for patients with hepatic or renal failure because it is mainly eliminated via the lungs.

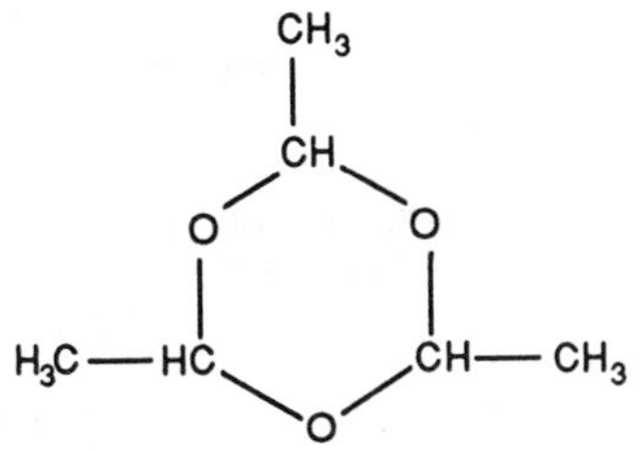

Figure 3-2. Paraldehyde.

e. Adverse effects
  (1) Its strong odor and disagreeable taste limit its use mainly to hospitals.
  (2) It is a gastrointestinal irritant.
  (3) Pulmonary disease and peptic ulcer disease are relative contraindications to paraldehyde administration.
  (4) It should not be used with disulfiram.

3. Glutethimide
  a. Pharmacokinetics. Glutethimide is erratically absorbed from the gastrointestinal tract and is chiefly metabolized in the liver. After metabolism, most is excreted by the kidney.
  b. Therapeutic uses. The use of glutethimide as a therapeutic agent is hard to justify. Its clinical use is now limited by its high addiction potential, the severity of withdrawal symptoms, and the problems caused by acute intoxication.
  c. Adverse effects
  (1) Chronic abuse of glutethimide can lead to toxic psychoses, convulsions, and hyperpyrexia.
  (2) Prolonged use of glutethimide can result in habituation and physical dependence.
  (3) Acute intoxication
    (a) Symptoms similar to those of barbiturate poisoning occur with respiratory depression and severe circulatory failure. In addition, atropine-like effects are observed, including persistent hyperpyrexia and convulsions.
    (b) The plasma half-life during acute intoxication can be as long as 4 days but can be reduced to 12 hours by hemodialysis.
    (c) Although the plasma levels decline after dialysis, a secondary rise in plasma levels is then observed. This is thought to result from additional intestinal absorption of glutethimide.

4. Methyprylon
  a. Pharmacokinetics. Methyprylon is used as an oral hypnotic, which closely resembles secobarbital in its onset and duration of action. It is absorbed from the gastrointestinal tract. Acute intoxication resembles that of barbiturates; treatment is supportive.
  b. Adverse effects
  (1) Suppression of REM sleep
  (2) Hangover-like effects
  (3) Skin rashes
  (4) Addictive potential

5. Etchchlorvynol
  a. Pharmacokinetics
  (1) Etchchlorvynol is classified as a tertiary alcohol. In addition to its sedative–hypnotic properties, it possesses muscle-relaxant and anticonvulsant properties.
  (2) It is absorbed from the gastrointestinal tract and shows an onset of action in 30 minutes and a 5-hour duration of action.
  b. Adverse effects
  (1) Suppression of REM sleep
  (2) Ataxia
  (3) Hypotension
  (4) Facial numbness
  (5) Physical dependence. An acute overdose is treated as barbiturate poisoning is treated.

6. Benzodiazepine derivatives (see VI C). The benzodiazepines at present are generally considered to be the preferred drugs for sedation–hypnosis. In contrast to the various other sedative–hypnotics, the benzodiazepines are not general neuronal depressants. They act on the allosteric site of the GABA receptor, facilitating chloride entry into the neuron, which produces an inhibitory effect on neuronal conduction. Whether the antianxiety properties of the benzodiazepines are distinct from their sedative–hypnotic effects is presently unclear.

a. Flurazepam

    (1) Pharmacologic effects. Flurazepam produces hypnotic effects within 20–40 minutes after an oral dose, which may last for 6–8 hours. The major metabolite has a long half-life and may cause daytime sedation and motor impairment.

    (2) Adverse effects

        (a) Flurazepam causes less suppression of REM sleep than other benzodiazepines.

        (b) Overdosage can occur and is treated as for other benzodiazepines (see VI C 4 b).

        (c) At moderate dosage, addiction potential is low, as is withdrawal (rebound) insomnia, which is often seen with many of the other hypnotics.

b. Triazolam

    (1) Pharmacokinetics. It has the shortest latency period before sleep, but because of its short duration of action, its effects may not persist through the night.

    (2) Therapeutic uses. Triazolam is used for the short-term treatment of insomnia.

    (3) Adverse effects

        (a) It is least likely to cause residual drowsiness but may cause daytime anxiety.

        (b) Rebound insomnia may occur.

        (c) Profound anterograde amnesia and toxic psychosis have been reported.

c. Temazepam

    (1) Pharmacokinetics

        (a) It is conjugated with glucuronic acid and is excreted in the urine; therefore, hepatic dysfunction has little effect on its elimination.

        (b) While it has a short elimination half-life, temazepam has an intermediate-to-slow onset and may accumulate with repeated use.

    (2) Pharmacologic effects. Temazepam decreases awakenings and increases sleep time. It does not affect sleep latency.

III. AGENTS USED IN THE TREATMENT OF SEIZURES

A. Barbiturates (see II A)

  1. Pharmacologic effects

    a. As antiseizure agents, the barbiturates have a narrow margin of safety. However, phenobarbital possesses more selectivity in its anticonvulsant action than in its sedative effect.

    b. If a barbiturate is used as an anticonvulsant during pregnancy, the neonate can experience withdrawal symptoms.

  2. Therapeutic uses

    a. Barbiturates are the drugs of choice for status epilepticus in infants and children.

    b. They are no longer a preferred treatment for the prophylactic control of general seizure states (generalized tonic–clonic seizures, simple and complex partial seizures).

  3. Adverse effects

    a. Sedation

    b. Physical and psychological dependence (see II A 7)

B. Deoxybarbiturates

  1. Pharmacokinetics and therapeutic uses

    a. The prototype agent of this class is **primidone,** which is useful for generalized tonic–clonic seizures and simple partial seizures.

    b. Primidone does not have a true barbituric acid ring structure but bears a close resemblance to the barbiturates (Figure 3-3).

    c. It is well absorbed from the gastrointestinal tract. Two major metabolites are seen, one of which is phenobarbital.

  2. Adverse effects

    a. Exacerbates petit mal epilepsy

    b. Skin rashes, which are also common to the barbiturates

    c. Leukopenia and thrombocytopenia

    d. Systemic lupus erythematosus

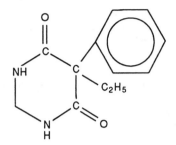

Figure 3-3. Primidone.

   e. Acute psychotic reactions
   f. Sedation, which decreases with continued use

C. Hydantoins. All hydantoins are highly fat-soluble and are insoluble in water. **Phenytoin** (diphenylhydantoin) is the most commonly prescribed hydantoin; **mephenytoin** and **ethotoin** are less frequently used.

   1. Phenytoin
      a. Pharmacokinetics
         (1) Phenytoin acts by stabilizing membranes by decreasing Na^+ conductance during high-frequency repetitive firing.
         (2) Phenytoin exerts its dampening effect only when neuronal activity is abnormally high. It allows the normal conduction of action potentials but halts seizure activity.
         (3) Because phenytoin is a weak acid (pK_a 8.3), its intestinal absorption is variable, incomplete, and slow. Nearly all (90%) is bound to plasma protein. The drug is metabolized by the microsomal system and is excreted first in the bile and then in the urine.
      b. Therapeutic uses
         (1) Phenytoin is used in the treatment of grand mal epilepsy and tonic–clonic seizure disorders.
         (2) Its use is contraindicated in liver disease and in patients with absence seizures (petit mal epilepsy) or with convulsions resulting from fever or barbiturate withdrawal.
      c. Adverse effects
         (1) Gastrointestinal irritation; thus, it should be taken with meals.
         (2) Ataxia and diplopia
         (3) Blood dyscrasias
         (4) Hypersensitivity reactions, including the Stevens-Johnson syndrome and systemic lupus erythematosus: Phenytoin should be stopped if a rash occurs.
         (5) Gingival hyperplasia, hirsutism, increased collagen proliferation, and bone growth
         (6) Hepatitis
         (7) Cardiovascular collapse and CNS depression, which may occur with intravenous administration exceeding 50 mg/min
         (8) Drug interactions: Increased plasma concentrations of phenytoin can occur due to inhibition of its inactivation by concurrent administration of chloramphenicol, isoniazid, cimetidine, dicumarol, disulfiram, and certain sulfonamides.
         (9) Fetal malformations: Phenytoin is teratogenic.

   2. Mephenytoin has a much higher incidence of blood dyscrasias than phenytoin and greater CNS depressant activity, which limit its usefulness.

   3. Ethotoin is safer but is much less effective than phenytoin.

D. Succinimides

   1. Ethosuximide
      a. Mechanism of action. Although the mechanism of action is unknown, it may involve the release of GABA.
      b. Pharmacokinetics. Ethosuximide is absorbed from the gastrointestinal tract. About 80% is metabolized in the hepatic microsomal metabolizing system; 20% is unchanged. Both unchanged drug and hepatic metabolites appear in the urine.
      c. Therapeutic uses. Ethosuximide is considered the drug of first choice in the treatment of petit mal epilepsy (absence seizures).
      d. Adverse effects
         (1) Exacerbates grand mal epilepsy

(2) Gastrointestinal reactions, such as anorexia and nausea
(3) CNS effects, such as drowsiness, headache, and hiccup; extrapyramidal symptoms and photophobia have also been reported.
(4) Hypersensitivity reactions
(5) Psychotic episodes

2. Both **methsuximide** and **phensuximide** have been useful antiepileptic agents with adverse experience profiles similar to that of ethosuximide. They appear to have a lower efficacy than the prototype agent, ethosuximide. Methsuximide is effective against absence seizures; however, it is not commonly used because it can cause ataxia.

E. Benzodiazepines

1. General considerations
  a. Besides the value of these agents as sedative–hypnotics and mild tranquilizers, some are also very effective in seizure control.
  b. Benzodiazepines enhance a variety of GABA-mediated synaptic systems involving both presynaptic and postsynaptic inhibition.
  c. When any benzodiazepine is used intravenously, cardiovascular and respiratory collapse can occur.

2. Diazepam, given intravenously, is now considered the drug of choice for status epilepticus in adults. It should be used with great caution in patients who have received barbiturates. It is also effective against all other types of seizures, particularly petit mal and other minor motor seizures. Its usefulness as a long-term antiepileptic agent is limited by the development of refractoriness within a few months.

3. Clonazepam is useful in the treatment of absence seizures and myoclonic seizures in children. It is absorbed well from the gastrointestinal tract, and its central effects develop rapidly. Its chief therapeutic limitation is the development of tolerance, which can be overcome by increasing the dose. At higher doses, however, sedation is induced.

4. Clorazepate is a useful adjunctive drug in the treatment of complex partial seizures.

F. Other anticonvulsants

1. Carbamazepine is an iminostilbene and is related chemically to the tricyclic antidepressants.
  a. It is used in the treatment of grand mal epilepsy, often as an adjunct to phenytoin therapy.
  b. Its anticonvulsant actions are similar to those of phenytoin.
  c. Other uses include the treatment of trigeminal neuralgia and occasionally the treatment of bipolar illness.
  d. Chronic use results in induction of drug-metabolizing enzymes, thereby reducing serum levels.
  e. Adverse effects
    (1) Diplopia, ataxia, and nausea
    (2) Bone marrow depression, including aplastic anemia
    (3) Congestive heart failure
    (4) Atropine-like symptoms
    (5) Kidney and liver toxicity

2. Valproic acid (dipropylacetic acid) had been used as a solvent in the screening of certain compounds for antiepileptic activity. It was itself found to possess antiseizure activity.
  a. Valproate has proved most effective in seizure states with a subcortical focus (e.g., absence seizures). It has also been somewhat effective in grand mal seizures but much less so in partial seizures.
  b. Valproate is rapidly absorbed from the gastrointestinal tract. Its mechanism of anticonvulsant action is unclear but is thought to involve inhibition of GABA transaminase, the enzyme responsible for the breakdown of GABA; valproate also inhibits succinic aldehyde dehydrogenase. Valproate antagonizes pentylenetetrazol-induced convulsions, suggesting an additional postsynaptic site of action.
  c. Adverse effects
    (1) Teratogenicity
    (2) Pancreatitis and hepatic failure, especially when the drug is used in combination with other antiseizure medication
    (3) Anorexia and nausea

(4) Sedation and ataxia

(5) Alopecia

(6) Drug interactions, including a 40% rise in plasma phenobarbital concentration with concurrent administration

G. Dantrolene

1. **Mechanism of action.** Dantrolene is an antispasticity drug, which works peripherally in the muscle by decreasing Ca^{2+} release from the sarcoplasmic reticulum.

2. **Therapeutic uses.** It is used in the treatment of malignant hyperthermia and for controlling the manifestations of clinical spasticity, resulting from upper motor neuron disorder.

3. **Adverse effects.** Dantrolene may cause generalized skeletal muscle weakness. Another major potential adverse reaction is life-threatening hepatic dysfunction of an idiosyncratic or hypersensitivity type.

IV. AGENTS USED IN THE TREATMENT OF PARKINSONIAN DISORDERS

A. Levodopa (L-dopa)

1. **Mechanism of action.** A dopamine deficiency in the striatum needs to be corrected in the treatment of parkinsonism.

   a. Dopamine does not cross the blood–brain barrier; thus, levodopa, the precursor of dopamine, is given instead.

   b. Levodopa is formed from L-tyrosine and is an intermediate in the synthesis of catecholamines.

   c. Levodopa itself has minimal pharmacologic activity, in contrast to its decarboxylated product, dopamine.

   d. Levodopa is rapidly decarboxylated in the gastrointestinal tract. Prior to the advent of decarboxylase inhibitors (carbidopa), large oral doses of levodopa were required; thus, toxicity from dopamine was a limiting factor.

2. **Pharmacokinetics**

   a. Levodopa is well absorbed from the small bowel; however, 95% is rapidly decarboxylated in the periphery.

   b. Peripheral dopamine is metabolized in the liver to dihydroxyphenylacetic acid (DOPAC) and homovanillic acid (HVA), which are then excreted in the urine.

3. **Pharmacologic effects**

   a. The effects on bradykinesia and rigidity are more rapid and complete than the effects on tremor. Other motor defects in Parkinson's disease improve. The psychological well-being of the patient is also improved.

   b. Tolerance to both beneficial and adverse effects (e.g., nausea) occurs with time.

4. **Adverse effects**

   a. Since the decarboxylation of levodopa increases peripheral concentrations of dopamine, prominent α- and β-adrenergic effects are seen, but these effects are significantly less severe than those seen with epinephrine, norepinephrine, or isoproterenol.

   b. Principal adverse effects include:

      (1) Anorexia, nausea, and vomiting upon initial administration, which often limit the initial dosage

      (2) Cardiovascular effects, including tachycardia, arrhythmias, and orthostatic hypotension

      (3) Mental disturbances, including delusions and hallucinations

      (4) A decrease in prolactin secretion

      (5) Dyskinesia upon long-term administration

5. **Drug interactions**

   a. Pyridoxine reduces the beneficial effects of levodopa by enhancing its extracerebral metabolism. The decarboxylation of levodopa to dopamine is mediated by an enzyme that is pyridoxine-dependent.

   b. Phenothiazines, reserpine, and butyrophenones antagonize the effects of levodopa because they lead to a junctional blockade of dopamine action.

    c. Therapy with monoamine oxidase (MAO) inhibitors must be stopped 14 days prior to the initiation of levodopa therapy.

    d. Anticholinergic agents act synergistically with levodopa, further improving many of the symptoms of parkinsonism.

B. Carbidopa

1. Pharmacokinetics. Carbidopa is an inhibitor of dopa decarboxylase. Since it is unable to penetrate the blood–brain barrier, it acts to reduce the peripheral conversion of levodopa to dopamine. As a result, when carbidopa and levodopa are given concomitantly, then:

    a. Levodopa blood levels are increased, and drug half-life is lengthened.

    b. The dose of levodopa can be significantly reduced, also reducing toxic side effects.

    c. A shorter latency period precedes the occurrence of beneficial effects.

    d. If the patient has been taking levodopa alone, it should be withheld for 8 hours before starting combined carbidopa–levodopa therapy, and the dosage of levodopa should be reduced by 75%.

2. Preparations. Sinemet is the trade name of a preparation that combines carbidopa and levodopa in fixed proportions (1:10 and 1:4). It is considered the most effective treatment for Parkinson's disease.

3. Adverse effects of the combination are similar to those seen with high doses of levodopa.

C. Amantadine

1. Therapeutic uses and mechanism of action

    a. Amantadine is an antiviral agent used in the prophylaxis of influenza A_2 (see Chapter 12 VIII A). It was found to improve parkinsonian symptoms by stimulating the release of dopamine from dopaminergic nerve terminals in the nigrostriatum and delaying its reuptake.

    b. Amantadine may be more efficacious in parkinsonism than the anticholinergic atropine derivatives (see IV E) but is less effective than levodopa.

2. Excretion. Amantadine is well absorbed orally and is excreted unchanged in the urine.

3. Adverse effects are infrequent; however, long-term use can produce livedo reticularis in the lower extremities. Tolerance is observed in 6–8 weeks.

D. Bromocriptine

1. Mechanism of action

    a. An ergot derivative, bromocriptine mimics the action of dopamine.

    b. Bromocriptine is expensive but probably provides additional therapeutic benefit when added to levodopa therapy.

2. Adverse effects such as hallucinations, hypotension, and livedo reticularis are more common with bromocriptine than with levodopa; however, it induces less dyskinesia than levodopa.

E. Anticholinergic agents

1. Mechanism of action

    a. Since the deficiency of dopamine in the striatum augments the excitatory cholinergic system in the striatum, the blockade of this system by anticholinergic agents, such as trihexyphenidyl, helps to alleviate the motor dysfunction.

    b. Improvement in the parkinsonian tremor is more pronounced than improvement in bradykinesia and rigidity.

2. Therapeutic uses. While not as effective as levodopa or bromocriptine, anticholinergic agents may have an additive therapeutic effect at any stage of the disease when taken concurrently.

3. Adverse effects, such as mental confusion and hallucinations due to central muscarinic toxicity, can occur as can peripheral atropine-like toxicity (e.g., cycloplegia, urinary retention, constipation).

F. Antihistamines (e.g., diphenhydramine) are less effective therapeutically but are better tolerated than anticholinergic agents.

G. Selegiline is a new drug currently under clinical investigation. It is a selective MAO type B inhibitor also known as deprenyl.

1. **Therapeutic uses.** The drug is used concurrently with levodopa and prevents catabolism of dopamine in the brain.

2. **Adverse effects.** MAO-B inhibitors, unlike MAO-A inhibitors used for depression, do not cause hypertension after the ingestion of tyramine-rich foods.

V. ANTIPSYCHOTIC AGENTS

A. General considerations

1. These agents are prescribed for the management of psychotic symptoms; they are sometimes referred to as **major tranquilizers**.

2. They are useful in both acute and chronic psychoses and in nonpsychotic individuals who are delusional or excited. They improve mood and behavior without producing excessive sedation.

3. As a group, these agents produce little physical dependence or habituation but, notably, are capable of causing extrapyramidal symptoms, both reversible (parkinsonian symptoms, akathisia) and irreversible (tardive dyskinesia).

B. Phenothiazines (Table 3-2)

1. **Chemistry.** The phenothiazines have a three-ring structure in which two benzene rings are linked by a sulfur and a nitrogen atom (Figure 3-4). Differences within this group result from substitution on the nitrogen.

2. **Pharmacokinetics**
   a. The phenothiazines are erratically absorbed from the gastrointestinal tract.
   b. They are highly protein-bound and enter the fetal circulation.
   c. Their biologic effects last 24 hours, allowing once-daily dosing.
   d. Phenothiazines are metabolized in the hepatic microsomal system by hydroxylation, followed by conjugation with glucuronic acid. In addition, the formation of sulfoxides is an important metabolic pathway.
   e. At least five metabolites ultimately appear in the urine.

3. **Pharmacologic effects**
   a. **CNS effects**
      (1) The psychotic patient has fewer hallucinations and delusions. Improvements in behavior are most often noted with long-term therapy.
         (a) Tolerance to these effects is rarely seen.
         (b) The antipsychotic effects are believed to be due to antagonism of dopaminergic neurotransmission in the limbic, nigrostriatal, and hypothalamic systems.
      (2) Extrapyramidal symptoms occur most often with chronic administration.
         (a) These effects arise, presumably, because of antidopaminergic effects in the basal ganglia.
         (b) Phenothiazines having the greatest antihistaminic and anticholinergic properties will exhibit the fewest extrapyramidal effects.

Table 3-2. Common Phenothiazine Derivatives

Drug	Major Use	Frequency of Adverse Effects	
		Orthostatic Hypotension	**Extrapyramidal Symptoms**
Chlorpromazine (Thorazine)	Antipsychotic Antiemetic	Moderate	Moderate
Clozapine (Clozaril)	Antipsychotic Anticholinergic Antihistaminic	Low	Low
Thioridazine (Mellaril)	Antipsychotic	Moderate	Low
Triflupromazine (Vesprin)	Antipsychotic	Moderate	High
Fluphenazine (Prolixin)	Antipsychotic	Low	High
Prochlorperazine (Compazine)	Antiemetic	Low	Low–moderate
Promethazine (Phenergan)	Antihistaminic	Moderate	Low

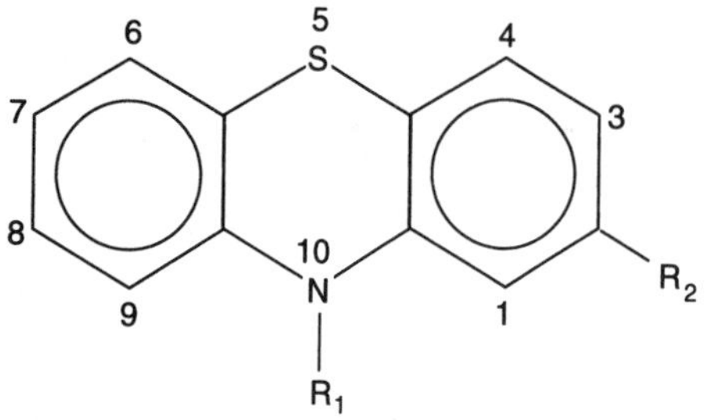

Figure 3-4. Phenothiazine nucleus.

- **(3)** The **neuroleptic effects** of the antipsychotic drugs consist of emotional quieting, reduced physical movement, and a potential for neurologic side effects. The drugs have little effect on the intellectual functioning of the patient.
- **(4)** Most phenothiazines are antiemetic. They antagonize agents, such as apomorphine, which stimulate the chemoreceptor trigger zone. In high doses, phenothiazines may directly depress the medullary vomiting center.
- **(5)** Phenothiazines are capable of altering temperature-regulating mechanisms. Normally, they produce hypothermia; however, in a hot climate they can cause hyperthermia because of failure to lose body heat.
- **(6)** Since phenothiazines depress the hypothalamus, endocrine alterations may occur.
  - **(a)** This includes the release of lactogenic hormone (prolactin), inducing lactation.
  - **(b)** Abnormal pigmentation can occur because of an increased release of melanocyte-stimulating hormone from the pituitary.
  - **(c)** Increased levels of prolactin may lead to galactorrhea and gynecomastia.
  - **(d)** In addition, phenothiazines decrease corticotropin release and secretion of pituitary growth hormone.
  - **(e)** Weight gain and increased appetite are seen with phenothiazine use.
- **b. Peripheral effects**
  - **(1)** An α-adrenergic blocking activity is seen, especially with the prototypic phenothiazine, chlorpromazine.
  - **(2)** Adrenergic potentiation, especially with chronic administration, is probably a result of the ability of phenothiazines to inhibit the reuptake of norepinephrine.
  - **(3)** Anticholinergic effects can result in blurred vision, constipation, dry mouth, decreased sweating, and, rarely, urinary retention. Miosis is seen with chlorpromazine and is probably due to α-adrenergic blockade. Other phenothiazines can produce mydriasis.
  - **(4)** Chlorpromazine is a potent local anesthetic.
  - **(5)** Antihistaminic activity is seen with most phenothiazine derivatives.
  - **(6)** Inhibition of ejaculation without interference with erection can occur, especially with thioridazine.
  - **(7)** Inhibition of antidiuretic hormone (ADH) secretion by chlorpromazine can result in a weak diuretic effect.
  - **(8)** Orthostatic hypotension can occur as a result of both the central action of phenothiazines and inhibition of norepinephrine uptake mechanisms. In addition, chlorpromazine has an antiarrhythmic effect upon the heart.
  - **(9)** Phenothiazines are known to enhance the pharmacologic actions of barbiturates, narcotics, and ethyl alcohol.

- **4. Therapeutic uses**
  - **a.** Phenothiazines are used chiefly in the treatment of psychotic disorders, including mania, paranoid states, schizophrenia, and psychoses associated with chronic alcoholism (alcoholic hallucinosis).
  - **b.** In addition, several phenothiazines have proven effective in the treatment of nausea and vomiting of certain etiologies, such as drug-induced nausea.
  - **c.** Some phenothiazines, due to their H_1 antihistaminic activity, are useful as antipruritics.
  - **d.** Chlorpromazine has proved useful in the control of intractable hiccup.

- **5. Adverse effects**
  - **a. CNS effects**
    - **(1)** A parkinsonian syndrome may occur in which patients display rigidity and tremor at rest.
    - **(2)** Acute dystonic reactions may be seen with initial drug therapy. Patients display facial grimacing and torticollis.

(3) Tardive dyskinesia may be seen with chronic therapy. Patients display sucking and smacking of the lips and other involuntary facial movements. The dyskinesia may persist far after discontinuation of therapy.

(4) Lethargy and drowsiness also may occur.

b. **Cardiovascular effects** include orthostatic hypotension, which can result in syncope, and reflex tachycardia.

c. **Allergic reactions** most often occur during the first few months of therapy.

(1) Cholestatic jaundice can occur; it resolves with discontinuation of drug therapy.

(2) Blood dyscrasias (e.g., agranulocytosis) and eosinophilia can occur but are rare.

(3) Various forms of dermatitis may occur, including a photosensitivity reaction that resembles a severe sunburn.

d. Children exhibit extrapyramidal symptoms and, less commonly, may develop jaundice, blood dyscrasias, or hyperpyrexia.

e. Somnolence and hypotension are prominent adverse effects of acute intoxication.

C. **Thioxanthene derivatives** are similar chemically and pharmacologically to the phenothiazine derivatives. They differ chemically in that a carbon is substituted for a nitrogen in the central ring of the phenothiazine nucleus (position 10). The thioxanthenes in clinical use are **chlorprothixene** and **thiothixene**.

D. **Butyrophenones**

1. The prototype is **haloperidol,** which resembles the phenothiazine derivatives pharmacologically. It has potent antiemetic properties, antagonizing stimulation of the chemoreceptor trigger zone. Significant extrapyramidal symptoms are associated with its use.

2. Another butyrophenone, **droperidol,** is often combined with a potent narcotic analgesic, such as fentanyl, to produce neuroleptanalgesia. This combination is known by the trade name Innovar.

E. **Clozapine**

1. **Chemistry.** It is a tetracyclic *N*-methyl-piperazinyl-dibenzodiazepine analog.

2. **Pharmacokinetics.** At least 80% of orally administered clozapine appears in the urine or feces as metabolites. The $t_{1/2}$ is 12 hours.

3. **Pharmacologic effects**

a. Unlike standard neuroleptic and antipsychotic agents, clozapine lacks extrapyramidal side effects.

b. It also differs from typical neuroleptic agents by having low affinity for D_1 and D_2 dopamine receptors.

c. It does have relatively potent anticholinergic activity.

d. Other activities include antiadrenergic, antiserotoninergic, and possible antihistiminergic activities.

4. **Therapeutic uses**

a. Although clozapine was developed 30 years ago as an antipsychotic agent, development was slowed by the recognition that it caused agranulocytosis.

b. Clozapine can be effective in treating some patients with psychosis who are unresponsive to standard neuroleptic drugs. It can be used safely if granulocyte counts are monitored closely.

5. **Adverse effects.** Because of the high risk of potentially fatal agranulocytosis, risk of seizures at high doses, inconvenience of weekly white cell counts, and the extraordinarily high cost of the drug, it is important to consider risk-benefit and cost-benefit relations.

VI. AGENTS USED IN THE TREATMENT OF ANXIETY

A. **General considerations.** Unlike the antipsychotic agents, these agents are used to treat anxiety or neurosis. They are not used in the treatment of psychosis. These drugs, therefore, are known as **antianxiety agents** or **minor tranquilizers**.

1. In addition, antianxiety agents have sedative and even hypnotic properties and also possess some central skeletal muscle relaxant activity.

2. They have a habituation and physical dependence liability.

3. Generally, the antianxiety agents have a lower incidence of adverse effects than the antipsychotic agents.

B. Meprobamate is a propyl alcohol derivative (propanediol carbamate). At one time, meprobamate was a widely used antianxiety agent; however, it has largely been replaced by the benzodiazepines.

1. Pharmacokinetics. Meprobamate is well absorbed from the gastrointestinal tract, and its peak serum concentration is reached in about 1½ hours. Metabolism occurs in the liver, and the inactive metabolites are excreted via the kidney.

2. Pharmacologic effects
a. It depresses the CNS in a fashion similar to that of the barbiturates, especially phenobarbital, but meprobamate is shorter-acting.
b. It is capable of promoting sleep, but, like phenobarbital, it decreases the REM phase.
c. The skeletal muscle relaxant activity demonstrated by meprobamate is probably a combination of its sedative effect and specific central skeletal muscle relaxant activity.

3. Adverse effects
a. Drowsiness, often seen with full therapeutic doses
b. Blood dyscrasias, including purpura, but these are rare
c. Habituation and physical dependence with long-term administration (withdrawal from drug therapy should, therefore, be gradual)

C. Benzodiazepines are considered the drugs of choice in the treatment of anxiety, partly because of their high therapeutic index. The first benzodiazepine developed was **chlordiazepoxide** (Figure 3-5). Others include **diazepam, clonazepam, lorazepam, oxazepam, clorazepate, halezapam, prazepam, alprazolam,** the anesthetic **midazolam,** and the sedative–hypnotics **flurazepam, triazolam,** and **temazepam** (see II B 6).

1. Pharmacokinetics (see Table 3-3)
a. Diazepam, flurazepam, and clorazepate are relatively rapidly absorbed, while oxazepam, prazepam, and temazepam are more slowly absorbed. Triazolam, midazolam, alprazolam, and clonazepam have an intermediate onset of action.
b. All benzodiazepines are soluble in lipids and cross the blood–brain barrier. Plasma levels reflect brain levels.
c. Benzodiazepines are metabolized primarily by microsomal oxidation and glucuronide conjugation.

2. Pharmacologic effects
a. CNS effects
(1) Benzodiazepines potentiate the binding of GABA to receptors. The benzodiazepine receptor that helps to potentiate the GABA binding is as yet unidentified.

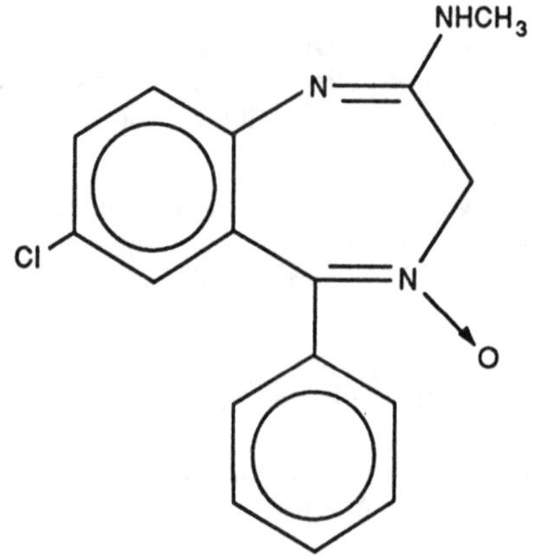

Figure 3-5. Chlordiazepoxide.

Table 3-3. Pharmacokinetics of Benzodiazepines

Agent	Duration of Action	Gastrointestinal Absorption Rate	Active Metabolite	Elimination Half-life
Midazolam	Short	Intermediate	No	2.5 hours
Triazolam	Short	Intermediate	No	3 hours
Alprazolam	Intermediate	Intermediate	No	14 hours
Lorazepam	Intermediate	Intermediate	No	15 hours
Oxazepam	Intermediate	Slow	No	10 hours
Temazepam	Intermediate	Slow	No	15 hours
Chlordiazepoxide	Long	Intermediate	Yes	2–4 days
Clonazepam	Long	Intermediate	Yes	2–3 days
Clorazepate	Long	Rapid	Yes	2–4 days
Diazepam	Long	Rapid	Yes	2–4 days
Flurazepam	Long	Intermediate	Yes	2–3 days
Halazepam	Long	Slow	Yes	2–4 days
Prazepam	Long	Slow	Yes	2–4 days

    (2) Because they increase the seizure threshold, benzodiazepines are useful as anticonvulsants, especially diazepam in status epilepticus. They prevent convulsions caused by strychnine or pentylenetetrazole.

    (3) Benzodiazepines are also effective hypnotics, and flurazepam, temazepam, and triazolam are promoted as such.

  b. At therapeutic doses, the benzodiazepines have minimal effects on the cardiovascular system.

  c. Although the benzodiazepines, especially diazepam, are widely used as central skeletal muscle relaxants, their effectiveness has not been firmly established.

3. Therapeutic uses

  a. Treatment of anxiety

  b. Anesthetic premedication (midazolam is a parenteral benzodiazepine that will replace diazepam for perioperative use; its advantages include less tissue irritation, faster onset of action, and more rapid elimination)

  c. Use as amnestics, such as in cardioversion

  d. Use as sedative–hypnotics

  e. Management of seizure disorders

  f. Treatment of alcohol withdrawal syndromes

  g. Use as central skeletal muscle relaxants

  h. Treatment of night terrors

4. Adverse effects

  a. Adverse effects are partially age- and dose-dependent. These effects include:

    (1) Ataxia, drowsiness, and sedation (additive depressant effects are seen when benzodiazepines are combined with other agents possessing CNS depressant activity)

    (2) Paradoxically increased anxiety, including psychoses, especially with high doses

    (3) Reversible confusion in the elderly

    (4) Menstrual irregularities, including anovulation

  b. Overdoses, although frequent, are seldom fatal. Treatment is supportive. Owing to the high plasma-protein–binding characteristics of benzodiazepines, the benefit from dialysis is limited.

  c. Withdrawal symptoms are influenza-like muscle aches and nausea. These symptoms are rare, except in the case of alprazolam.

  d. Agent-specific effects include:

    (1) Triazolam may cause rebound insomnia.

    (2) Lorazepam and triazolam have a greater risk of inducing anterograde amnesia.

    (3) Flurazepam at higher doses (30 mg) is associated with daytime residual sedation.

D. Buspirone is an antianxiety agent that is not chemically or pharmacologically related to the benzodiazepines, barbiturates, or other sedative–anxiolytic drugs.

  1. Mechanism of action. Although the exact mechanism of action is unknown, buspirone can bind to dopamine and serotonin receptors. It does not bind to benzodiazepine receptors and does not have muscle-relaxant, anticonvulsant, or hypnotic activity.

2. Pharmacokinetics
   a. Buspirone is rapidly and completely absorbed from the gastrointestinal tract.
   b. The drug undergoes an extensive first-pass effect. One hydroxylated metabolite is pharmacologically active.
   c. Buspirone is highly protein-bound.
   d. It is partly excreted in the urine and has an elimination half-life of 4.8 hours.

3. Therapeutic uses. Buspirone is used for the short-term treatment of generalized anxiety. It may require 1–2 weeks for a therapeutic effect to take place.

4. Adverse effects include restlessness and dysphoria with high doses. Buspirone is remarkably free of other adverse effects. It has little potential for abuse.

VII. MOOD-ALTERING DRUGS

A. Lithium carbonate is used in the treatment of mania and manic episodes of bipolar disorder (manic–depressive illness).

1. Mechanism of action. This is thought to be related to lithium's inhibition of hormone-sensitive adenylate cyclase and the greater stabilization of dopamine and β-adrenergic receptors.

2. Pharmacokinetics. Lithium ion is well-absorbed from the gastrointestinal tract and eventually reaches equilibrium between plasma and tissues. It is eliminated by renal excretion; 80% of the lithium is reabsorbed in the proximal tubule. Lithium ion is secreted into breast milk.

3. Route of administration. Lithium is given orally. Since lithium has a low therapeutic index, serum concentrations must be carefully maintained between 0.8 and 1.5 mEq/L.

4. Therapeutic uses
   a. The major therapeutic indications are the prevention of bipolar illness and the treatment of acute mania.
   b. Lithium may also be useful in reducing the intensity of depression and increasing the duration between bouts of depression in unipolar depression.
   c. Lithium has no effect on schizophrenia and does not produce psychotropic effects in normal individuals.

5. Adverse effects
   a. High serum concentrations of lithium are associated with anorexia, vomiting, diarrhea, excessive thirst, and polyuria. The latter two symptoms probably involve the ability of lithium to inhibit the action of ADH on renal adenylate cyclase. This ultimately can result in diabetes insipidus; in fact, lithium is the most common cause of nephrogenic diabetes insipidus.
   b. Epileptic seizures have been reported, as well as somnolence, confusion, and psychomotor disturbances.
   c. The use of lithium during early pregnancy can result in cardiovascular anomalies in the newborn.
   d. Adverse cardiovascular effects include hypotension and cardiac arrhythmias.
   e. Chronic lithium use can result in thyroid enlargement.
   f. Lithium intoxication can usually be reversed by osmotic diuresis or, in more severe cases, by dialysis.

B. Antidepressant agents

1. General considerations
   a. Depression is an alteration of mood characterized by sadness, worry, and anxiety. The patient may suffer from losses of weight and libido.
   b. Most antidepressants are believed to improve mood by increasing catecholamine stores, although recent evidence suggests that there may be a correlation between improvement in mood and a decrease in adenylate cyclase.
   c. There are various pharmacologic modalities that may be useful, and selection often depends on the patient's history and symptomatology.

2. Monoamine oxidase (MAO) inhibitors
   a. Chemistry. Chemically, the MAO inhibitors consist of two major groups, the hydrazides and the nonhydrazides.

(1) The **hydrazide derivatives** include **isocarboxazid, phenelzine,** and **iproniazid.** The latter is no longer used because of its hepatotoxicity.

(2) The prototypic **nonhydrazide** is **tranylcypromine** (Figure 3-6), which structurally resembles dextroamphetamine.

b. Mechanism of action

(1) The MAO inhibitors form stable complexes with the enzyme monoamine oxidase, irreversibly inactivating it, thereby preventing the oxidative deamination of biogenic amines, such as norepinephrine, epinephrine, dopamine, serotonin, and tyramine.

    (a) These biogenic amines are, thus, increased significantly in the brain, intestines, heart, and blood.

    (b) The increase of biogenic amine levels in the brain is thought to underlie the observed antidepressant effects.

(2) There are two types of MAO inhibitors, which are distinguished by differing responses to specific inhibitors and by differing preferences for substrates.

    (a) Type A deaminates serotonin and norepinephrine but not phenylethylamine.

    (b) Type B deaminates phenylethylamine better than serotonin or norepinephrine, and it is inhibited by deprenyl. MAO-B is the type found largely in the CNS.

(3) The nonhydrazide, tranylcypromine, by way of its amphetamine-like action, releases norepinephrine centrally. This probably accounts for the relative rapidity of action with tranylcypromine (action can occur in 48 hours) in contrast to the other MAO inhibitors, which have latency periods of 2–3 weeks.

c. Pharmacokinetics

(1) All MAO inhibitors are rapidly absorbed from the gastrointestinal tract, but, inexplicably, the observed therapeutic response does not occur for 2–3 weeks.

(2) The hydrazide derivatives are cleaved, resulting in biologically active products. Inactivation occurs by acetylation, and in patients who are genetically slow acetylators, conventional doses of agents, such as phenelzine, may produce exaggerated effects.

(3) Enzyme regeneration terminates the drug effect, but this frequently takes weeks after use of the drug is stopped.

(4) When switching antidepressant therapy, a minimum of 2 weeks' delay is required after termination of MAO-inhibitor therapy [see VII B 3 g (3)].

d. Pharmacologic effects

(1) CNS effects

    (a) Besides their effect on depression, MAO inhibitors are effective in sleep disorders, including narcolepsy. They suppress REM sleep.

    (b) Except for tranylcypromine, which has a stimulant effect on the electroencephalogram (EEG), other MAO inhibitors have minimal EEG effects.

(2) Cardiovascular effects

    (a) Hypotension, especially postural, can result from the ability of MAO inhibitors to affect ganglionic transmission and reduce the release of norepinephrine in certain organ systems. This effect is believed to be due to the uptake and release of "false transmitters," such as tyramine.

    (b) MAO inhibitors can **interact with foods containing a high tyramine content,** such as cheese, beer, and chicken liver.

        (i) The high concentrations of tyramine absorbed from these foods cannot undergo oxidative deamination.

        (ii) The tyramine can, therefore, induce the release of large amounts of stored catecholamines from nerve terminals. This can precipitate a **hypertensive crisis,** which is the most serious adverse effect of MAO inhibitors.

(3) Hepatic effects

    (a) MAO inhibitors interfere with the detoxification of many drugs.

    (b) They enhance the action of general anesthetics, sedatives, atropine-like agents, narcotics (especially meperidine, which can result in hyperpyrexia), and tricyclic antidepressants.

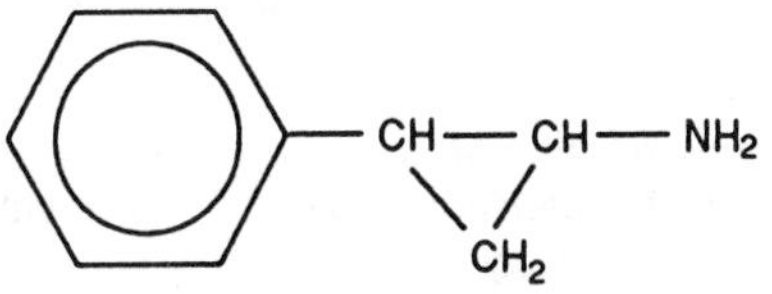

Figure 3-6. Tranylcypromine.

      e. Therapeutic uses. MAO-A inhibitors are especially effective in the treatment of atypical depression, characterized by symptoms such as hypersomnolence, hyperphagia, and hyperanxiety. Deprenyl (see IV G) is a MAO-B inhibitor, which may be useful in the treatment of Parkinson's disease.

      f. Adverse effects

         (1) The most serious effect is marked hypertension from an interaction between a MAO-A inhibitor and certain amines or their precursors (see VII B 2 b).

         (2) Hydrazide-derived MAO inhibitors can cause hepatocellular damage.

         (3) Excessive CNS stimulation has occurred, resulting in insomnia and convulsions.

         (4) Overdosage can result in agitation, headache, hallucinations, convulsions, and hypotension or hypertension. Treatment of overdosage is usually supportive. Since the effects of MAO inhibitors are lengthy, patients should be observed in the hospital for at least 1 week.

3. Tricyclic antidepressants

      a. Chemistry. Chemically, the tricyclic antidepressants and their desmethyl derivatives are similar to the phenothiazines. The basic structure is shown in Figure 3-7.

      b. Specific agents

         (1) Imipramine is closely related to the phenothiazines.

         (2) Amitriptyline is thought to be better tolerated than imipramine in older psychotic or depressed patients. Amitriptyline is effective in multiple sclerosis patients with **pseudobulbar palsy,** the syndrome of pathologic laughing and weeping.

         (3) Desipramine, the monodesmethyl derivative of imipramine, is less sedating than its parent compound.

         (4) Nortriptyline, like desipramine, produces less sedation than its parent compound amitriptyline.

         (5) Doxepin is also effective in treating depression when anxiety is present.

         (6) Protriptyline has a 3- to 5-day half-life and causes little sedation.

      c. Mechanism of action

         (1) Tricyclic antidepressants potentiate the action of biogenic amines, presumably by blocking the inactivating reuptake of the amines after release from the presynaptic neuron. It is thought that the demethylated antidepressants (secondary amines) are more selective in blocking the uptake of norepinephrine.

         (2) Tricyclic antidepressants have both antihistaminic (H_1-receptor–blocking) and α-adrenergic properties.

         (3) In addition, the tricyclic antidepressants possess antimuscarinic action and block the reuptake of serotonin. Tertiary amines (imipramine, amitriptyline) are more effective at blocking serotonin uptake.

      d. Pharmacokinetics

         (1) The tricyclic antidepressants are well absorbed from the gastrointestinal tract.

         (2) Because of their lipophilic nature, these agents become widely distributed and have relatively long half-lives. They are metabolized in the microsomal metabolizing system. Hydroxylation, *N*-demethylation, and conjugation with glucuronic acid are the major metabolic pathways.

         (3) The demethylated metabolites of both amitriptyline and imipramine have antidepressant activity.

         (4) Excretion of metabolites is via the kidney.

      e. Pharmacologic effects

         (1) CNS effects

            (a) A nondepressed person experiences sleepiness when a tricyclic antidepressant is administered. In addition, anxiety and toxic anticholinergic effects may be experienced.

            (b) In the depressed patient, an elevation of mood occurs 2–3 weeks after administration begins. The latency period can be as long as 4 weeks.

            (c) Tricyclic antidepressants can cause extrapyramidal symptoms and ataxia.

            (d) High doses of tricyclic antidepressants are capable of producing seizures and coma.

         (2) Cardiovascular effects

            (a) Orthostatic hypotension and arrhythmias are two common effects.

            (b) Tachycardia in response to the hypotension and interference with atrioventricular conduction similar to that produced by quinidine can occur.

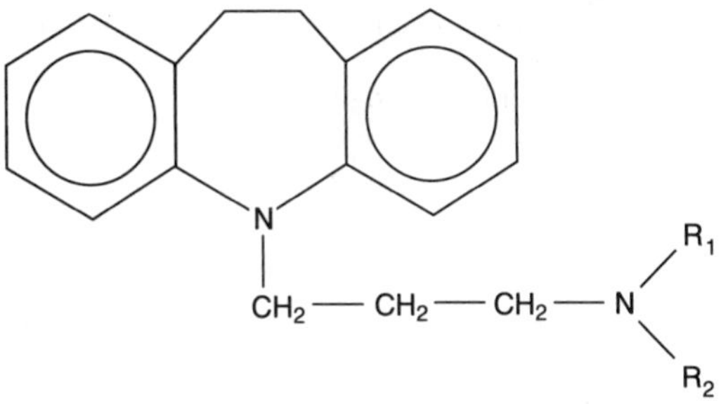

Figure 3-7. Basic structure of tricyclic antidepressants.

(3) The most common **autonomic nervous system effect** is anticholinergic. Amitriptyline possesses the most potent antimuscarinic effects.

f. Therapeutic uses

(1) These agents are considered the treatment of choice for severe endogenous depression (characterized by regression and inactivity). In terms of overall efficacy, the various tricyclic antidepressants are equivalent at appropriate dosages.

(2) Enuresis has been successfully treated with imipramine.

(3) Obsessive–compulsive neurosis accompanied by depression, and phobic–anxiety syndromes, chronic pain, and neuralgia may respond to tricyclic agents; it should be noted that these indications are investigational.

g. Adverse effects

(1) The adverse effects of tricyclic antidepressants often resemble those seen with phenothiazines, owing to the common structural features of the two groups of drugs.

(a) Anticholinergic effects can be prominent and occur both peripherally and centrally. Amitriptyline produces the highest incidence of antimuscarinic effects. Because of these actions, caution is required in treating patients with prostatic hypertrophy and glaucoma. Tolerance often develops to these effects.

(b) Sweating is common, although its mechanism is unknown.

(c) The elderly may suffer from dizziness and muscle tremor.

(d) As with phenothiazines, cardiac arrhythmias can occur. In addition, hypotension is frequent and results from a down-regulation of adrenergic receptors.

(e) Manic excitement and delirium can occur in patients with bipolar illness.

(f) Other, less common adverse effects include skin rashes, cholestatic jaundice, and orgasmic impotence.

(2) Acute poisoning is often treated with activated charcoal, although gastric lavage and physostigmine have been used successfully as adjuncts. Vital functions need to be supported and constantly monitored, since seizures, ventricular arrhythmias, and death can result from overdoses.

(3) The combination of a MAO inhibitor with a tricyclic antidepressant should be avoided, since hyperpyrexia, convulsions, and coma can result.

4. Second-generation antidepressants differ from the older tricyclic agents primarily in terms of their more favorable side-effect profiles. Specific agents include **amoxapine,** a member of the dibenzoxapine class, and **maprotiline**. These drugs have few anticholinergic effects.

5. Atypical antidepressants

a. Trazodone has perhaps the least anticholinergic side effects but should be used sparingly in men because priapism can occur.

b. Fluoxetine

(1) Chemistry. Chemically, fluoxetine is a phenyltolylpropylamine that inhibits the uptake of serotonin.

(2) Mechanism of action

(a) It is a selective inhibitor of serotonin uptake in the CNS.

(b) It has little effect on central norepinephrine or dopamine function.

(c) It has less adverse effects because of minimal binding to cholinergic, histaminic, and α-adrenergic receptors.

(3) Pharmacokinetics

(a) Fluoxetine is well absorbed after oral ingestion.

(b) It undergoes extensive hepatic biotransformation to the active metabolite norfluoxetine. The inactive metabolites are excreted in the urine.

(c) The elimination half-life is 1–3 days for fluoxetine and 7–15 days for norfluoxetine.

(d) The onset of action is within 1–3 weeks after beginning treatment.

(4) Therapeutic uses

(a) Fluoxetine is used for treatment of endogenous depression.

(b) It may be useful in treating obsessive–compulsive disorder, obesity, and alcoholism.

(5) Adverse effects

(a) Fluoxetine has caused anorexia and, unlike the tricyclics, does not cause weight gain.

(b) It may precipitate mania or hypomania.

(c) Nausea, nervousness, headache, and insomnia occur more frequently with fluoxetine than with tricyclics.

(d) Uticaria or some other rash develops in 4% of patients.

c. Bupropion

(1) Chemistry. Chemically, bupropion is a trimethylated monocyclic phenylaminoketone.

(2) Mechanism of action. Although the exact mechanism of action is unknown, the drug does weakly block dopamine reuptake.

(3) Pharmacokinetics

(a) Bupropion is rapidly absorbed from the gastrointestinal tract and undergoes extensive first-pass metabolism.

(b) It is eliminated primarily in the urine.

(4) Therapeutic uses. Bupropion is used for the treatment of major depression. Significant improvement is often seen within a week of treatment. Bupropion is sometimes effective in depressed patients who do not respond to tricyclics.

(5) Adverse effects. Bupropion does not produce sedation, orthostatic hypotension, weight gain, or the sexual dysfunction associated with other antidepressants; however, it is contraindicated in patients with eating disorders, seizures, or major head trauma as it may produce or exacerbate grand mal seizures.

VIII. CNS STIMULANTS

A. Amphetamine (β-phenylisopropylamine)

1. CNS effects

a. In addition to its peripheral sympathomimetic action (see Chapter 2 II G), amphetamine is a powerful CNS stimulant, presumably acting by releasing biogenic amines from storage sites in the nerve terminals.

b. Amphetamine stimulates the medullary respiratory center and has analeptic action, counteracting the central depression produced by other drugs (e.g., barbiturates).

c. Increased alertness, decreased sense of fatigue, increased motor and speech activity, and elevation of mood are often produced.

2. Therapeutic uses

a. Amphetamine is an anorectic and has been used in weight control of obese individuals. Since tolerance develops rapidly, psychologically driven food intake is not affected, and abuse potential is significant, this therapeutic use is of questionable merit.

b. The stimulant effect of amphetamine is useful in the treatment of narcolepsy.

c. A paradoxical calming effect is produced with long-term therapy in many abnormally hyperactive children (i.e., those with hyperkinetic syndrome).

3. Adverse effects

a. Some individuals experience dysphoria, headache, confusion, dizziness, fatigue, or delirium.

b. Blood pressure is usually raised, and cardiac arrhythmias may occur.

c. Larger doses or prolonged usage are usually followed by fatigue and mental depression.

d. The toxic dose of amphetamine shows wide variation.

(1) Overdosage results in psychotic reactions, marked cardiovascular effects, such as hypertension or hypotension and circulatory collapse, and, eventually, convulsions and coma.

(2) Treatment of acute intoxication is facilitated by acidification of the urine to increase excretion.

B. Dextroamphetamine and methamphetamine are preferred to amphetamine because of their increased CNS action and reduced peripheral effects.

C. Cocaine

1. **Chemistry.** Cocaine is benzoylmethylecgonine; its sole clinical use is as a local anesthetic (see Chapter 4 II C 1).

2. **Pharmacokinetics**
   a. Cocaine is well absorbed across mucous membranes and the mucosa of the gastrointestinal tract.
   b. Cocaine is degraded by plasma esterases and, in some animals, by hepatic enzymes.
   c. The half-life of cocaine is approximately 1 hour.

3. **Pharmacologic effects**
   a. Cocaine is a CNS stimulant that blocks neuronal uptake of norepinephrine. Initially, there is an intense euphoric experience followed in minutes by dysphoria.
      (1) Alkaloidal cocaine (free base) is a form of the drug that is suitable for smoking. When the cocaine crystals are heated, a cracking sound is produced, thus, the moniker "crack." "Freebasing" or smoking delivers cocaine to the vascular bed of the lung, producing an effect comparable to that achieved by intravenous injection.
      (2) Intranasal use of cocaine hydrochloride does not provide the rush generally associated with freebasing. Vasoconstriction of the nasal mucous membranes limits the absorption of the drug when it is snorted.
   b. Blocking neuronal uptake of norepinephrine increases heart rate and blood pressure.
   c. At higher doses, central depression occurs, followed by respiratory failure.

4. **Adverse effects**
   a. Increased heart rate and blood pressure occur, which may produce or exacerbate angina pectoris, myocardial infarction, and ventricular arrhythmias.
   b. High doses may cause hyperpyrexia, seizures, and cardiac arrhythmias.
   c. Cocaine crosses the placenta and may accumulate in the fetus. Exposure to cocaine during pregnancy increases the incidence of spontaneous abortion, fetal growth retardation, and possibly congenital anomalies.
   d. Cocaine intoxication can occur in breast-fed babies via maternal use.

IX. NARCOTIC ANALGESICS

A. General considerations

1. **Definitions**
   a. **Analgesia** is the relief of pain without loss of consciousness, as opposed to anesthesia. The chief action of opiates and similar compounds is to impair the normal sensory awareness and response to tissue injury.
   b. **Opiates** are derived from the poppy plant. The exudate of the seed capsule contains morphine, codeine, thebaine, and papaverine. The term **opioid** refers to both naturally occurring opiates and synthetic drugs with similar actions.

2. **Mechanism of action**
   a. Through the use of ligand-binding techniques, **opiate receptors** of several types have been identified and quantitated within the CNS (Table 3-4). These receptors are found in the following sites:
      (1) The limbic system, including the amygdaloid nucleus and the hypothalamus
      (2) The medial and lateral thalamus and the area postrema, which is the site of the chemoreceptor trigger zone governing nausea and emesis
      (3) The nucleus of the solitary tract, which is the location of the cough center
      (4) The substantia gelatinosa and, to a lesser degree, other areas of the spinal cord
   b. Endogenous ligands known as **enkephalins** are pentapeptides that are localized in some nerve endings. Their distribution closely parallels the distribution of opioid receptors. It is thought that the enkephalins may be involved in the modulation of the pain response.

Table 3-4. Classification of Opiate Receptors

Receptor type	Action
Mu (μ)	Supraspinal analgesia, respiratory depression, euphoria, physical dependence
μ₁	Analgesia
μ₂	Respiratory depression
Kappa (κ)	Spinal analgesia, miosis, sedation
Sigma (σ)	Dysphoria, hallucinations, respiratory and vasomotor stimulation

    c. In addition, longer polypeptides called **endorphins** possess potent analgesic activity and are found in the anterior pituitary and hypothalamus.

    d. Analgesia produced at opioid receptors requires binding by a molecule that has a terminal quaternary nitrogen that is capable of being charged at physiologic pH and resides four or five atoms from an aromatic group.

    e. The interruption of pain impulses may be mediated by calcium gating via endorphin receptors, enkephalin receptors, or both.

  B. Morphine and related opioids

    1. Morphine (Figure 3-8) is a member of the phenanthrene series of alkaloids.

      a. Pharmacokinetics

        (1) Morphine is well absorbed from the gastrointestinal tract. However, the analgesic effect is greater when the drug is administered intramuscularly or intravenously, rather than orally.

        (2) Morphine is metabolized in the liver, where it is transformed into inactive metabolites by conjugation with glucuronide. It undergoes a significant first-pass effect.

        (3) Ninety percent of a given dose is excreted in the urine; the remaining 10% is excreted in the feces. This latter component is derived from bile as conjugated morphine.

      b. Pharmacologic effects

        (1) CNS effects

          (a) Dose-related analgesia and increased tolerance of pain are the most prominent effects of morphine. Consciousness is not lost, and the patient can usually still locate the source of pain. Some patients become euphoric. If morphine is given to a person who is pain-free, dysphoria, anxiety, or mental clouding may be produced.

          (b) Morphine stimulates the chemoreceptor trigger zone, producing nausea and vomiting. In most cases, after the first therapeutic dose, subsequent doses of morphine do not produce vomiting.

          (c) Morphine produces miosis by stimulating the Edinger-Westphal nucleus, and pinpoint pupils are indicative of toxic dosage prior to asphyxia. The miosis can be blocked with atropine.

          (d) Morphine is a powerful respiratory depressant, which acts by reducing the responsiveness of the respiratory centers in the brain stem to blood levels of carbon dioxide.

            (i) Both alveolar and serum carbon dioxide tension (Pco_2) are increased because of the depression of medullary responsiveness.

            (ii) Due to the depressed respiration and increased arterial carbon dioxide retention, cerebral vasodilation can occur, causing an increase in intracranial pressure.

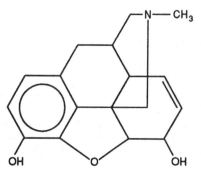

Figure 3-8. Morphine.

(e) Morphine is believed to stimulate the release of ADH, producing oliguria.

(f) Morphine is a potent cough suppressant.

(g) Morphine has a biphasic, dose-dependent effect on body temperature. Low doses of morphine cause a decrease in body temperature; higher doses cause an increase.

(2) Cardiovascular effects. Orthostatic hypotension can occur due to vasomotor medullary depression and histamine release.

(3) Gastrointestinal effects

    (a) Constipation results from reduced peristalsis and stomach motility. In addition, spasmodic nonpropulsive contractions of gastrointestinal smooth muscle are produced.

    (b) Both biliary and pancreatic secretions are decreased.

    (c) Constriction at the sphincter of Oddi causes an increase in biliary pressure.

(4) Other systemic effects

    (a) Morphine increases detrusor muscle tone in the urinary bladder, producing a feeling of urinary urgency. Vesical sphincter tone is also increased, making voiding difficult.

    (b) Prolongation of labor can occur by an undefined uterine mechanism.

    (c) Bronchoconstriction can occur because morphine causes the release of histamine and causes vagal stimulation.

    (d) Cutaneous vasodilation secondary to histamine release can result in pruritus and sweating.

c. Therapeutic uses

    (1) Analgesia, such as the relief of pain from myocardial infarction, terminal illness, surgery, and obstetrical procedures, is the major use of morphine.

    (2) It is also used for the acute treatment of dyspnea due to pulmonary edema, in which morphine produces decreased peripheral resistance and increased capacity of peripheral and splanchnic vascular compartments.

    (3) Because of their constipating effects, the morphine-like drugs can be useful in treating severe diarrhea.

d. Adverse effects

    (1) Respiratory depression is the most important effect and is dose-dependent.

    (2) Nausea and sometimes dysphoria can occur.

    (3) Increased biliary tract pressure can occur, and caution should be exercised in giving opiates to patients with gallbladder disease.

    (4) Long-term chronic administration can result in physical dependence. Pinpoint pupils are a consistent finding in addiction.

    (5) Allergic reactions can occur, and skin rashes are a common manifestation.

    (6) Due to morphine's bronchoconstrictive action, the drug is contraindicated for asthmatic patients.

    (7) Some phenothiazines are capable of producing antianalgesia when combined with an opiate such as morphine, whereas other phenothiazines can enhance the analgesic action of morphine. However, phenothiazines are likely to increase the sedative and respiratory depressant effects of opioids.

e. Tolerance and dependence

    (1) Tolerance may develop to the analgesia, the euphoria, and the respiratory depression.

    (2) Tolerance to the miosis and to the delayed gastric emptying and constipation also develops, but to a much lesser extent.

    (3) Physical addiction occurs, although the morphine withdrawal syndrome is not as severe as barbiturate withdrawal.

2. Codeine

    a. Codeine is the 3-methyl ether of morphine. It can be obtained from opium or synthesized by methylation of morphine.

    b. Although the pharmacologic effects of codeine are similar to those of morphine, it has about one-twelfth the analgesic potency of morphine, and it is generally used for somewhat milder pain.

    c. Codeine has a high oral–parenteral potency ratio so that when it is administered orally, it is 60% as potent as when injected intramuscularly.

    d. An oral dose of 30 mg of codeine is equivalent in analgesia to 600 mg of aspirin.

    e. Codeine is also very useful as a cough suppressant.

    f. Codeine produces less sedation or respiratory depression than morphine and fewer gastrointestinal effects.

    g. Addiction liability is lower than with morphine, and withdrawal is less severe.

3. Hydrocodone and oxycodone

    a. Although these agents are codeine derivatives, they possess an analgesic potency closer to that of morphine.

    b. Their potential for causing respiratory depression is also greater than that of codeine; this is especially true of oxycodone.

    c. They possess a significant addiction liability.

4. Heroin

    a. Heroin is diacetylated morphine.

    b. Heroin has a more rapid onset and shorter duration of action than morphine.

    c. It has an analgesic potency greater than that of morphine: 3 mg of heroin is equivalent to 10 mg of morphine.

    d. Heroin is not used clinically in the United States.

5. Hydromorphone

    a. Hydromorphone is 10 times more potent than morphine in producing analgesia with correspondingly more respiratory depressant activity.

    b. Hydromorphone is less nauseating and less constipating than morphine.

    c. It is highly physically addicting.

    d. Hydromorphone can be administered orally, parenterally, or rectally.

6. Levorphanol produces effects similar to those of morphine but with a lower incidence of nausea and vomiting.

C. Meperidine and congeners

1. Meperidine, a phenylpiperidine derivative, is an entirely synthetic analgesic.

    a. It is about one-eighth as potent as morphine, 100 mg of meperidine being equivalent to 15 mg of morphine.

    b. Meperidine is well absorbed by all routes of administration and is better absorbed orally than morphine is. Excretion is mainly in the urine.

    c. Meperidine causes respiratory depression and possesses addiction liability, although withdrawal effects are less severe than with morphine.

    d. Meperidine causes histamine release and smooth muscle spasm, including bronchospasm.

    e. It possesses weak, atropine-like activity and tends to cause mydriasis. In toxic doses, the pharmacologic effects are, in part, atropine-like.

    f. With intravenous administration, the incidence of adverse effects is increased. Repeated intramuscular administration can produce tissue irritation.

    g. Meperidine has no gastrointestinal or antitussive action.

2. Diphenoxylate, a derivative of meperidine, is available in combination with atropine (e.g., Lomotil).

    a. Its principal use is to control diarrhea.

    b. In the recommended dosage, it causes few morphine-like subjective effects and has low addiction liability.

    c. Due to the atropine in the combination, adverse effects, such as dry mouth and blurred vision, curtail abuse.

3. Fentanyl, like diphenoxylate, is a congener of meperidine.

    a. It has 80 times the analgesic potency and respiratory depressant properties of morphine, and is more effective than morphine in maintaining hemodynamic stability.

    b. When combined with droperidol, it produces dissociative analgesia, or neuroleptanalgesia (see Chapter 4 I B 2).

    c. Its principal use is in anesthesia, where it is administered parenterally. It has a rapid onset and short duration of action.

    d. High doses of fentanyl are capable of producing muscular rigidity.

4. Sufentanil is used as a short-acting anesthetic adjunct; it has a shorter onset of action than fentanyl.

5. Alfentanil is a synthetic opioid analgesic related to fentanyl and sufentanil.

    a. It has a more rapid onset of action and shorter duration of narcotic effect than fentanyl.

    b. It is used as an adjunct to general anesthetics and as an anesthetic induction agent.

D. Methadone and congeners

1. **Methadone** is a modified diphenylheptane (Figure 3-9).
   a. This synthetic analgesic has pharmacologic properties similar to those of morphine, but it is more effective orally than morphine.
   b. The duration of analgesia with methadone is equal to that of morphine, although the half-life of methadone is longer. This can result in cumulative toxicity.
   c. Methadone is well absorbed from the gastrointestinal tract, undergoes extensive biotransformation in the liver, and is excreted in both the urine and bile.
   d. Its principal uses are in analgesia, in the suppression of withdrawal symptoms due to opiate addiction, and in treatment of heroin users.
      (1) In methadone maintenance, opiate addicts receive periodic oral doses of methadone.
      (2) In appropriate doses, methadone will satisfy the craving for heroin without producing euphoria or somnolence.
      (3) Because of cross-tolerance, the effects of other self-administered opiates will be blocked.
   e. Adverse effects are similar to those caused by morphine.
   f. Both tolerance and physical dependence can occur with methadone administration. Methadone withdrawal is less severe than the withdrawal from other opiates.

2. **Propoxyphene** is a structural analog of methadone with a spectrum of pharmacologic activity similar to that of codeine.
   a. Propoxyphene is not an anti-inflammatory agent; therefore, it is less effective in treating pain associated with inflammation. In analgesic potency, it closely resembles codeine. When combined with aspirin, propoxyphene produces more analgesia than either drug alone; however the combination of aspirin and codeine is less costly than that of aspirin and propoxyphene.
   b. The water-soluble hydrochloride is absorbed more rapidly than the water-insoluble napsylate.
   c. The *N*-demethylated metabolites are slowly excreted in the urine.
   d. Propoxyphene depresses respiration about one-third as much as codeine.
   e. The incidence of abuse is comparable to that seen with codeine.
   f. Physical dependence and tolerance can occur but usually are seen only after chronic high-dose administration.

E. Opioid receptor antagonists and partial antagonists

1. **Nalorphine** was originally used as an opioid antagonist.
   a. It became recognized that it possessed analgesic properties with less respiratory depression than morphine.
   b. Nalorphine then became classified as a partial antagonist.
   c. Nalorphine can lead to withdrawal symptoms when it is given to narcotic-dependent patients.

2. **Pentazocine** is a benzomorphan derivative with moderate agonistic and weak antagonistic activity.
   a. Due to its antagonistic activity, pentazocine is capable of precipitating withdrawal in addicts.

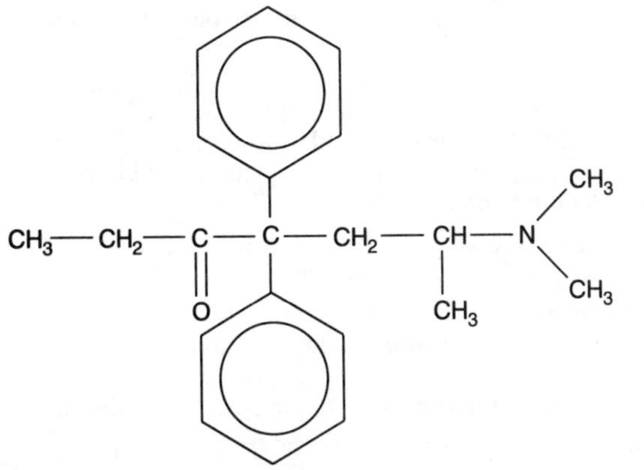

Figure 3-9. Methadone.

   b. Although pentazocine is similar to morphine in pharmacologic properties, it has one-fifth the analgesic potency. A dose of 50 mg, given parenterally, produces analgesia equivalent to 10 mg of morphine; given orally, 50 mg is equivalent to 60 mg of codeine.
   c. Pentazocine is well absorbed from the gastrointestinal tract as well as from subcutaneous and intramuscular sites. Pentazocine is biotransformed in the liver and excreted via the kidney.
   d. Adverse effects
      (1) Pentazocine can produce psychotomimetic effects, such as anxiety and hallucinations.
      (2) There may be less nausea associated with its use than with other opioids.
      (3) Analgesic doses are capable of increasing the pulmonary artery pressure and cardiac work.
      (4) Respiratory depression with higher doses is less pronounced than with comparable doses of morphine.
      (5) Tolerance to the analgesia can develop.
      (6) Pentazocine possesses both physical dependence potential and abuse potential.

3. Butorphanol has actions similar to those of pentazocine.
   a. As with pentazocine, but in contrast to morphine, as the analgesic dose is increased, respiratory depression is not increased proportionately.
   b. Pulmonary artery pressure and myocardial work are increased at analgesic doses.
   c. Unlike pentazocine, butorphanol does not precipitate a withdrawal syndrome in opioid addicts.

4. Nalbuphine, although structurally similar to naloxone, is equivalent (on a weight basis) to morphine in producing analgesia.
   a. It is considered to be a partial antagonist. Although its antagonistic properties are weak, it precipitates withdrawal in the opioid addict.
   b. Nalbuphine produces respiratory depression, but doses beyond 30 mg produce no further depression.
   c. Unlike pentazocine and butorphanol, nalbuphine does not cause adverse cardiac effects.
   d. Nalbuphine possesses abuse potential, and physical dependence has been reported.

5. Naloxone, an *N*-allyl derivative of oxymorphone, is a full **antagonist**.
   a. Naloxone, like other competitive receptor antagonists, blocks the opioid receptor.
   b. The sedative effects, respiratory depression, and adverse cardiovascular effects of opioid agonists are reversed within 1–2 minutes after parenteral administration of naloxone. There may be an "overshoot," producing increased respiration for a short period of time.
   c. The duration of the antagonistic effect is dose-dependent and usually lasts 1–4 hours.
   d. If naloxone is administered to opioid-addicted patients, a withdrawal syndrome is easily precipitated.
   e. Tolerance to the antagonistic effects does not develop.
   f. Naloxone is usually administered parenterally. It is metabolized in the liver via glucuronide conjugation.
   g. In obstetrics, mothers who have received opioids during labor may be given a dose of naloxone just prior to delivery to minimize neonatal respiratory depression. Alternatively, naloxone can be administered to the neonate via the umbilical vein.

6. Naltrexone
   a. Naltrexone, another full antagonist, is now the treatment of choice for patients addicted to heroin or other opioids.
   b. It can be administered orally.
   c. It has twice the potency of naloxone and three times the duration of action.
   d. An opioid abstinence syndrome can result if naltrexone is administered too vigorously.
   e. Naltrexone may cause insomnia, anxiety, abdominal cramping, nausea, and joint pain.
   f. It is **contraindicated** in patients with acute hepatitis or hepatic failure.

7. Buprenorphine is a partial antagonist with low potential for abuse (it is a schedule V drug).
   a. Its onset of action is within 15 minutes when given parenterally.
   b. It is metabolized in the liver and excreted in the feces and urine.
   c. The respiratory depression caused by buprenorphine is quantitatively similar to that caused by morphine.
   d. Buprenorphine can precipitate withdrawal symptoms in narcotic-addicted patients.

    e. Buprenorphine's pharmacologic activity is not easily reversed, even with high doses of naloxone.

F. Nonopioid antitussives (dextromethorphan)

    1. Dextromethorphan is the *d* isomer of the codeine analog of levorphanol.

    2. In contrast to the *l* isomer, dextromethorphan does not possess analgesic or addictive properties, and its principal use is as a cough suppressant.

    3. Although it is as effective as codeine in cough suppression, it is not beset with codeine's adverse effects, although at high doses, CNS depression may occur.

    4. It is commonly found in over-the-counter formulations.

STUDY QUESTIONS

Directions: Each of the numbered items or incomplete statements in this section is followed by answers or by completions of the statement. Select the **one** lettered answer or completion that is **best** in each case.

1. All of the following statements about sedative–hypnotics are true EXCEPT

(A) chloral hydrate is a relatively hazardous hypnotic drug
(B) they can activate GABA receptors, resulting in decreased neuronal excitation
(C) alcohol potentiates the CNS depressant effects of ethchlorvynol
(D) habituation and physical dependence develop with prolonged use of glutethimide
(E) thiopental is a useful anesthetic induction agent

2. Barbiturates are being replaced by benzodiazepines for use as sedative–hypnotic agents because of the shortcomings of barbiturate therapy, which include all of the following EXCEPT

(A) a narrow therapeutic index
(B) suppression of REM sleep
(C) induction of seizures
(D) high potential for physical dependence

3. Among the nonbarbiturate sedative–hypnotics, a certain agent can produce a particularly hazardous condition involving CNS depression, hyperpyrexia, and profound cardiovascular shock upon acute overdosage. The agent capable of producing this condition is

(A) methyprylon
(B) glutethimide
(C) chloral hydrate
(D) ethchlorvynol
(E) methaqualone

4. Granulocytopenia, gastrointestinal irritation, gingival hyperplasia, and facial hirsutism are all possible side effects of which one of the following anticonvulsant drugs?

(A) Phenobarbital
(B) Carbamazepine
(C) Dantrolene
(D) Phenytoin
(E) Valproate

5. Which of the following drugs could be prescribed for a child who suffers from night terrors?

(A) Meprobamate
(B) Clonazepam
(C) Droperidol
(D) Lithium
(E) Amphetamine

6. A patient undergoing general anesthesia experiences muscle rigidity upon intravenous injection of succinylcholine for tracheal intubation. The body temperature rises precipitously. A drug that may be useful in this situation is

(A) carbamazepine
(B) valproic acid
(C) dantrolene
(D) clonazepam
(E) clorazepate

7. The antianxiety agents, such as diazepam and lorazepam, differ from antipsychotic agents, such as triflupromazine, in all of the following ways EXCEPT

(A) they do not cause parkinsonian tremor
(B) they are better skeletal muscle relaxants
(C) they are good anticonvulsant agents
(D) they are ineffective in treating psychotic symptoms
(E) their adverse effects are not dose- and age-dependent

8. An adverse effect that is common to most phenothiazines is

(A) a marked increase in blood pressure
(B) rigidity and tremor at rest, particularly with prolonged use
(C) suppression of prolactin
(D) a diminished response to CNS depressants, such as barbiturates
(E) nausea

1-A	4-D	7-E
2-C	5-B	8-B
3-B	6-C	

9. The least likely side effect seen in patients taking chlorpromazine for 2 months would be

(A) extrapyramidal symptoms
(B) hypotension
(C) lethargy
(D) weight gain
(E) nausea and vomiting

10. Side effects most frequently seen with benzo-diazepines include all of the following EXCEPT

(A) drowsiness
(B) ataxia
(C) lethargy
(D) seizures
(E) amnesia

11. A physician prescribes buspirone for short-term treatment for a patient with generalized anx-iety. All of the following statements about this ther-apy are true EXCEPT

(A) it is chemically related to the benzodiazepines
(B) it is rapidly absorbed from the gastrointestinal tract
(C) it undergoes extensive first-pass metabolism
(D) it has little abuse potential
(E) dysphoria has been reported with high doses

12. Type A MAO inhibitors and tricyclic antide-pressants have which of the following features in common?

(A) Both are useful for the manic phase of bipolar disorder
(B) Both are useful for enuresis
(C) Both can precipitate hypotensive crises if cer-tain foods are ingested
(D) Both act postsynaptically to produce their ef-fect
(E) Both drugs increase levels of biogenic amines

13. A new antidepressant that is chemically a phenyltolypropylamide and causes fewer side ef-fects than the older agents is

(A) trazodone
(B) amoxapine
(C) maprotiline
(D) alprazolam
(E) fluoxetene

14. All of the following opiate receptors are cor-rectly matched with their physiologic effect EX-CEPT

(A) μ_1—analgesia
(B) μ_2—respiratory stimulation
(C) κ—spinal analgesia
(D) σ—dysphoria
(E) κ—miosis

15. Pentazocine is a partial agonist–antagonist opioid agent that is best characterized by

(A) severe nausea as a side effect
(B) a notably increased potency compared to morphine
(C) an increase in pulmonary artery pressure and cardiac work
(D) a lack of constipating effects
(E) absence of tolerance to the analgesic effect

16. A patient has returned from a skiing holiday with a painful sprained ankle as well as a bad cough. Which of the following agents would re-lieve both the pain and the cough?

(A) Meperidine
(B) Naloxone
(C) Dextromethorphan
(D) Codeine
(E) Buspirone

9-E	12-E	15-C
10-D	13-E	16-D
11-A	14-B	

Directions: Each item below contains four suggested answers of which **one or more** is correct. Choose the answer

  A   if **1, 2, and 3** are correct
  B   if **1 and 3** are correct
  C   if **2 and 4** are correct
  D   if **4** is correct
  E   if **1, 2, 3, and 4** are correct

17. Dopamine can be used to treat which of the following conditions?

(1) Parkinson's disease
(2) Cardiogenic shock
(3) Side effects of phenothiazines
(4) Congestive heart failure

18. Drugs that are useful in the treatment of schizophrenia include which of the following?

(1) Diphenhydramine
(2) Fluphenazine
(3) Promethazine
(4) Haloperidol

17-C
18-C

ANSWERS AND EXPLANATIONS

1. The answer is A *[II A 2 a, 3 b, B 1 b, 3, 5]*
Chloral hydrate is a relatively safe hypnotic agent. When GABA receptors are activated, chloride channels open. Chloride enters the cell, resulting in hyperpolarization and decreased excitation. Alcohol is a CNS depressant and would potentiate the effects of any other CNS depressant drug. Glutethimide does possess habituation and physical dependence liabilities. These and other undesirable properties limit its usefulness. Thiopental is an excellent anesthetic induction agent.

2. The answer is C *[II A 7 a–c]*
Although still used as sedative–hypnotic agents, barbiturates are being replaced by benzodiazepines because they have a narrow therapeutic index, they suppress REM sleep, and they have a high potential for physical dependence. Barbiturates do not induce seizures. Certain barbiturates, because of their rapid onset of action, can be used in the emergency treatment of convulsions.

3. The answer is B *[II B 3 c]*
Glutethimide can produce all of the adverse effects listed in the question (i.e., CNS depression, hyperpyrexia, profound cardiovascular shock with acute overdosage). In addition, its plasma half-life during acute intoxication can be as long as 4 days. Even with hemodialysis, a secondary rise in glutethimide plasma levels can result from additional intestinal absorption.

4. The answer is D *[III C 1 c]*
Phenytoin can induce blood dyscrasias. Other adverse effects include gastrointestinal irritation, ataxia and diplopia, gingival hyperplasia, hypersensitivity reactions, hirsutism, hepatitis, and drug interactions.

5. The answer is B *[III E 3; V D 2; VI B; VII A 4 a; VIII A 2 c]*
Clonazepam is a benzodiazepine. Besides being useful for seizure disorders, including petit mal, it is an antianxiety agent and helps to relieve night terrors. Meprobamate, one of the earliest, antianxiety agents, has been largely replaced by the benzodiazepines. Droperidol, a butyrophenone, is used in anesthesiology. Lithium is used for the treatment of bipolar disease. Amphetamine can produce a calming effect with long-term therapy in hyperkinetic syndrome.

6. The answer is C *[III G 1–3]*
Dantrolene is an antispasticity drug, which works peripherally in the muscle by decreasing Ca^{2+} release from the sarcoplasmic reticulum. It is used in the treatment of malignant hyperthermia. Carbamazepine is often used as an adjunct to phenytoin therapy for grand mal epilepsy. Valproic acid is useful in absence seizures. Clonazepam is useful in the treatment of absence seizures and myoclonic seizures in children. Clorazepate is a useful adjunctive drug in the treatment of complex partial seizures.

7. The answer is E *[V; VI]*
The benzodiazepine antianxiety agents, such as diazepam and lorazepam, do not produce parkinsonian tremor, are better skeletal muscle relaxants, and are good anticonvulsant agents compared to antipsychotic agents, such as the phenothiazines. Antianxiety agents are not used in the treatment of psychosis. Adverse effects of benzodiazepine therapy are partially dose- and age-dependent.

8. The answer is B *[V B 3; Table 3-2]*
Extrapyramidal symptoms, such as parkinsonian rigidity and rest tremors, are characteristic unwanted effects of the phenothiazines, and of other antipsychotic agents as well. Clozapine is one of the first effective antipsychotic agents to have few of the extrapyramidal side effects. The phenothiazines are apt to cause orthostatic hypotension, rather than a rise in blood pressure, due to their α-adrenergic blocking activity. Since the phenothiazines affect the hypothalamus, endocrine changes can occur; these include an increase, not a decrease, in prolactin levels. The combination of a phenothiazine and another CNS depressant, such as a barbiturate, can result in severe CNS depression. Most phenothiazines are antiemetic; they suppress, not cause, nausea.

9. The answer is E *[V B 3 a (4), (6) (e), 5]*
Chlorpromazine can cause hypotension due to its α-adrenergic blocking properties. Lethargy and increased weight are adverse effects. The most distinguishing adverse effects seen with administration of a phenothiazine, such as chlorpromazine, are extrapyramidal symptoms. Several phenothiazines have proven effective in the treatment of nausea and vomiting of certain etiologies, such as drug-induced nausea.

10. The answer is D *[VI C 4]*
Drowsiness, ataxia, and lethargy all can be seen with benzodiazepine ingestion. Drugs of this class possess significant anticonvulsant activity, however, and do not cause seizures. Other side effects can include confusion, dysarthria, anterograde amnesia, and various psychological manifestations, such as nightmares, hallucinations, euphoria, and anxiety.

11. The answer is A *[VI D]*
Buspirone is an antianxiety agent that is not chemically or pharmacologically related to the benzodiazepines, barbiturates, or other sedative–anxiolytic drugs. It is rapidly and completely absorbed from the gastrointestinal tract and undergoes an extensive first-pass metabolism. Buspirone is used for the short-term treatment of generalized anxiety. While there are few adverse effects, dysphoria has been reported with high doses. It has little potential for abuse.

12. The answer is E *[VII B 2 b, e, 3 c, f]*
MAO inhibitors are classified as follows: Type A deaminates serotonin and norepinephrine but not phenylethylamine, and type B deaminates phenylethylamine better than serotonin or norepinephrine. They are not useful in the manic phase of bipolar illness and can precipitate a hypertensive crisis if certain foods (e.g., cheese, beer, chicken livers) are ingested. Tricyclic antidepressants act presynaptically by preventing the reuptake of biogenic amines. Only the tricyclic imipramine is used to treat enuresis. Both groups of antidepressants produce an absolute increase in biogenic amine levels. In addition, they have a considerable lag time prior to the onset of clinically useful effects. This latency period is usually 2 weeks or more, although it may be as short as 48 hours with the nonhydrazide MAO inhibitor tranylcypromine.

13. The answer is E *[VII B 5 b]*
Fluoxetene is a phenyltolylpropylamide, which inhibits the reuptake of serotonin in the CNS and, therefore, has fewer adverse effects. The antidepressants trazodone, amoxapine, and maprotiline also cause fewer anticholinergic side effects than the older antidepressants but otherwise appear to be pharmacologically similar to the older agents. Of the three, trazodone probably causes fewest anticholinergic effects; however, trazodone should be used sparingly in men because it can cause priapism. Alprazolam is a benzodiazepine that is considered effective for the treatment of anxiety.

14. The answer is B *[IX A 2; Table 3-4]*
Mu (μ) receptors are associated with supraspinal analgesia (μ_1), respiratory depression (μ_2) as well as euphoria and physical dependence. Kappa receptors are associated with spinal analgesia, miosis, and sedation. Sigma receptors, when stimulated cause dysphoria, hallucinations, and respiratory and vasomotor stimulation.

15. The answer is C *[IX E 2]*
Pentazocine produces less nausea than other opioids and shows only one-fifth the analgesic potency of morphine. Pentazocine can cause constipation like other narcotics, and tolerance to the analgesic effect can occur. Pentazocine can cause an increase in cardiac work by increasing pulmonary and peripheral vascular resistance.

16. The answer is D *[IX B 2 b, e, C 1 g, E 5, F 2]*
Of the drugs listed in the question, only codeine has both antitussive and analgesic effects. The analgesic meperidine has no antitussive activity; the cough suppressant dextromethorphan has no analgesic activity. Naloxone has neither effect: It is a pure opioid antagonist and is used to reverse the unwanted effects of opioids (e.g., in neonates whose mothers received morphine during labor). Buspirone is an antianxiety agent, which is remarkably free of adverse effects.

17. The answer is C (2, 4) *[IV A 1 a; Ch 2 II C 4]*
Dopamine, an intermediate in the biosynthesis of norepinephrine, is an important neurotransmitter in the CNS. Dopamine is a β_1-adrenergic agonist with positive inotropic effects on the myocardium and is, therefore, used in the treatment of cardiogenic and septic shock and in chronic refractory congestive heart failure. In Parkinson's disease, a dopamine deficiency in the striatum appears to cause the neurologic symptoms. However, the drug dopamine does not cross the blood–brain barrier, and therefore, levodopa, the precursor of dopamine, is given instead. The neurologic side effects of antipsychotic agents, such as the phenothiazines, resemble the symptoms of Parkinson's disease, but again dopamine would be ineffective as therapy.

18. The answer is C (2, 4) *[V B, D; Table 3-2]*
Fluphenazine, a phenothiazine, and haloperidol, a butyrophenone, are useful for the control of psychotic symptoms. Fluphenazine can be given by depot injection, a useful form of therapy for patients who are prone to neglect taking their medication. Haloperidol is also useful for Gilles de la Tourette's syndrome and some other neurologic motor disorders. Promethazine, although it is a phenothiazine derivative, has antihistaminic and antiemetic properties rather than antipsychotic effects. Diphenhydramine, an antihistamine, is useful for treating the extrapyramidal symptoms that can develop with antipsychotic agents.

4

Anesthetic Agents

I. INTRODUCTION

A. Local anesthetics

1. Local anesthetic agents act by blocking both sensory and motor nerve conduction to produce a temporary loss of sensation without a loss of consciousness.

2. Unlike general anesthetics, they normally do not cause central nervous system (CNS) depression.

B. General anesthetics act on the CNS or autonomic nervous system (ANS) to produce analgesia, amnesia, or hypnosis. Used alone or in combination with other agents (e.g., preanesthetic medication), an optimum depth of anesthesia may be obtained for a variety of surgical procedures.

1. **Inhalation anesthetics,** notably ether and nitrous oxide, revolutionized surgery after 1846, when their anesthetic properties were accepted by the medical community.

2. **Intravenous anesthetics** are mostly used for induction of anesthesia (e.g., thiopental) before administration of more potent anesthetic agents; however, they can be used for some procedures of longer duration.
   a. **Neuroleptanesthesia** is induced by combining a powerful narcotic analgesic with a neuroleptic agent together with the inhalation of nitrous oxide and oxygen.
   b. **Dissociative anesthesia,** such as that caused by ketamine, produces rapid analgesia and amnesia while maintaining laryngeal reflexes.
   c. **Preanesthetic medication** may include sedatives, opioids, tranquilizers, and anticholinergic agents.

II. LOCAL ANESTHETICS

A. Chemistry

1. Structurally, all local anesthetics consist of a hydrophilic amino group linked through a connecting group to a lipophilic aromatic residue.
   a. If the **connecting link** between the intermediate group and the aromatic residue is an **ester group,** the site of metabolism is hydrolysis by plasma pseudocholinesterase.
   b. If the link is an **amide bond,** hydrolysis occurs in the liver.
   c. The greater the length of the connecting and amino groups, the greater the potency and the toxicity of the local anesthetic.

2. Local anesthetics are weak bases and, thus, are usually water-insoluble. The drug may be dispensed as a crystal but usually is prepared as an acidic salt solution, which is highly water-soluble and stable.

3. At tissue pH, depending upon the pK_a of the agent, the drug will exist as either an uncharged tertiary or secondary amine or a positively charged ammonium cation. The former state is lipophilic and crosses connective tissue and enters nerve cells; the cation is thought to block the generation of action potentials via a membrane–receptor complex.

B. Mechanism of action

1. Local anesthetics slow the propagation of nerve impulses by reducing the rate of rise of the action potential and the rate of repolarization.

2. The increased threshold for electrical excitability results in a complete block of conduction.

3. Local anesthetics specifically block nerve conduction by interfering with cell membrane permeability to sodium, particularly voltage-dependent Na^+ channels. Two theories may explain the mechanism of interference with membrane permeability.

    a. The **specific receptor theory** postulates that the local anesthetic displaces Ca^{2+} from a site near the Na^+ channel and then blocks the adjacent Na^+ channel.

    b. The **membrane expansion theory** hypothesizes that local anesthetics, because of their lipophilic properties, incorporate into the cell membrane, preventing the opening of pores and, thus, interfering with the passage of electrolytes.

4. A differential sensitivity of nerve fibers to local anesthetics has been identified and characterized.

    a. The smallest unmyelinated fibers, which conduct impulses for pain, temperature, and autonomic activity, conduct slowly and are the first to be blocked by local anesthetics.

    b. This sensitivity is a reflection of the **critical length** necessary to be exposed for an anesthetic action; smaller nerve fibers have a proportionally smaller critical length required to result in this action.

C. Agents

1. Cocaine (see Chapter 3 VIII C)

    a. Chemistry. Cocaine is an ester of benzoic acid; its structure is shown in Figure 4-1.

    b. Pharmacokinetics

        (1) Cocaine is quickly degraded by plasma esterases and has a half-life of approximately 1 hour.

        (2) Tolerance, abuse, and poisoning can occur with cocaine overuse.

        (3) Cocaine is metabolized in the blood by ester hydrolysis using pseudocholinesterase.

    c. Pharmacologic effects. In addition to local anesthetic activity, the spectrum of activity of cocaine includes the following:

        (1) CNS effects

            (a) Cocaine initially produces euphoria and sometimes dysphoria.

            (b) The initial effect is followed by poststimulatory depression.

        (2) Cardiovascular effects

            (a) Cocaine blocks the uptake of catecholamines at adrenergic nerve terminals.

            (b) This causes sympathetically mediated tachycardia and vasoconstriction, leading to hypertension. (The vasoconstriction also decreases intraoperative mucous membrane bleeding.)

        (3) Hyperpyrexia

        (4) Anorexia

    d. Preparations and therapeutic uses

        (1) Cocaine hydrochloride is used in 4%–10% concentrations and as crystals for topical anesthesia of the nose, pharynx, and tracheobronchial tree.

        (2) While cocaine has the dubious distinction of being the first identified local anesthetic, its CNS effects (abuse potential) and the development of more potent agents have resulted in a decline in its clinical use.

2. Procaine

    a. Chemistry. This local anesthetic is an ester of diethylaminoethanol and para-aminobenzoic acid (PABA). Its structure is shown in Figure 4-2.

    b. Pharmacokinetics

        (1) Procaine is well-absorbed following parenteral administration and is rapidly metabolized by pseudocholinesterase. It has a short duration of action.

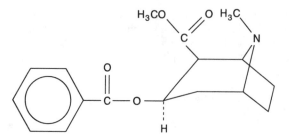

Figure 4-1. Cocaine.

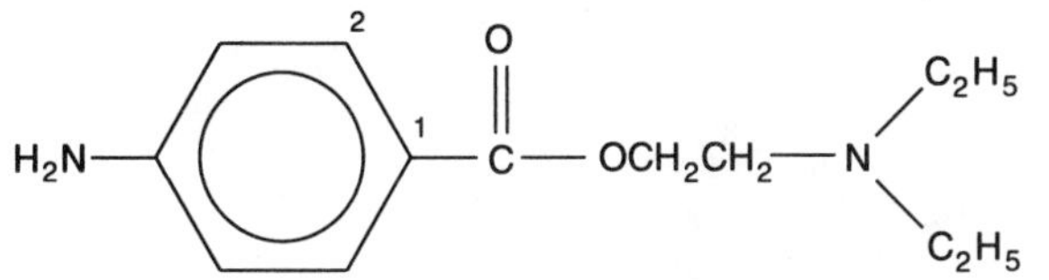

Figure 4-2. Procaine.

    (2) The drug lacks topical activity.

    (3) Procaine administration causes minimal systemic toxicity and no local irritation.

  c. Pharmacologic effects, in addition to local anesthetic activity, include a procaine–sulfonamide antagonism. The metabolic product of procaine hydrolysis is PABA, which inhibits the action of sulfonamides.

  d. Preparations and therapeutic uses. Procaine hydrochloride is available with and without epinephrine. **Epinephrine** decreases the rate of anesthetic absorption in the bloodstream and so approximately doubles the duration of anesthesia produced by a given dose.

    (1) A 1%–2% solution is used for nerve block and infiltration anesthesia.

    (2) A 5%–20% solution is used for spinal anesthesia.

3. Tetracaine

  a. Chemistry. This local anesthetic is an ester and derivative of PABA. Its structure is shown in Figure 4-3.

  b. Pharmacokinetics

    (1) It is approximately 10 times more potent (and more toxic) than procaine.

    (2) Its onset of action is approximately 5 minutes, and its duration of action is between 2 and 3 hours.

  c. Preparations and therapeutic uses

    (1) Tetracaine hydrochloride is a commonly used local anesthetic for spinal anesthesia and, in this context, usually is combined with 10% dextrose to increase the specific gravity so that the solution is heavier than cerebrospinal fluid.

    (2) A 2% solution is used topically on mucous membranes.

4. Lidocaine

  a. Chemistry. This drug is an amide local anesthetic and an acetanilid derivative. Its structure is shown in Figure 4-4.

  b. Pharmacokinetics. Lidocaine is rapidly absorbed after parenteral administration and is metabolized in the liver by microsomal mixed-function oxidases.

  c. Pharmacologic effects include:

    (1) Rapid onset of anesthesia

    (2) Minimal local irritation

    (3) A greater potency and longer duration of action than procaine

    (4) Moderate topical activity

  d. Preparations and therapeutic uses

    (1) The major clinical uses of lidocaine are as a local anesthetic and, intravenously, as an antiarrhythmic agent (see Chapter 5 II C).

    (2) Lidocaine hydrochloride can be administered with or without epinephrine.

    (3) A 0.5% solution is used for infiltrative anesthesia.

    (4) A 1%–2% solution is used for topical mucosal and nerve block anesthesia.

    (5) For spinal anesthesia, the concentration of lidocaine used is 5% or less.

    (6) For topical anesthesia, lidocaine is available as an ointment, jelly, cream, and solution.

5. Dibucaine

  a. Chemistry. This drug is a substituted amide and a quinoline derivative.

  b. Pharmacokinetics

    (1) Dibucaine is a potent anesthetic with a long duration of action.

    (2) It has a very high systemic toxicity and is currently used only as a topical anesthetic.

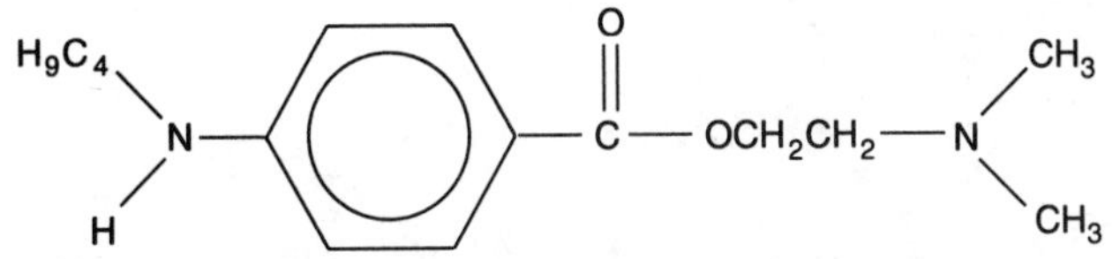

Figure 4-3. Tetracaine.

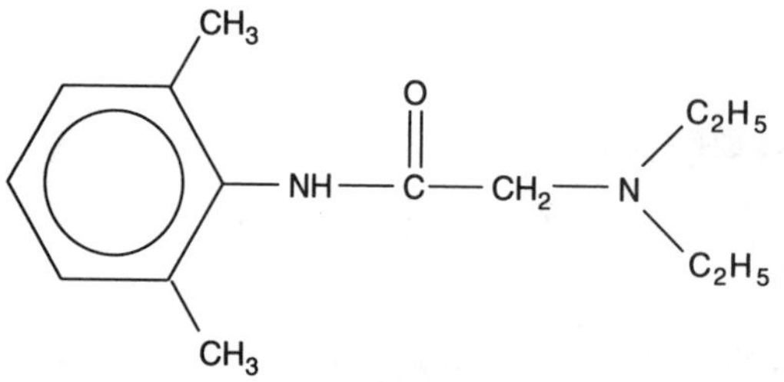

Figure 4-4. Lidocaine.

    c. Preparations and therapeutic uses. Dibucaine hydrochloride is used for anesthesia of mucous membranes in a 0.2% concentration.

6. Prilocaine
    a. Chemistry. Like lidocaine, prilocaine is an amide local anesthetic.
    b. Pharmacokinetics
        (1) Its onset and duration of action are slightly longer than those of lidocaine.
        (2) The major disadvantage of prilocaine is the production of methemoglobinemia and a shift of the oxygen-dissociation curve for hemoglobin to the left.
    c. Preparations and therapeutic uses. Prilocaine hydrochloride has been used for infiltrative, regional, and spinal anesthesia and is available in a 1%–3% solution.

7. Etidocaine
    a. Chemistry. The structure of etidocaine is shown in Figure 4-5.
    b. Pharmacokinetics. Etidocaine is similar to lidocaine except for its greater potency and longer duration of action.
    c. Preparations and therapeutic uses
        (1) Etidocaine is used clinically in epidural, infiltrative, and regional anesthesia. The drug usually blocks motor fibers before sensory fibers.
        (2) Etidocaine hydrochloride is available both with and without epinephrine, in concentrations ranging from 0.5%–1.5%.

8. Mepivacaine
    a. Chemistry. Like lidocaine, mepivacaine is an amide-type local anesthetic. The structure of mepivacaine is shown in Figure 4-6.
    b. Pharmacokinetics
        (1) Mepivacaine is similar to lidocaine. However, it does not have antiarrhythmic activity.
        (2) In onset of action, mepivacaine is more rapid than lidocaine, and its duration of action is about 20% longer.
        (3) Epinephrine is rarely used with this drug.
    c. Preparations and therapeutic uses
        (1) Major uses of mepivacaine are for infiltrative and regional nerve block anesthesia. It also can be used for spinal anesthesia.
        (2) Mepivacaine hydrochloride is used in concentrations ranging from 1%–4%.

9. Bupivacaine
    a. Chemistry. An amide local anesthetic, bupivacaine is structurally similar to mepivacaine.
    b. Pharmacokinetics
        (1) It is more potent and has a longer duration of action than mepivacaine, lasting for more than 24 hours in some situations, possibly as a result of increased tissue binding. The onset of action is slower than that of mepivacaine.
        (2) Toxicity is similar to that of tetracaine; however, cardiac arrest has been reported in association with a 0.75% solution of bupivacaine used for obstetric epidural anesthesia.

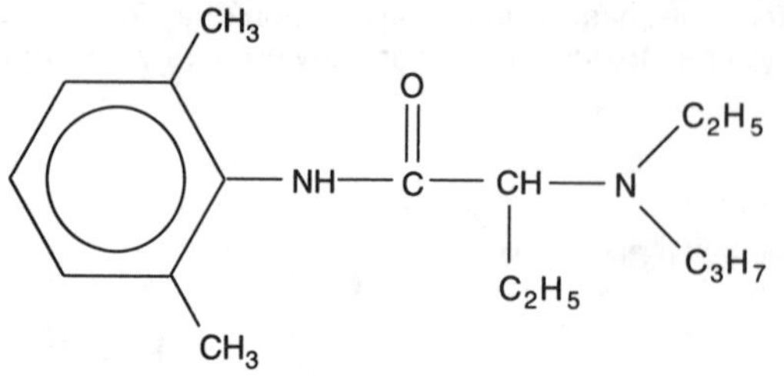

Figure 4-5. Etidocaine.

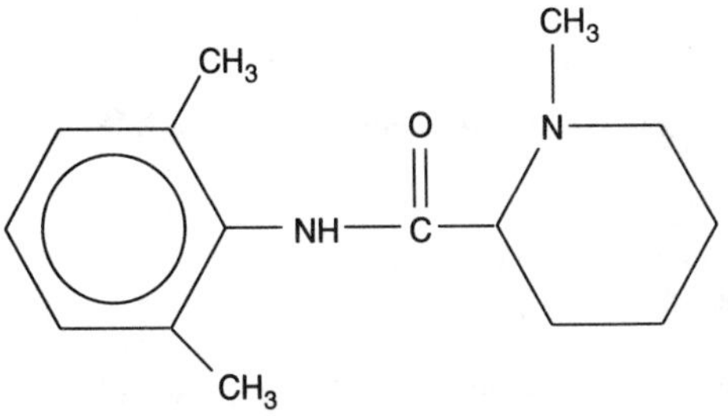

Figure 4-6. Mepivacaine.

    c. Preparations and therapeutic uses. Bupivacaine hydrochloride is used mainly for regional nerve block anesthesia in concentrations ranging from 0.25%–0.75%.

  10. Several drugs that are chemically related to local anesthetics—**procainamide, tocainide,** and **flecainide**—are, like lidocaine, used as antiarrhythmic agents and are discussed in Chapter 5 II B 2, C 3, D.

D. Adverse systemic effects of local anesthetics result from absorption of toxic amounts of these agents into the bloodstream. Adding epinephrine, a vasoconstrictor, to the optimal concentration of a local anesthetic reduces the rate of systemic absorption of the anesthetic and so can decrease systemic toxicity.

  1. Seizures, the result of absorption of the local anesthetic and stimulation of the CNS, are the most serious adverse effect. Convulsions, if they occur, are treated with basic supportive measures, including ventilation and oxygenation, and with intravenous diazepam.

  2. Respiratory failure secondary to CNS depression is a late stage of intoxication.

  3. A quinidine-like effect on the myocardium can be produced by local anesthetics.

  4. Hypotension is a late effect that can occur as the result of myocardial depression and peripheral arterial vasodilation; affected patients are treated with appropriate parenteral vasopressor agents.

  5. Allergic reactions to local anesthetic agents rarely occur.

III. GENERAL ANESTHETICS

A. Inhalation anesthetics

  1. General considerations
    a. The relationship between the administered dose of an inhalation anesthetic and the quantitative effect produced is described as the **minimum alveolar concentration (MAC)** of the anesthetic at 1 atm that will produce loss of movement in 50% of subjects exposed to a noxious stimulus. The MAC is used as the **measure of potency** for all inhalation anesthetics.
    b. The concentration of an inhalation anesthetic in blood or tissue is the product of its solubility and partial pressure. The **solubility** of an agent is expressed most commonly in terms of a blood:gas or a tissue:blood partition coefficient.
      (1) An agent with a **blood:gas partition coefficient** of 2 will reach twice the concentration in the blood phase as in the gas phase when the partial pressure is the same in both phases (i.e., at equilibrium). Very soluble agents (e.g., ether) have a blood:gas partition coefficient as high as 12; relatively insoluble agents (e.g., nitrous oxide) have a coefficient of less than 1. **The lower the blood:gas partition coefficient of an anesthetic, the more rapid the induction of anesthesia** with that agent, because high blood solubility constantly lowers the alveolar gas pressure.
      (2) Most inhalation agents are equally soluble in lean tissue and in blood, so that the **tissue:blood partition coefficient** often approximates 1. On the other hand, most anesthetics have a far greater concentration in fatty tissues than in blood at equilibrium.

  2. Halothane
    a. Pharmacokinetics
      (1) Halothane, with a MAC of 0.75%, is a potent anesthetic agent.
      (2) Halothane lacks significant analgesic potency and, thus, is most frequently used with another anesthetic.

b. Pharmacologic effects
   (1) Respiratory effects
      (a) Respirations become rapid and shallow, and there is a reduction in the minute volume.
      (b) It causes a reduction in the ventilatory response to carbon dioxide. This effect appears to be due to depression of central chemoreceptors.
      (c) Halothane produces bronchiolar dilation.
   (2) Cardiovascular effects
      (a) Halothane causes a dose-dependent decrease in arterial blood pressure.
      (b) Cutaneous blood flow may increase as blood vessels dilate.
      (c) Myocardial contractility is depressed with halothane administration.
      (d) Halothane interferes with the action of norepinephrine and, thus, antagonizes the sympathetic response to arterial hypotension.
      (e) Halothane anesthesia depresses cardiac sympathetic activity, which can result in a slow heart rate.
      (f) Although arrhythmias are uncommon, halothane can increase the automaticity of the heart. This condition is exacerbated by adrenergic agonists, cardiac disease, hypoxia, and electrolyte abnormalities.
   (3) CNS effects
      (a) As halothane anesthesia deepens, fast, low-voltage electroencephalographic waves are replaced by slow, high-voltage waves.
      (b) Cerebral blood vessels dilate, increasing cerebral blood flow and cerebrospinal fluid pressure. A maldistribution of cerebral blood flow and altered metabolism can occur.
      (c) Shivering during recovery is common.
   (4) Renal effects
      (a) At a level of 1 MAC, halothane causes renal blood flow and glomerular filtration to drop to about 50% of normal.
      (b) These effects are mitigated by adequate hydration.
   (5) Hepatic effects
      (a) Halothane depresses liver function. This effect is rapidly reversed when administration of the anesthetic is stopped.
      (b) **Hepatic necrosis** that cannot be attributed to known etiologies can occur with halothane anesthesia.
         (i) Two to five days postoperatively, an affected patient develops fever, anorexia, and vomiting. This syndrome is known as **halothane hepatitis**.
         (ii) Eosinophilia and biochemical abnormalities characteristic of hepatitis occur.
         (iii) Halothane hepatitis has an incidence of 1 in 7000 individuals receiving halothane anesthesia, and it is associated with a 20%–50% mortality rate.
         (iv) It is likely that halothane-induced hepatic damage is metabolic in origin. The possibility of genetic susceptibility has been suggested and would provide evidence that the rate of halothane metabolism is genetically determined.
         (v) Patient characteristics that increase the potential for liver damage include middle age; closely spaced, repeated administration of halothane; obesity; and female sex. Preexisting liver disease is not exacerbated by halothane.
         (vi) Children do not appear to be susceptible to the liver damage associated with halothane.
   (6) Muscular effects
      (a) Halothane causes skeletal muscle relaxation by both central and peripheral mechanisms.
      (b) It appears to increase the sensitivity of end-plates to the action of competitive neuromuscular blocking agents.
      (c) It relaxes uterine smooth muscle.
      (d) Halothane, like all potent inhalation agents, can trigger **malignant hyperthermia,** a potentially fatal condition believed to be autosomal dominant, in which, in response to anesthesia, a sudden, rapid rise in body temperature and signs of increased muscle metabolism occur.
c. Excretion
   (1) Approximately 70% of halothane is eliminated unchanged in exhaled gas in the first 24 hours after administration.

(2) Approximately 5% is biotransformed by the cytochrome P-450 system in the endoplasmic reticulum of the liver.

d. Therapeutic uses

   (1) Halothane is a highly potent, nonflammable general anesthetic with a relatively high blood:gas partition coefficient; thus, induction of and recovery from anesthesia with this agent may be prolonged.

   (2) Halothane is not irritating to the larynx, and thus, induction of anesthesia with this agent is smooth and bronchospasm is uncommon.

   (3) Halothane administration is often supplemented with thiopental for induction of anesthesia. Nitrous oxide, oxygen, and muscle relaxants are normally used with halothane.

   (4) Halothane is a safe anesthetic for children.

3. Enflurane

a. Pharmacokinetics

   (1) Enflurane has a MAC of 1.68%.

   (2) Enflurane causes mild stimulation of salivation and tracheobronchial secretions. It suppresses laryngeal reflexes.

b. Pharmacologic effects

   (1) Respiratory effects

   (a) Enflurane produces dose-dependent respiratory depression.

   (b) With enflurane at a level of 1 MAC, respiratory responses to hypoxia and hypercapnia are less than with halothane.

   (c) Enflurane causes bronchodilation and inhibits bronchoconstriction.

   (2) Cardiovascular effects

   (a) Dose-dependent depression of the arterial blood pressure and depressed baroreceptor responses are similar to those caused by halothane.

   (b) Dose-dependent myocardial depression also occurs and is similar to that caused by halothane.

   (c) Bradycardia usually does not occur with enflurane, and cardiac output is not decreased as much as with halothane.

   (d) Enflurane causes a lower incidence of arrhythmias and less sensitization of the myocardium to catecholamines than does halothane.

   (3) CNS effects

   (a) Enflurane anesthesia can lead to an electroencephalographic pattern characteristic of seizure activity or to frank seizures.

   (i) The seizures are self-limited and can be prevented by avoiding both high concentrations of enflurane and hyperventilation, which leads to hypocapnia.

   (ii) Enflurane is contraindicated in patients who have known seizure disorders.

   (b) Enflurane causes cerebral vasodilation and increased intracranial pressure as long as the arterial blood pressure remains normal.

   (4) Renal effects

   (a) At a level of 1 MAC, enflurane anesthesia causes a reduction in renal blood flow and glomerular filtration that is similar to that caused by halothane.

   (b) Although fluoride is a metabolic product of enflurane biotransformation, it poses little, if any, danger of renal toxicity.

   (5) Hepatic effects

   (a) Liver impairment has been reported but usually is reversible.

   (b) Hepatic necrosis also has been reported, especially after repeated administration of enflurane.

   (6) Muscular effects

   (a) Enflurane provides adequate muscular relaxation for most surgical procedures. The agent acts directly on the neuromuscular junction.

   (b) Enflurane relaxes uterine smooth muscle.

c. Excretion

   (1) Approximately 80% of enflurane is eliminated unchanged as expired gas.

   (2) Because enflurane's oil:gas partition coefficient is less than that of other halogenated anesthetics, enflurane leaves fatty tissues more rapidly.

   (3) About 5% of enflurane is metabolized in the liver. Free fluoride ion is released.

d. Therapeutic uses

   (1) Enflurane is a potent general anesthetic that causes a lower incidence of arrhythmias than halothane.

(2) Enflurane is a better skeletal muscle relaxant than halothane but, unlike halothane, can cause seizure activity.

4. Isoflurane is the anesthetic of choice among the dialkyl-haloethers (volatile anesthetics such as enflurane and isoflurane having the general structure shown in Figure 4-7).

a. Pharmacologic effects

(1) Isoflurane is an isomer of enflurane and has similar physical properties.

(2) It produces significant respiratory depression.

(3) Because of hypercapnia resulting from respiratory depression, cardiac output may increase.

(4) Peripheral vascular resistance is decreased by isoflurane, resulting in a fall in arterial blood pressure.

(5) Isoflurane does not sensitize the heart to catecholamines and rarely causes cardiac arrhythmias.

(6) It is a better muscle relaxant than either halothane or enflurane.

b. Therapeutic use. Unlike enflurane, isoflurane does not cause seizure activity; unlike halothane, isoflurane does not sensitize the myocardium to epinephrine or induce arrhythmias.

5. Nitrous oxide

a. Pharmacokinetics

(1) Nitrous oxide (N_2O) is an inorganic inert gas that supports combustion.

(2) The MAC for nitrous oxide is 105.2%, meaning that hyperbaric conditions would be required to reach a level of 1 MAC with this drug. For maintaining anesthesia, a concentration of 75%–80% nitrous oxide is required.

(3) Nitrous oxide is not effective for anesthesia as a single agent, and attempting to use it in this manner is likely to induce hypoxia. To achieve "complete" anesthesia with this agent, administration of opioids to supplement analgesia, the use of thiopental for narcosis, and a neuromuscular blocking agent for muscular relaxation are all required.

(4) When nitrous oxide is combined with more potent inhalation agents, such as enflurane or halothane, it provides significant analgesia.

b. Pharmacologic effects

(1) Respiratory effects

(a) The effects of nitrous oxide on respiration are minimal when a concentration of 50% is used.

(b) However, when nitrous oxide is combined with thiopental or another anesthetic agent for induction of anesthesia, the respiratory stimulant response to carbon dioxide is depressed more than when thiopental or the other anesthetic agent is used alone.

(2) Cardiovascular effects. When nitrous oxide is combined with a potent inhalation anesthetic, activation of the sympathetic nervous system results; blood pressure and total peripheral vascular resistance rise, and cardiac output is reduced.

c. Excretion

(1) Nitrous oxide is eliminated primarily as an expired gas.

(2) The amount of nitrous oxide subject to biotransformation is not known.

d. Therapeutic uses

(1) Nitrous oxide is an important and powerful **analgesic** that is well-tolerated. Its onset of action is rapid, as is recovery from its effects. Because of this, it is frequently used for outpatient dental procedures.

(2) Nitrous oxide is used as a supplement to more potent anesthetic agents and, in this capacity, is probably the most widely used general anesthetic agent.

e. Adverse effects

(1) Because of its high partial pressure in blood and its low blood:gas partition coefficient, nitrous oxide diffuses into air-containing body cavities and can increase the pressure or expand the volume of gas in air pockets. This action can result in:

(a) Distention of the bowel

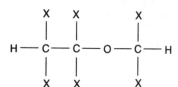

Figure 4-7. Structure of the dialkyl-haloethers. The halide (*X*) can be either chlorine or fluorine.

(b) Expansion or rupture of a pulmonary cyst

(c) Rupture of the tympanic membrane in an occluded middle ear

(d) Pneumocephalus

(2) When nitrous oxide is dissolved in blood, it can enlarge the volume of air emboli.

(3) **Diffusion hypoxia** can occur at the termination of nitrous oxide anesthesia if a patient abruptly begins to breathe room air. This hypoxia is caused by a rapid outward diffusion of nitrous oxide from tissues into the bloodstream and then into the alveoli, where it decreases alveolar tension and consequently lowers arterial oxygen levels. This problem can be avoided by administration of 100% oxygen for a short period at the termination of nitrous oxide anesthesia.

(4) Nitrous oxide is associated with a high incidence of postoperative nausea and vomiting.

(5) Inactivation of vitamin B_{12} can occur.

(6) Leukopenia has been reported with chronic nitrous oxide abuse.

(7) Nitrous oxide is contraindicated in pregnant women, immunosuppressed patients, and patients with pernicious anemia.

6. **Diethyl ether**
   a. **Pharmacokinetics.** Diethyl ether is a highly flammable and explosive anesthetic agent, which essentially has been replaced by halogenated anesthetics.
   b. **Pharmacologic effects**
      (1) **Respiratory effects**
         (a) Increased sympathetic activity produced by diethyl ether results in bronchodilation.
         (b) The respiratory response to carbon dioxide, although reduced, is maintained spontaneously by reflex excitation at peripheral sites.
      (2) **Cardiovascular effects**
         (a) Although diethyl ether is a myocardial depressant, cardiac output and arterial blood pressure are maintained because of sympathetic activation.
         (b) Vagal blockade also occurs with diethyl ether administration, resulting in tachycardia.
      (3) **Renal effects.** Diethyl ether is a strong stimulant of antidiuretic hormone.
      (4) **Hepatic effects.** Sympathetic activation results in increased hepatic glycogenolysis.
      (5) **Muscular effects**
         (a) Diethyl ether is a good skeletal muscle relaxant because it causes CNS depression at synaptic pathways in the spinal cord.
         (b) In addition, diethyl ether has a curare-like action, allowing a lower dose of neuromuscular blockers; several aminoglycoside antibiotics augment this effect.
   c. **Adverse effects.** When used as a sole agent to induce anesthesia, diethyl ether causes increased salivary secretions, vomiting, and laryngospasm.

B. **Intravenous anesthetics**

1. **Neuroleptanesthesia**
   a. **General considerations**
      (1) When a neuroleptic agent is combined with a powerful narcotic, **neuroleptanalgesia** is produced. The addition of nitrous oxide and oxygen to this combination produces **neuroleptanesthesia**.
      (2) The agents most frequently used to achieve neuroleptanalgesia are **droperidol** (a butyrophenone derivative—see Chapter 3 V D) and **fentanyl** (an opioid—see Chapter 3 IX C 3). A premixed combination of the two drugs is available as a product called **Innovar**.
   b. **Pharmacologic effects**
      (1) **Respiratory effects**
         (a) Droperidol slightly decreases the respiratory rate but increases tidal volume.
         (b) Fentanyl reduces both respiratory rate and tidal volume.
         (c) The marked respiratory depressant effect of the two drugs outlasts the analgesic effect.
      (2) **Cardiovascular effects**
         (a) Droperidol can produce mild α-adrenergic blockade, causing some hypotension.
         (b) Fentanyl has a parasympathomimetic effect that can cause bradycardia and hypotension.

(c) Innovar can cause bradycardia. However, it rarely causes other cardiac arrhythmias, and in general, it has little effect on the cardiovascular system.

c. Therapeutic uses

(1) Fentanyl should be administered as a slow intravenous infusion (given over 5–10 minutes) since rapid injection may cause respiratory muscle spasm.

(2) Respiratory depression is a frequent occurrence, and adequate ventilation and oxygenation may require use of mechanical measures.

(3) After induction of neuroleptanalgesia, nitrous oxide administration is begun. Supplementary fentanyl may be required for prolonged analgesia because fentanyl has a short duration of action.

d. Adverse effects

(1) Confusion and mental depression are the most common complaints after neuroleptanesthesia.

(2) Extrapyramidal symptoms occur rarely.

2. Dissociative anesthesia

a. General considerations

(1) Dissociative anesthesia is a state similar to neuroleptanalgesia in which anesthetized patients feel totally dissociated from their surroundings. **Phencyclidine** was the original dissociative anesthetic; the structurally similar **ketamine** is the only drug used at present to produce this state.

(2) Ketamine produces profound analgesia and amnesia.

(3) It has no effect on laryngeal reflexes.

(4) Skeletal muscle tone, heart rate, arterial blood pressure, and cerebrospinal fluid pressure can be increased by ketamine.

(5) The respiratory cycle is maintained near normal.

b. Therapeutic uses

(1) Premedication with atropine reduces salivary secretions; premedication with a narcotic analgesic decreases the dose of ketamine needed for anesthesia.

(2) Ketamine is used mainly for children and young adults, for diagnostic procedures of short duration.

c. Adverse effects

(1) Because of its hallucinogen-like structure, ketamine frequently produces unpleasant dreams, especially in adults. Recovery from ketamine anesthesia often is accompanied by emergence delirium and psychomotor activity.

(2) Contraindications to the use of ketamine include psychiatric disorders, a history of cerebrovascular disease (to avoid the risk of hypertension-induced stroke), and respiratory infections.

3. Barbiturates

a. General considerations

(1) **Thiopental** is the barbiturate most frequently used for general anesthesia. It provides rapid and pleasant induction and, thus, often is used before administration of stronger agents. It can be used alone to provide anesthesia for short procedures, but thiopental and other barbiturates are poor analgesics.

(2) Once a barbiturate has been injected, little can be done to facilitate its removal. Termination of its effects depends on redistribution of the drug from the brain to other tissues and, to a lesser extent, on biotransformation.

b. The pharmacology and therapeutic uses of barbiturates are presented in Chapter 3 II A.

4. Propofol

a. General considerations

(1) Propofol is a short-acting intravenous anesthetic that can be used for induction of anesthesia or maintenance as part of a balanced anesthesia regimen.

(2) Onset of unconsciousness occurs within 1 minute, and duration of action is only 3–5 minutes due to rapid redistribution.

(3) The clarity of mental status upon recovery makes propofol particularly useful for ambulatory surgical patients.

b. Pharmacologic effects. The hemodynamic and respiratory effects are similar to those occurring with barbiturate induction.

c. Adverse effects. Hypotension can be particularly severe in older patients.

5. Medazolam
  a. General considerations
  (1) Medazolam is a parenteral benzodiazepine used for sedation during short procedures, sedation before general anesthesia, induction of general anesthesia, and as a hypnotic drug in balanced anesthesia regimens.
  (2) Medazolam is three to four times as potent as diazepam, but unlike diazepam, it does not cause local irritation after intramuscular or intravenous injection.
  b. Pharmacokinetics
  (1) It is highly lipid soluble and rapidly crosses the blood–brain barrier.
  (2) It is metabolized in the liver and has a half-life of 1–4 hours.
  c. Adverse effects. It can cause respiratory depression, and anterograde amnesia lasts for at least 2 hours.

6. Etomidate
  a. General considerations
  (1) Etomidate is an ultra-–short-acting hypnotic used for induction of anesthesia.
  (2) Cardiovascular effects are virtually absent.
  b. Adverse effects
  (1) Pain on injection; myoclonic movements; and postoperative nausea and vomiting, especially with opioid use, are common adverse effects.
  (2) Etomidate has embryocidal activity.

C. Preanesthetic medications can foster an uncomplicated anesthetic and operative course by improving the rapidity and smoothness of induction, reducing anxiety, providing analgesia and amnesia, and compensating for the salivation, bradycardia, and some of the other side effects of anesthesia. Agents used as preanesthetic medications include sedatives, opioids, tranquilizers, and anticholinergic agents. The pharmacology, therapeutic uses, and undesirable effects of barbiturates, opioids, and tranquilizers are discussed in Chapter 3; anticholinergic agents are discussed in Chapter 2.

  1. Barbiturates, such as **secobarbital** and **pentobarbital,** are the preoperative sedatives most frequently employed. These agents produce less postoperative nausea and vomiting than opioids.

  2. Opioids, such as **morphine, fentanyl,** or **alfentanil,** often are given to patients who are to be anesthetized with general anesthetics of fairly low potency, such as the combination of nitrous oxide and thiopental. In addition, they can be administered with a barbiturate or diazepam for regional anesthesia. In both instances, they provide analgesia. Alfentanil may offer advantages over fentanyl for longer procedures. Response and recovery appear to be more rapid.

  3. Phenothiazine derivatives, such as **promethazine** and the antihistamine **hydroxyzine,** often are administered concomitantly with opioids because they potentiate the analgesic effect without increasing side effects.

  4. Tranquilizers, such as **diazepam,** are useful in a wide variety of anesthetic situations. They can provide preoperative sedation, help to prevent and treat the CNS stimulation caused by local anesthetics, and provide amnesia.

  5. Anticholinergic agents. Atropine and **scopolamine,** as well as the quaternary ammonium compound **glycopyrrolate,** are used routinely to decrease the flow of saliva. Because of a lower incidence of undesirable side effects, glycopyrrolate is recommended as the anticholinergic agent of choice for bronchoscopy.

STUDY QUESTIONS

Directions: Each of the numbered items or incomplete statements in this section is followed by answers or by completions of the statement. Select the **one** lettered answer or completion that is **best** in each case.

1. A patient who has an untreatable hepatic carcinoma must undergo foot surgery. All of the following local anesthetic agents may be deleterious to this patient based on his history EXCEPT

(A) lidocaine
(B) prilocaine
(C) mepivacaine
(D) procaine
(E) etidocaine

2. Correct statements concerning procaine include all of the following EXCEPT

(A) it has an ester linkage
(B) it interferes with sodium influx during depolarization
(C) it is relatively short acting
(D) it can produce a lupus-like syndrome
(E) its metabolic product can inhibit the action of sulfonamides

3. The local anesthetic with the shortest duration of action is

(A) procaine
(B) bupivacaine
(C) lidocaine
(D) mepivacaine
(E) tetracaine

4. A patient with a pseudocholinesterase deficiency requires minor surgery. A local anesthetic will be used. The choice of an anesthetic agent will depend on all of the following factors EXCEPT

(A) procaine should not be used in this patient because a pseudocholinesterase deficiency would lengthen its duration of action
(B) tetracaine should not be used because it is most commonly used for spinal anesthesia
(C) the chemical structure of lidocaine would most likely explain its therapeutic usefulness in this case
(D) dibucaine would not be contraindicated since it is a surface anesthetic
(E) although cocaine has abuse potential, because it is metabolized in the liver, it would be of therapeutic value in this case

5. Lidocaine has all of the following properties EXCEPT

(A) it is a therapeutically useful local anesthetic
(B) it has a rapid onset of activity
(C) it has an esteratic linkage
(D) it is metabolized in the liver
(E) epinephrine is not required when lidocaine is administered

6. A toxic dose of lidocaine is inadvertently administered locally into the dorsalis pedis artery of a patient. All of the following effects may occur EXCEPT

(A) convulsions
(B) respiratory depression
(C) hypotension
(D) increased inotropic effect
(E) reduced P_{O_2}

1-D   4-E
2-D   5-C
3-A   6-D

7. All of the following statements concerning the inhalation anesthetic halothane are true EXCEPT that

(A) it may profoundly depress myocardial force of contraction
(B) it can cause temporary depression of renal and hepatic function
(C) it may cause respiratory depression to the extent that respiratory acidosis will ensue unless ventilation is artificially supported
(D) it possesses significant analgesic potency
(E) it does not possess pulmonary anti-inflammatory activity

8. All of the following factors enhance the potential for halothane-induced liver damage EXCEPT

(A) preexisting liver disease
(B) recent previous administrations of halothane
(C) obesity
(D) female sex
(E) middle age

9. A patient is given an inhalation anesthetic, an inert gas that supports combustion. Though it is not effective as a single agent, when combined with more potent inhalation agents, it provides significant analgesia. Because of its high partial pressure in blood, this agent could result in all of the following EXCEPT

(A) distention of the bowel
(B) leukocytosis
(C) pneumocephalus
(D) rupture of a pulmonary cyst
(E) rupture of a tympanic membrane in an occluded middle ear

10. Neuroleptanalgesia has all of the following properties EXCEPT

(A) it is used chiefly for diagnostic and minor surgical procedures
(B) droperidol and fentanyl are commonly used agents
(C) hypertension is a common consequence
(D) it can be used with nitrous oxide
(E) confusion can occur as an adverse effect

11. All of the following agents are frequently used as preanesthetic medication EXCEPT

(A) diazepam
(B) morphine
(C) neostigmine
(D) scopolamine
(E) secobarbital

7-D   10-C
8-A   11-C
9-B

Directions: The question below contains four suggested answers of which **one or more** is correct. Choose the answer

      A   if **1, 2, and 3** are correct
      B   if **1 and 3** are correct
      C   if **2 and 4** are correct
      D   if **4** is correct
      E   if **1, 2, 3, and 4** are correct

12. Properties of inhalation anesthetics are found to correlate well (directly or inversely) with an index of solubility (a ratio) called a "partition coefficient." Which of the following pharmacologic factors relate to the blood:gas partition coefficient?

(1) Anesthetic efficacy
(2) Minimum alveolar concentration
(3) Respiratory rate
(4) Induction rate

Directions: Each group of items in this section consists of lettered options followed by a set of numbered items. For each item, select the **one** lettered option that is most closely associated with it. Each lettered option may be selected once, more than once, or not at all.

Questions 13–16

Match each type of anesthesia with the correct anesthetic agent.

(A) Ketamine
(B) Halothane
(C) Droperidol plus fentanyl plus nitrous oxide and oxygen
(D) Thiopental

13. Dissociative anesthesia

14. Neuroleptanesthesia

15. Inhalation anesthesia

16. Intravenous induction anesthesia

Questions 17–20

For each of the descriptions that follows, select the anesthetic drug most likely to be associated with it.

(A) Halothane
(B) Diethyl ether
(C) Nitrous oxide
(D) Isoflurane
(E) Thiopental

17. Given intravenously and not adequate for prolonged surgery

18. Has the highest minimum alveolar concentration value

19. Highly explosive agent

20. Widely used inhalation agent that can cause liver necrosis

12-C	15-B	18-C
13-A	16-D	19-B
14-C	17-E	20-A

ANSWERS AND EXPLANATIONS

1. The answer is D *[II A 1, C 2 b, 4 b, 6 a, 7 b]*
Procaine is metabolized systemically by pseudocholinesterase while lidocaine, prilocaine, mepivacaine, and etidocaine are metabolized in the liver by microsomal mixed-function oxidases. Thus, procaine would be the anesthetic agent of choice among this group.

2. The answer is D *[II B 3, C 2]*
Procaine is an ester of diethylaminoethanol and PABA, which can inhibit the action of sulfonamides. It does interfere with sodium influx during depolarization. It has a short duration of action and is metabolized by pseudocholinesterase. Unlike procainamide, procaine does not cause a lupus-like syndrome.

3. The answer is A *[II C 2]*
The duration of action (shortest to longest) is procaine, lidocaine, tetracaine, mepivacaine, bupivacaine. Procaine is rapidly metabolized by pseudocholinesterase and lacks topical activity.

4. The answer is E *[II C 2, 3 c, 4 a, b, 5 c]*
Patients with cholinesterase deficiency would have difficulty metabolizing local anesthetics possessing ester linkages. Thus, cocaine, which is an ester of benzoic acid, is metabolized via ester hydrolysis in the blood by pseudocholinesterase; it is not metabolized in the liver.

5. The answer is C *[II C 4]*
Lidocaine has an amide, not an esteratic, linkage. Possessing an amide linkage gives it a greater duration of action than procaine, which is metabolized by ester hydrolysis. Lidocaine is a therapeutically useful local anesthetic with a rapid onset of activity. Metabolism of the drug takes place in the liver. It can be administered with or without epinephrine.

6. The answer is D *[II C 4, D]*
Lidocaine toxicity can cause convulsions, followed by a CNS depression that results in respiratory depression, reduced oxygen levels, and hypotension. Local anesthetic toxicity can also produce myocardial depression (a negative inotropic effect).

7. The answer is D *[III A 2 a, b]*
All general inhalation anesthetics are myocardial depressants. They can temporarily depress renal and hepatic function. Unless ventilation is supported, respiratory acidosis can occur. They do not possess any anti-inflammatory activity. Halothane lacks significant analgesic potency and, thus, is most frequently used with another anesthetic.

8. The answer is A *[III A 2 b (5)]*
Preexisting liver disease is not exacerbated by halothane. Also, children do not appear to be susceptible to liver damage after administration of halothane. Important patient characteristics that do enhance the potential for liver damage include middle age; closely spaced, repeated administrations of halothane; obesity; and female sex. It is likely that halothane-induced hepatic damage is metabolic in origin.

9. The answer is B *[III A 5 e (1)–(7)]*
The inhalation anesthetic described in the question is nitrous oxide. Because of its high partial pressure in blood and its low blood:gas partition coefficient, nitrous oxide diffuses into air-containing body cavities and can increase the pressure or expand the volume of gas in air pockets, resulting in distention of the bowel, rupture of a tympanic membrane in an occluded middle ear, or rupture of a pulmonary cyst, and pneumocephalus. Leukopenia has been reported with chronic nitrous oxide abuse.

10. The answer is C *[III B 1]*
Neuroleptanalgesia is produced when a neuroleptic agent is combined with a powerful narcotic. The agents most commonly used are droperidol (a butyrophenone) and fentanyl (an opioid). When nitrous oxide and oxygen are added after neuroleptanalgesia is achieved, neuroleptanesthesia results. Droperidol and fentanyl can both cause hypotension, not hypertension; however, use of these agents for neuroleptanalgesia generally has little effect on the cardiovascular system. Confusion and mental depression are the most common complaints. Neuroleptanalgesia is used chiefly for diagnostic procedures (e.g., endoscopy) and minor surgical procedures.

11. The answer is C *[III C 1, 2, 4, 5]*
Agents used as preanesthetic medications include sedatives, opioids, tranquilizers, and anticholinergic agents. Secobarbital is a commonly used preoperative sedative. Morphine is often given when low-potency general anesthesia is planned. It can also be given in combination with a barbiturate or diazepam for regional anesthesia. Diazepam or other tranquilizers are given for a variety of pharmacologic effects: They provide sedation, relieve anxiety, counteract the stimulant effects of local anesthetics, and provide postoperative amnesia. Anticholinergic agents (atropine, scopolamine) are used preoperatively to reduce respiratory tract secretions and nausea. Neostigmine is an anticholinesterase agent, which is a postanesthetic agent used to reverse neuromuscular blockade produced by curare and its derivatives.

12. The answer is C (2, 4) *[III A 1]*
The minimum alveolar concentration (MAC) necessary to anesthetize 50% of patients relates to the blood:gas partition coefficient. This MAC is also a good index of potency. The induction rate is inversely proportional to the blood:gas partition coefficient because low blood:gas partitioning means only limited amounts of anesthetic must enter the blood. Moreover, the blood:tissue partition coefficient is usually not greater than 2 with the exception of fat so that blood levels grossly approximate total body load.

13–16. The answers are: 13-A *[III B 2]*, **14-C** *[III B 1]*, **15-B** *[III A 2]*, **16-D** *[III B 3]*
Dissociative anesthesia, such as that caused by ketamine, produces rapid analgesia and amnesia while maintaining laryngeal reflexes. Neuroleptanesthesia is induced by combining a powerful narcotic analgesic (fentanyl) with a neuroleptic agent (droperidol) together with the inhalation of nitrous oxide and oxygen. Inhalation anesthesia (halothane) transfers across the alveolus and depresses the CNS. Intravenous anesthetics are mostly used for induction of anesthesia (thiopental) before the administration of more potent anesthetic agents.

17–20. The answers are: 17-E *[III B 3]*, **18-C** *[III A 5]*, **19-B** *[III A 6]*, **20-A** *[III A 2]*
Thiopental is administered intravenously for induction of anesthesia but is not adequate alone except for short procedures. Nitrous oxide has a minimum alveolar concentration (MAC) of 105.2%, making it the least potent inhalation anesthetic agent used. Diethyl ether is a highly explosive anesthetic agent and, thus, has limited usefulness. Halothane is the most widely used anesthetic agent in the United States; it has been associated with hepatitis and liver necrosis that may be due to toxic or immunogenic products.

5
Cardiovascular Agents

I. DRUGS USED IN THE TREATMENT OF CONGESTIVE HEART FAILURE

A. Introduction

1. **Definition.** Congestive heart failure (CHF) is defined as the inability of the heart to meet the metabolic requirements of the peripheral systems.

2. **Pathophysiology**
   a. Myocardial cell loss due to regional ischemia or myopathy results in deterioration of systolic and diastolic performance.
   b. When confronted by an increased load, the remaining normal heart hypertrophies to maintain adequate cardiac performance.
      (1) Hypertrophy results in a fall in stroke volume index and a rise in left ventricular filling pressure.
      (2) Peripheral vascular resistance increases and pulmonary congestion develops.
   c. Vasoconstrictor compensatory mechanisms develop to maintain cerebral and coronary perfusion. These include:
      (1) Stimulation of the sympathetic nervous system
      (2) Stimulation of the renin–angiotensin system

3. **Symptoms.** Major symptoms include weakness, fatigue, and dyspnea.

B. Cardiac glycosides

1. **Chemistry**
   a. **Cardiac** glycosides are the combination of an aglycone, or genin, and one to four sugars.
      (1) The **aglycone** is chemically similar to bile acids and to steroids, such as adrenocortical and sex hormones. It is the pharmacologically active portion of the glycosides.
      (2) The **sugars** modify the water- and lipid-solubility of the glycoside molecule and, thus, affect its potency and duration of action.
   b. Glycosides are obtained from dried leaves of the foxglove, *Digitalis purpurea* (digitoxin) or *Digitalis lanata* (digitoxin, digoxin), and from the seeds of *Strophanthus gratus* (ouabain).
   c. The term **digitalis** is frequently used to refer to the entire group of cardiac glycosides.

2. **Pharmacokinetics** (Table 5-1)
   a. **Digoxin** is the most commonly used digitalis glycoside.
      (1) The bioavailability varies widely for different proprietary preparations of digoxin; intestinal absorption of the drug may be as low as 40%.
      (2) The serum half-life is normally about 36 hours but is significantly prolonged by impaired renal function.
      (3) Digoxin is not metabolized and is eliminated principally by the kidneys in almost unchanged form.
   b. **Digitoxin**
      (1) Digitoxin is well absorbed (90%–100%) from the gastrointestinal tract and does not have the variable bioavailability seen with digoxin.
      (2) The serum half-life of digitoxin is 5–7 days.
      (3) Digitoxin is metabolized by the liver, and drugs that increase the activity of hepatic microsomal enzymes, such as phenobarbital and phenytoin, accelerate its metabolism.
      (4) In contrast to digoxin, digitoxin is about 97% bound to plasma albumin.

Table 5-1. Pharmacokinetics of Commonly Used Cardiac Glycoside Preparations

Drug	Gastrointestinal Absorption	Protein Binding	$t_{1/2}$	Principal Metabolic Route	Serum Concentration (ng/ml)
Digoxin	Approx. 75%	< 30%	36 hours	Kidney	Therapeutic: 0.5–2.5 Toxic: > 2
Digitoxin	90%–100%	97%	5–7 days	Liver	Therapeutic: 10–35 Toxic: > 35

3. Pharmacologic effects
    a. General considerations
        (1) The most important property of cardiac glycosides is the **positive inotropic effect;** that is, their ability to increase the force of myocardial contraction. The result is increased cardiac work at reduced metabolic cost.
        (2) Glycosides also have effects on the electrophysiologic properties of the heart (conductivity, refractory period, automaticity).
        (3) In addition, glycosides have extracardiac effects on vascular smooth muscle, neural tissue, and other tissues.
        (4) Factors that influence the effects of cardiac glycosides on the heart include:
            (a) The dose of the agent (see I B 5)
            (b) The interaction of direct cardiac effects with reflex changes in the autonomic and hormonal regulation of cardiovascular function
            (c) The underlying cardiovascular pathophysiology
    b. Effects of digitalis glycosides on the heart (Table 5-2)
        (1) Myocardial contractility
            (a) Cardiac glycosides **increase the contractility of cardiac muscle** by increasing both the velocity of muscle contraction and the maximum force that is developed. Cardiac glycosides do not prolong the duration of the contraction.
            (b) In CHF patients, glycosides cause a shift in the ventricular function curve, which **increases cardiac output, decreases cardiac filling pressures, decreases heart size,** and **decreases venous and capillary pressures**.
            (c) Cardiac glycosides appear to exert their **positive inotropic effect** by two mechanisms:
                (i) Digitalis inhibits membrane-bound Na^+,K^+-activated adenosine triphosphatase (Na^+,K^+-ATPase), thus increasing intracellular Ca^{2+} levels.
                (ii) The movement of Ca^{2+} into the cell causes an increase in the slow inward Ca^{2+} current during the action potential (see II A 2 a).
            (d) Cardiac glycosides do not directly affect myocardial contractile proteins or alter cellular mechanisms that provide energy for contraction. However, digitalis may interfere with Ca^{2+} binding to the sarcoplasmic reticulum, making more Ca^{2+} available for interaction with contractile proteins.

Table 5-2. Effects of Cardiac Glycosides on the Heart

Effects	Atria	A-V Node	Ventricles
Direct effects	Contractility ↑ ERP ↑ Conduction velocity ↓	ERP ↑ Conduction velocity ↓	Contractility ↑ ERP ↓ Automaticity ↑
Indirect effects	ERP ↓ Conduction velocity ↑	ERP ↑ Conduction velocity ↓	No effect
Effects on electrocardiogram	P changes	P–R ↑	Q–T ↓ T and S–T depressed
Adverse effects	Extrasystole Tachycardia	A-V depression or block	Fibrillation Extrasystole Tachycardia

ERP = Effective refractory period. Arrows indicate changes: ↑ = increased; ↓ = decreased.

    (2) Myocardial oxygen consumption (MVO$_2$)
        (a) The digitalis-induced increase in myocardial contractility causes an increase in MVO$_2$.
        (b) Decreased ventricular volume, resulting from the digitalis-induced increase in muscle tone and cardiac output, decreases the MVO$_2$.
    (3) Electrophysiologic activity
        (a) The electrophysiologic effects of cardiac glycosides vary in different parts of the heart (see Table 5-2).
        (b) Cardiac glycosides indirectly increase the vagal tone of the heart. They prolong the refractory period of the atrioventricular (A-V) node and decrease conduction velocity (direct and indirect effects) through the A-V node.
    (4) Heart rate
        (a) In CHF patients, digitalis slows the heart rate (a **negative chronotropic effect**). This is due to a combination of vagal and sinoatrial (S-A) nodes.
        (b) Tachycardia is seen with excessive doses of digitalis (a **positive chronotropic effect**) [see I B 6 e (6)].
        (c) In normal individuals, digitalis has little effect on the heart rate.
  c. Extracardiac effects
    (1) When cardiac glycosides increase the cardiac output in CHF patients, there is a drop in peripheral vascular resistance and venomotor tone as well as an increase in blood flow. In normal individuals, digitalis produces venous and arterial constriction.
    (2) Because digitalis increases the stroke volume in CHF patients, systolic blood pressure may rise.
    (3) Diastolic pressure may fall because of improved circulation, increased tissue oxygenation, and diminished reflex vasoconstriction.
    (4) A diuretic effect occurs because the increased cardiac output and renal blood flow combine to reduce the neurohumoral factors that inhibit the excretion of salt and water.

4. Therapeutic uses and contraindications
  a. Cardiac glycosides are of greatest value for treating **low-output cardiac failure**.
  b. They are also of great value in the **control of atrial fibrillation and flutter** because of the ability to reduce the ventricular rate by prolonging the refractory period of conduction tissue. Digitalis may convert atrial flutter to atrial fibrillation.
  c. Paroxysmal atrial tachycardia frequently responds to digitalis therapy, presumably as a result of reflex vagal stimulation.
  d. The use of cardiac glycosides is **contraindicated** in **cardiac tamponade, high-output CHF, constrictive pericarditis,** and **idiopathic hypertrophic subaortic stenosis** with outlet obstruction.

5. Digitalization and maintenance dosage
  a. General considerations
    (1) Since digitalis glycosides are used almost exclusively either to restore adequate circulation in patients with CHF or to slow ventricular rate in patients with atrial fibrillation or flutter, long-term therapy is frequently necessary to maintain therapeutic myocardial concentrations.
    (2) The low margin of safety (see I B 6) increases the critical nature of dosage and administration.
  b. Digoxin
    (1) When there is no urgency, an **oral digitalizing dose** is first administered, and then the maintenance dose is adjusted on the basis of clinical and laboratory assessment. Usually, a steady-state level is achieved in 5 half-lives (about 8 days).
    (2) When digitalization must be achieved rapidly, digoxin can be administered intravenously over a period of several minutes. The onset of action is within 5–30 minutes; the maximal effect is reached within 1–5 hours.
  c. Digitoxin
    (1) The total **oral loading dose** of digitoxin is divided into doses given every 6 hours and administered over the course of 36–48 hours.
    (2) The maximal effect of a dose of digitoxin is reached approximately 9 hours after oral administration.
    (3) Once optimal benefit has been achieved, the maintenance dose usually is adjusted to 10% of the digitalizing dose.

(4) Although digitoxin is available for intravenous administration, its long latency period precludes its use in emergency situations.

6. Adverse effects

   a. Digitalis glycosides have a **low margin of safety,** and intoxication from an excess of the drug is a common and potentially fatal problem. In most CHF patients, the lethal dose of a digitalis glycoside is likely to be only 5–10 times the minimal effective dose.

   b. The **therapeutic:toxic ratio** does not vary from one glycoside to another, and the only difference among the drugs lies in the **duration of toxicity.**

   c. Intoxication is most frequently precipitated by depletion of serum K^+ due to diuretic therapy, but it can also occur from accumulation of maintenance glycoside doses taken over a long period of time. Intoxication due to hypokalemia may also occur as a result of:

   (1) Prolonged administration of corticosteroids

   (2) Protracted vomiting

   (3) Protracted diarrhea

   d. Decreased renal function and hypothyroidism predispose patients to digitalis glycoside toxicity because they reduce the excretion or the metabolism of the glycoside, and hence, they result in excessive accumulation of the glycoside.

   e. When the concentrations of digoxin and digitoxin rise above 2 ng/ml and 35 ng/ml of blood, respectively, **signs of systemic toxicity** often appear, and therapy must be discontinued. Signs of toxicity include:

   (1) Anorexia (often the earliest sign)

   (2) Nausea, vomiting, and diarrhea

   (3) Headache, fatigue, malaise, neuralgias, and delirium

   (4) Vision changes, including abnormal color perception

   (5) Gynecomastia (rare)

   (6) Cardiac effects

   (a) Premature ventricular contractions (PVCs) and ventricular tachycardia and fibrillation

   (b) A-V dissociation and block

   (c) Sinus arrhythmia and S-A block

   (d) Paroxysmal and nonparoxysmal atrial tachycardia, often with A-V block

7. Treatment of digitalis toxicity

   a. Cardiac glycosides and K^+-depleting diuretics are discontinued.

   b. KCl is administered orally or by slow, careful intravenous infusion if hypokalemia is present; K^+ is **not** given, however, if severe A-V block is found or if serum K^+ levels are high.

   c. Because hypomagnesemia may accompany hypokalemia, magnesium replacement may also be necessary.

   d. Phenytoin can be given for ventricular and atrial arrhythmias.

   e. Lidocaine and procainamide can be used to treat ventricular tachyarrhythmias.

   f. Propranolol can be used for ventricular and supraventricular tachycardia but **not** in the presence of A-V block.

   g. Atropine can be used to control sinus bradycardia and various degrees of A-V block.

   h. Cholestyramine binds to cardiac glycosides and has been used to hasten their elimination.

   i. A digoxin-specific antibody fragment from immunized sheep is available for the treatment of life-threatening digoxin or digitoxin overdosage. Its use is reserved for patients exhibiting shock or cardiac arrest, ventricular arrhythmias, progressive bradyarrhythmias, or severe hyperkalemia.

   j. Electrical conversion is often hazardous in the treatment of digitalis-induced arrhythmias because it can precipitate ventricular fibrillation.

C. Angiotensin-converting enzyme (ACE) inhibitors (see IV I 1; Chapter 8 V C 2)

   1. Chemistry, mechanism of action, and pharmacokinetics (see IV I)

   2. Pharmacologic effects

   a. ACE inhibitors (i.e., captopril, enalapril, lisinopril) produce beneficial hemodynamic effects by decreasing the conversion of angiotensin I to angiotensin II. They also inhibit the degradation of bradykinin.

b. Hemodynamically, these agents increase cardiac output by reducing afterload and by decreasing total peripheral resistance, pulmonary resistance, and preload.

3. Therapeutic uses
   a. Initially, these agents were used in patients not responding adequately to digitalis and diuretics. More recently, captopril and enalapril are being used as first-line agents for CHF.
   b. Adding an ACE inhibitor to therapy with diuretics and digitalis has increased the survival rate among patients with moderate to severe CHF.
   c. After myocardial infarction, ACE inhibitors may lessen the progressive enlargement of the left ventricle.

4. Adverse effects
   a. Severe persistent cough occasionally occurs.
   b. Hypotension and deterioration of renal function can occur with an ACE inhibitor–diuretic combination.
   c. Hypokalemia and ventricular arrhythmias occur less frequently in CHF patients given an ACE inhibitor combined with a diuretic than in those treated with digoxin.
   d. Adverse effects associated with captopril, such as rash, taste disturbances, proteinuria, and leukopenia, may be related to the sulfhydryl moiety of captopril.

D. Other drugs used in CHF

1. Diuretic therapy (see Chapter 6) **and Na$^+$ restriction** play an important role in reducing extracellular fluid volume. Diuretics relieve symptoms of heart failure more rapidly than any other oral agent and along with digoxin are first-line drugs in the treatment of CHF.

2. Alpha-adrenergic blocking agents (see Chapter 2 III A) may be used in CHF to improve cardiac function by inducing vasodilation through both direct and reflex actions.

3. Other vasodilators (see III) may be used for patients not responding to digitalis glycosides and diuretics.
   a. Arteriolar dilators decrease afterload, whereas **venous vasodilators** reduce preload. The decrease in preload and afterload serves to increase cardiac output while reducing pulmonary congestion.
   b. Isosorbide dinitrate, hydralazine, and **prazosin** (see III A; IV E 2, F 2) have all been used in the treatment of CHF. Isosorbide improves cardiac function, but it has not been shown to improve survival rates when used alone. Increased survival rates have been demonstrated with isosorbide and hydralazine used together.

4. Amrinone is a bipyridine derivative, which inhibits phosphodiesterase type III. It is reserved for the short-term therapy of CHF that is refractory to other agents.
   a. Pharmacologic effects. It exerts a positive inotropic effect and increases systemic vasodilation.
   b. Route of administration. This agent is administered intravenously.
   c. Adverse effects
      (1) A dose-related thrombocytopenia may occur.
      (2) Amrinone may increase the ventricular rate in patients with atrial flutter or fibrillation.

II. DRUGS USED IN THE TREATMENT OF ARRHYTHMIA

A. General considerations

1. Cardiac arrhythmias
   a. Cardiac arrhythmias are abnormalities in the rate, regularity, or site of origin of the cardiac impulse, or a disturbance in conduction of the impulse such that the normal sequence of activation of atria and ventricles is altered.
   b. Arrhythmias may be due to:
      (1) Faulty impulse initiation
      (2) Faulty impulse conduction
      (3) Combinations of the above
   c. The change in the impulse upsets the normal relationship that exists between the duration of the refractory period and the conduction velocity in myocardial tissue. Changes in the normal relationship between refractoriness and conduction velocity may be critical, considering the heterogeneity of electrophysiologic and mechanical properties of the heart.

2. Cardiac electrophysiology
   a. Action potential phases
      (1) The action potential of cardiac cells is divided into phases.
      (2) The voltage changes of the action potential are associated with changes in ionic conductance across the cell membrane. The following list gives only the major ionic currents.
         (a) Phase 0. Rapid depolarization: Na^+ rapidly enters the cell through Na^+-specific channels ("fast" channels) in the cell membrane.
         (b) Phase 1. Rapid repolarization: K^+ briefly leaves the cell.
         (c) Phase 2. Sustained depolarization (plateau): Ca^{2+} enters the cell through Ca^{2+}-specific channels ("slow" channels) in the cell membrane.
         (d) Phase 3. Rapid repolarization: K^+ leaves the cell.
         (e) Phase 4. Slow depolarization (diastole): In cells capable of self-excitation (e.g., His–Purkinje cells), several ionic currents flow into and out of the cell until an impulse is fired off. Other cells remain resting until activated.
   b. Automaticity
      (1) Automaticity is the ability of a cardiac cell to reach threshold potential and generate impulses spontaneously.
      (2) In the cardiac cells, the resting potential depolarizes during phase 4 until a threshold potential is reached and an action potential is initiated.
      (3) In man, the S-A node is the **normal pacemaker** since it has the steepest slope of phase 4 and the most rapid firing rate. However, specialized atrial conduction fibers, distal cells of the A-V node, and His–Purkinje fibers are **latent pacemakers**.
      (4) Abnormalities in cardiac rhythms arise from alterations in the site of normal automaticity and abnormal generation of impulses.
      (5) Most antiarrhythmic agents depress the automaticity (i.e., decrease the rate of phase 4 depolarization) of latent pacemakers more effectively than of the S-A node.
      (6) Inhibition of automaticity may also be due to a decreased threshold potential or decreased excitability of pacemaker cells.
   c. Conduction velocity
      (1) Conduction velocity is the speed at which an impulse is propagated.
      (2) It is a function of:
         (a) The maximum rate ($\dot{V}_{max}$) of depolarization of phase 0
         (b) The threshold potential
         (c) The resting membrane potential
      (3) Depolarization of the membrane is associated with a decrease in conduction velocity.
      (4) The **effective refractory period (ERP)** is the period of repolarization during which no normal action potential can be elicited. Shortening of the ERP during tachycardia may produce arrhythmia, and an effective antiarrhythmic agent increases the **ERP/APD ratio (the effective refractory period/action potential duration ratio)**.
      (5) Disturbances in cardiac conductance may underlie supraventricular or ventricular arrhythmias.
      (6) In areas of injured myocardium, conduction may be slow, or refractoriness shortened, or both, resulting in the **reentry of aberrant impulses** and, hence, a cardiac arrhythmia.

3. Classes of antiarrhythmic drugs
   a. Class I antiarrhythmic agents depress phase 0 of the action potential by blocking Na^+ channels.
      (1) Class IA antiarrhythmics cause moderate phase 0 depression but prolong repolarization. Class IA drugs include quinidine, procainamide, and disopyramide.
      (2) Class IB antiarrhythmics cause minimal phase 0 depression and shorten repolarization. Class IB drugs include lidocaine, phenytoin, mexiletine, and tocainide.
      (3) Class IC antiarrhythmics cause marked phase 0 depression but have little effect on repolarization. Class IC drugs include flecainide and encainide.
   b. Class II antiarrhythmic agents act by β-adrenergic blockade. Class II drugs include propranolol, acebutolol, and esmolol.
   c. Class III antiarrhythmic agents prolong repolarization and lengthen phase 2 of the action potential. Class III drugs include amiodarone and bretylium.
   d. Class IV antiarrhythmic agents are Ca^+ antagonists (see III C). Class IV drugs include verapamil, diltiazem, and others. Verapamil is currently approved as an antiarrhythmic agent, while diltiazem is currently being evaluated for supraventricular arrhythmias.

B. Class IA antiarrhythmic agents

1. Quinidine
  a. Chemistry. Quinidine, an alkaloid isolated from cinchona bark, is the d isomer of quinine.
  b. Pharmacokinetics
   (1) Quinidine as the sulfate or gluconate is well absorbed after oral administration. It exerts a maximum effect within 1–2 hours after administration by this route.
   (2) Quinidine is given intramuscularly as the gluconate.
   (3) Approximately 80% of the drug is bound to plasma albumin.
   (4) Quinidine is metabolized in the liver and excreted by the kidneys.
  c. Pharmacologic effects
   (1) Effects on the heart (Table 5-3). At high concentrations, quinidine has direct effects on most cells of the heart. At lower concentrations, indirect (anticholinergic) effects may significantly contribute to the overall action of quinidine on the heart.
      (a) Responsiveness, conduction, and refractoriness. Quinidine is believed to block Na^+ channels. The major effect of quinidine is to reduce the $\dot{V}_{max}$ of depolarization during phase 0 at all transmembrane voltages in atrial, ventricular, and Purkinje fibers. Thus, conduction velocity decreases and ERP increases in all of these tissues.
      (b) Automaticity is decreased in ventricular tissue by depression of the slope of phase 4. Quinidine has little effect on automaticity of the sinus node.
      (c) Electrocardiographic effects (Table 5-4).
         (i) Because quinidine depresses conduction in the bundle of His and Purkinje fibers, it produces progressive prolongation of the QRS complex.
         (ii) Prolongation of the Q–T interval and alterations in T waves are related to delayed repolarization.
         (iii) Prolongation of the P–R interval is caused by the direct effect of the drug on A-V conduction and the refractoriness of the A-V system.
   (2) Extracardiac effects. Quinidine can depress vascular smooth muscle tone, in part by α-receptor blockade. This may contribute to a reduction in peripheral vascular resistance.
  d. Therapeutic uses (Table 5-5)
   (1) Supraventricular arrhythmias
      (a) Quinidine is primarily used chronically and prophylactically to prevent recurrences of paroxysmal supraventricular tachycardia due to A-V nodal reciprocating tachycardia or to Wolff-Parkinson-White syndrome.

Table 5-3. Effects of Antiarrhythmic Drugs on Electrophysiologic Properties of the Heart

| Drug | Automaticity | | Effective Refractory Period | | Membrane Responsiveness (Purkinje Fibers) |
	Sinus Node	Purkinje Fibers	A-V Node	Purkinje Fibers	
Quinidine Procainamide Amiodarone Disopyramide	→	↓	↑→↓	↓	↓
Lidocaine Phenytoin Tocainide Mexiletine	→	↓	↑→↓	↓	↓
Propranolol	↓	↓	↑	↑	↓
Esmolol	↓	↓	↑	↑	↓
Acebutolol	↓	↓	↑	↑	↓
Bretylium	↑↓	↑↓	↓→↑	↑	→
Verapamil	↓	→↓	↑	→	→

Arrows indicate changes: ↑ = increased; ↓ = decreased; → = no change.

Table 5-4. Major Effects of Antiarrhythmic Drugs on Electrocardiogram

Drug	QRS	Q–T	P–R*
Quinidine Procainamide Amiodarone	↑	↑	→ ↑
Disopyramide	↑	↑	→
Lidocaine Phenytoin Tocainide Mexiletine	→	↓	→ ↑ ↓
Propranolol	→	↓	→ ↑

Arrows indicate changes: ↑ = increased; ↓ = decreased; → = no change.

*P–R intervals: All antiarrhythmic drugs have a variable response, usually with little observable effect. However, lidocaine hardly ever affects the P–R interval, while phenytoin and propranolol usually increase the P–R interval.

    (b) Quinidine can also be used to convert atrial flutter or fibrillation to normal sinus rhythm, but direct-current cardioversion is now the procedure of choice for this problem. Quinidine is now more frequently used to prevent recurrence of this arrhythmia.

    (c) Quinidine should not be used without prior digitalization because its vagolytic action may increase the frequency of impulse transmission across the A-V node.

  (2) Ventricular arrhythmias. Quinidine is very useful for long-term treatment of ventricular premature depolarization or to prevent recurrences of ventricular tachycardia after cardioversion of this arrhythmia.

e. Route of administration

  (1) Quinidine is usually given orally three or four times a day.

  (2) For intravenous use, the dose must be diluted in glucose solution and injected slowly, and the patient's electrocardiogram must be carefully monitored.

f. Adverse effects

  (1) Cardiotoxicity includes A-V block, ventricular tachyarrhythmias, and depression of myocardial contractility.

    (a) A 50% increase in the QRS complex indicates the need for a prompt reduction in dosage.

    (b) Ventricular arrhythmias are life-threatening, and if the therapist can distinguish this adverse effect of quinidine from the underlying disease, treatment (besides cessation of quinidine) may be either of the following:

      (i) Na^+ lactate or $NaHCO_3$ catecholamines (see Chapter 2 II A) or glucagon

Table 5-5. Uses of Antiarrhythmic Drugs in Common Cardiac Arrhythmias

Arrhythmia	Treatment of Choice	Alternatives
I. Supraventricular		
Atrial fibrillation or flutter	Digitalis to control ventricular rate, DC shock for conversion	Quinidine to suppress recurrences after DC shock
Paroxysmal atrial or nodal tachycardia	Vagotonic maneuver; digitalis	Verapamil (quinidine, procainamide, disopyramide, and β-adrenergic antagonists may all be useful, especially prophylactically)
II. Ventricular		
Ventricular premature depolarization	Lidocaine	Procainamide, quinidine, or disopyramide for prolonged suppression
Ventricular tachycardia	DC shock	Lidocaine, procainamide, or mexiletine
III. Digitalis-induced	Lidocaine or phenytoin	Procainamide is somewhat useful; β-adrenergic antagonists are useful but have a high incidence of adverse effects

        (ii) Removal of quinidine by dialysis

    (c) "Quinidine syncope" due to ventricular tachyarrhythmias of polymorphic form (**"torsades de pointes"**) can occur, especially in patients whose Q–T interval is prolonged by the drug.

    (d) Quinidine increases serum levels of digitalis and can lead to digitalis toxicity.

  (2) Diarrhea, vomiting, nausea, and anorexia are the most common side effects and, when severe, may force discontinuation of quinidine.

  (3) Quinidine can cause cinchonism. Mild symptoms of this condition include tinnitus, hearing loss, vomiting, and diarrhea; severe symptoms include headache, diplopia, photophobia, altered perception of color, confusion, and psychosis.

  (4) Sensitivity phenomena, including thrombocytopenia, can occur.

  (5) Quinidine, especially when administered intravenously, can cause hypotension because of a decrease in arteriolar resistance. When arterial pressure declines by 20 mm Hg or more, the drug should be stopped.

2. Procainamide

a. Chemistry. Procainamide differs from procaine only in that it contains an amide structure rather than an ester linkage; this difference protects it from enzymatic hydrolysis and frees it from most of the central nervous system (CNS) effects of procaine.

b. Pharmacokinetics

  (1) Procainamide may be administered orally, intravenously, or intramuscularly.

  (2) It is rapidly absorbed after oral administration and, when capsules are used, normally has a peak effect in about 1 hour. However, absorption of the drug from the gastrointestinal tract may be impaired immediately after an acute myocardial infarction.

  (3) The half-life of procainamide is approximately 3 hours.

  (4) Approximately 15% of the drug is bound to plasma proteins.

  (5) Procainamide is eliminated by both hepatic metabolism and renal excretion, and renal failure can produce toxicity.

    (a) There is a rather marked variation among individuals in the rate of acetylation and excretion.

    (b) From 50%–60% of an administered dose is excreted unchanged in the urine.

c. Pharmacologic effects

  (1) **Effects on the heart** (see Table 5-3)

    (a) The direct cardiac effects of procainamide are quite similar to those of quinidine.

        (i) Procainamide decreases automaticity and lengthens the APD and the ERP in the atria and ventricles.

        (ii) It slows conduction in the atrium, A-V node, and ventricle.

    (b) **Electrocardiographic effects** are also very similar to those of quinidine (see Table 5-4).

        (i) Prolongation of the QRS complex is the most consistent finding.

        (ii) At high doses, prolongation of the P–R interval or heart block may appear.

  (2) **Extracardiac effects**

    (a) Procainamide, especially when given intravenously, can cause a drop in blood pressure, probably from peripheral vasodilation.

    (b) Unlike quinidine, procainamide does not have α-adrenergic blocking properties.

d. Therapeutic uses (see Table 5-5)

  (1) The clinical uses of procainamide are similar to those of quinidine. Patients may respond to one drug after failing to respond to the other.

  (2) **Ventricular arrhythmias.** Procainamide is particularly effective in promptly abolishing ventricular premature depolarizations and paroxysmal ventricular tachycardia.

  (3) **Supraventricular arrhythmias.** Procainamide is now believed to be as effective as quinidine for the management of atrial arrhythmias; however, higher doses of procainamide than of quinidine may be necessary.

e. Route of administration

  (1) Procainamide may be given orally, both initially and for maintenance.

  (2) The intravenous dose, which is reserved for life-threatening situations, must be administered slowly. When the arrhythmia has been interrupted, infusion is stopped.

f. Adverse effects

  (1) Acute procainamide toxicity can cause ventricular arrhythmia, ventricular fibrillation, and cardiac depression (see II B 1 f).

(2) Nausea, vomiting, diarrhea, and anorexia occur fairly frequently with oral administration of procainamide, but they occur much less commonly than with quinidine therapy.

(3) Mental confusion and psychosis have been reported but occur less commonly than with the chemically similar compounds procaine and lidocaine.

(4) Hypersensitivity reactions are much more common than with quinidine.

    (a) Fever, joint and muscle pain, and skin rashes can occur.

    (b) Fatal agranulocytosis has occurred.

    (c) A syndrome resembling systemic lupus erythematosus, which is reversible on discontinuation of procainamide, develops in as many as 30% of patients taking procainamide for long periods of time. As many as 70% of patients taking procainamide develop positive antinuclear antibody tests. The latter occurs more rapidly in slow acetylators.

(5) Hypotension can result, especially following intravenous administration.

(6) Procainamide can precipitate acute glaucoma and urinary retention.

3. Disopyramide

  a. Pharmacokinetics

    (1) Disopyramide is well absorbed (83%) following oral administration.

    (2) The free plasma concentration is a nonlinear function of the total amount of drug in the plasma. It varies from 5%–75% as the total increases from 0.1–8 μg/ml.

    (3) Approximately 50% of a dose of disopyramide is excreted in the urine in unchanged form. Disappearance from the plasma is a function of both renal and hepatic clearance.

    (4) The half-life of disopyramide in plasma is 5–7 hours but may be prolonged in patients with renal disease.

  b. Pharmacologic effects

    (1) Effects on the heart (see Table 5-3). Disopyramide has both direct and indirect actions on the heart, which resemble those of quinidine.

      (a) Responsiveness, conduction, and refractoriness

        (i) Disopyramide reduces membrane responsiveness, amplitude of the action potential, and excitability of atrial and ventricular muscle.

        (ii) Accordingly, conduction velocity is decreased and ERP is increased in these tissues.

        (iii) Unlike either quinidine or procainamide, disopyramide produces a greater reduction in the $\dot{V}_{max}$ of phase 0 depolarization at depressed membrane potentials than at normal resting membrane potentials.

      (b) Automaticity. Concentrations of disopyramide that do not affect conduction velocity or ERP can reduce automaticity in atrial and ventricular tissue.

      (c) Electrocardiographic changes are similar to but milder than those of quinidine and procainamide (see Table 5-4).

    (2) Extracardiac effects. Disopyramide has a mild atropine-like action. It is neither an α-receptor antagonist nor a β-receptor antagonist.

  c. Therapeutic uses (see Table 5-5)

    (1) Disopyramide is approved in the United States for oral administration in the treatment of ventricular arrhythmias as an alternative to quinidine and procainamide.

    (2) It may be as effective as quinidine and procainamide against atrial arrhythmias, but it has not been approved for this use.

  d. Adverse effects

    (1) Major untoward effects are related to the action of disopyramide on the heart and may include conduction disturbances, CHF, or hypotension. Disopyramide has a negative inotropic action that can be especially troublesome in patients with preexisting ventricular failure.

    (2) Other adverse effects relate to its anticholinergic action. These effects include dry mouth, constipation, blurred vision, and urinary retention. Consequently, patients with glaucoma or with conditions causing urinary retention should not take the drug.

C. Class IB antiarrhythmic agents

1. Lidocaine

  a. Chemistry. Lidocaine is an amide local anesthetic (see Chapter 4 II C 4).

b. Pharmacokinetics
  (1) Lidocaine is rapidly metabolized by the hepatic microsomal enzyme system with 70% of the amount that enters the liver being metabolized in a single pass **(first-pass metabolism)**. Reductions in hepatic blood flow or function will reduce lidocaine plasma clearance.
  (2) Oral administration of lidocaine results in a very low plasma concentration because of the high percentage of the drug that is removed by hepatic metabolism before reaching the general circulation.
  (3) Lidocaine has an elimination half-time of approximately 1½ hours.
  (4) Approximately 70% of the drug is bound to plasma albumin.
c. Pharmacologic effects
  (1) Effects on the heart (see Table 5-3)
    (a) Automaticity. Lidocaine does not affect sinus nodal pacemaker discharge. It will depress the rate of phase 4 depolarization of Purkinje and atrial muscle fibers and, thus, depresses automaticity at these sites.
    (b) Responsiveness, conduction, and refractoriness
        (i) Lidocaine has very little effect on these electrophysiologic properties of the atria.
        (ii) In the His–Purkinje system, lidocaine reduces action potential amplitude and membrane responsiveness.
        (iii) The $\dot{V}_{max}$ of phase 0 depolarization in normal Purkinje fibers is not as greatly depressed with lidocaine as it is with procainamide or quinidine. However, the $\dot{V}_{max}$ of phase 0 is severely depressed in fibers with reduced resting membrane potentials and elevated extracellular K^+.
        (iv) Lidocaine decreases the APD by blocking the Na^+ channel in depolarized cells; it also shortens the ERP of Purkinje fibers.
    (c) Electrocardiographic effects. Unlike quinidine and procainamide, lidocaine produces very few changes in the electrocardiogram (see Table 5-4).
  (2) Extracardiac effects. Lidocaine has little effect on autonomic tone.
d. Therapeutic uses (see Table 5-5). The use of lidocaine as an antiarrhythmic agent is limited, even though lidocaine is very effective in treating ventricular arrhythmias. Because of its rapid onset and short duration of action, the drug is particularly useful in treating these arrhythmias when they arise in emergency situations, such as:
  (1) Open-heart surgery
  (2) Digitalis intoxication
  (3) Myocardial infarction
e. Route of administration. Lidocaine can be administered intravenously or intramuscularly.
  (1) The usual intravenous dose is given until the arrhythmia is abolished.
  (2) Lidocaine can also be given by continuous intravenous infusion. Because its half-life is short, a steady-state plasma concentration can be reached quickly by this method.
  (3) Lidocaine may be given intramuscularly to achieve rapid plasma levels during emergencies.
f. Adverse effects
  (1) CNS side effects of lidocaine can include drowsiness, paresthesias, decreased auditory function, convulsions, and respiratory arrest.
  (2) Circulatory collapse can occur in patients with an acute myocardial infarction after a rapid, large intravenous injection.
  (3) Propranolol or cimetidine can decrease the plasma clearance of lidocaine.
  (4) The concurrent use of tocainide and lidocaine can cause seizures.

2. Mexiletine
  a. Chemistry. Mexiletine is an orally active congener of lidocaine.
  b. Pharmacokinetics
    (1) Mexiletine is well absorbed when given orally.
    (2) Unlike lidocaine, its first-pass metabolism is low.
    (3) Its plasma elimination half-time is 10–12 hours.
    (4) Mexiletine is metabolized in the liver. Only 10% is excreted unchanged in the urine.
  c. Pharmacologic effects (see Table 5-3). The prominent effects of mexiletine on the heart are similar to the effects of lidocaine, and like lidocaine, the electrocardiographic effects of mexiletine are minimal (see Table 5-4).
  d. Therapeutic uses (see Table 5-5). Mexiletine is most useful in suppressing symptomatic ventricular arrhythmias.

    e. Route of administration
      (1) Mexiletine is given orally; administration with food and antacid is recommended.
      (2) A minimum of 2–3 days between dose adjustments is recommended.
      (3) Patients with liver disease may require lower doses.
    f. Adverse effects
      (1) In controlled trials up to 40% of patients discontinued treatment because of gastrointestinal or neurologic adverse effects.
      (2) Mexiletine may aggravate preexisting sinus node or intraventricular conduction defects.
      (3) Hepatic enzyme inducers (e.g., phenobarbital) can lower mexiletine plasma levels.

  3. Tocainide, a lidocaine analog, is also an amide local anesthetic (see Chapter 4 II). Unlike lidocaine, tocainide can be given orally.
    a. Tocainide, like lidocaine, can suppress ventricular arrhythmias.
    b. It shortens the APD and the ERP.
    c. Uncommonly, tocainide may aggravate ventricular arrhythmias.
    d. Other side effects include gastrointestinal distress, CNS disturbances, and allergic reactions, most frequently a maculopapular rash.

  4. Phenytoin (diphenylhydantoin) is closely related in structure to phenobarbital and is effective in treating epileptic seizures (see Chapter 3 III C 1). As an antiarrhythmic agent, phenytoin resembles lidocaine in many respects.
    a. Pharmacokinetics
      (1) Phenytoin is slowly and somewhat variably absorbed following oral administration.
      (2) It is inactivated by microsomal enzymes in the liver with considerable variability in this process among individuals.
      (3) The plasma elimination half-time is prolonged with increasing doses and is about 17 hours for a single 300-mg dose.
      (4) Approximately 90% of a dose of phenytoin is bound to plasma proteins.
    b. Pharmacologic effects
      (1) Effects on the heart (see Table 5-3)
        (a) The prominent effects of phenytoin on the heart are very similar to the effects of lidocaine.
        (b) Electrocardiographic effects of phenytoin, like those of lidocaine, are minimal (see Table 5-4).
      (2) Extracardiac effects. Phenytoin exerts a depressant action on the sympathetic centers in the CNS that may contribute to its antiarrhythmic effects.
    c. Therapeutic uses (see Table 5-5). Phenytoin is most useful in treating ventricular arrhythmias. It is particularly useful for ventricular arrhythmias associated with digitalis toxicity or acute myocardial infarction.
    d. Route of administration
      (1) Phenytoin is most often administered by intermittent intravenous injection, until either a therapeutic effect is achieved or a toxic effect results. (Intravenous administration is dangerous and should be undertaken only in severe acute arrhythmia and with continuous monitoring of the patient.)
      (2) Orally, therapy is initiated with a loading dose, followed by maintenance oral therapy.
    e. Adverse effects (see Chapter 3 III C 1 c)
      (1) CNS side effects are the most common problems encountered with phenytoin and include nystagmus, vertigo, and loss of mental acuity.
      (2) Large intravenous doses can alter hemodynamic function and produce both a fall in cardiac output and hypotension, resulting in death.

D. Class IC antiarrhythmic agents

  1. Flecainide and **encainide** are indicated for use in patients with life-threatening arrhythmias, such as sustained ventricular tachycardia.

  2. These agents are no longer indicated for less severe ventricular arrhythmias because they can precipitate cardiac arrest.

  3. Both agents are administered orally.

E. Class II antiarrhythmic agents: β-adrenergic antagonists (β blockers)

1. **Propranolol** is a β-adrenergic receptor blocking agent and is discussed in this context in Chapter 2 III B 1. Its antiarrhythmic action is featured here, while its uses in treating angina and hypertension are discussed later in this chapter.

   a. **Pharmacokinetics.** Propranolol is a nonselective β-adrenergic antagonist, blocking both β_1 and β_2 receptors (see Chapter 2 III B 1 b).

   b. **Pharmacologic effects**

      (1) **Effects on the heart.** The antiarrhythmic effects of propranolol are due primarily to β-receptor blockade but also result from a direct membrane effect (see Table 5-3).

         (a) **Automaticity.** Propranolol, by blocking β receptors in the S-A node and blocking sympathetic and hormonal influences on this structure, depresses S-A node firing and causes bradycardia. Automaticity is also depressed in Purkinje fibers.

         (b) **Responsiveness and conduction velocity** are not greatly affected by propranolol.

         (c) **APD and refractoriness.** The major effect of propranolol, which underlies its use as an antiarrhythmic agent, is that it causes a substantial increase in the ERP of the A-V node due to β blockade. The refractoriness of the S-A node and of atrial and ventricular muscle is not greatly affected, whereas the ERP of Purkinje fibers is shortened substantially.

      (2) **Electrocardiographic effects.** Propranolol prolongs the P–R interval by its action on the A-V node (see Table 5-4).

      (3) **Hemodynamic effects** are discussed in Chapter 2 III B 1.

   c. **Route of administration**

      (1) For intravenous administration, propranolol is given slowly with additional doses usually given every 3–5 minutes.

      (2) Oral medication usually is begun with relatively small divided doses. The total amount may need to be increased significantly to produce a therapeutic effect.

   d. **Therapeutic uses** (see Table 5-5)

      (1) Propranolol is used to control supraventricular tachyarrhythmias, including atrial fibrillation, atrial flutter, and paroxysmal supraventricular tachycardia. By decreasing conduction through the A-V node, propranolol decreases the response of the ventricles to atrial flutter and fibrillation but does not usually convert these arrhythmias to sinus rhythm.

      (2) Propranolol is useful in ventricular arrhythmias that are due to enhanced adrenergic stimulation (from emotional stress, exercise).

      (3) Propranolol is sometimes used to abolish ventricular arrhythmias caused by digitalis excess, but it can cause conduction problems in this context, resulting in A-V dissociation. Furthermore, propranolol, by itself, can depress myocardial contractility.

   e. **Adverse effects**

      (1) Because propranolol decreases sympathetic activity, it can produce severe hypotension, significantly worsen congestive heart failure, and cause cardiac arrest.

      (2) Because it impairs A-V conduction and depresses ventricular pacemaker activity, propranolol can produce asystole.

      (3) Propranolol can induce significant bronchospasm in asthmatic patients and can mask signs and symptoms of acute hypoglycemia.

      (4) Sudden withdrawal of the drug can produce angina, arrhythmias, and infarction.

2. **Beta$_1$-selective (cardioselective) adrenergic antagonists**

   a. **Acebutolol** is a β_1-selective adrenergic receptor blocker with some sympathomimetic (adrenergic) activity.

      (1) **Therapeutic uses.** Acebutolol is used chiefly for controlling ventricular premature beats.

      (2) **Adverse effects** (see Chapter 2 III B 6)

   b. **Esmolol** is a cardioselective β-adrenergic blocking agent with a short duration of action.

      (1) **Therapeutic uses.** Esmolol is given by intravenous infusion to provide rapid control of supraventricular arrhythmias.

      (2) **Adverse effects.** Dose-related hypotension and bradyarrhythmias can occur.

F. Class III antiarrhythmic agents

1. **Bretylium**
   a. **Mechanism of action**
      (1) Bretylium, a quaternary ammonium salt, is an adrenergic neuronal blocking agent (see Chapter 2 III C 4). It accumulates in postganglionic adrenergic nerve terminals, where it initially stimulates norepinephrine release but then inhibits the release of norepinephrine in response to neuronal stimulation. Bretylium does not impair the postsynaptic response to exogenous catecholamines.
      (2) The drug also has direct electrophysiologic effects on the heart.
   b. **Pharmacokinetics**
      (1) Oral absorption of bretylium is poor; however, it is well absorbed after intramuscular administration.
      (2) The drug is excreted unchanged in the urine.
      (3) Its elimination half-time is approximately 6–10 hours.
   c. **Pharmacologic effects**
      (1) **Effects on the heart** (see Table 5-3)
         (a) **Automaticity.** Bretylium does not directly affect automaticity. It is one of the few antiarrhythmic agents that does not affect automaticity in His–Purkinje systems.
         (b) **Excitability and threshold.** Resting membrane potentials are not greatly affected in any cardiac cell. However, bretylium increases the ventricular fibrillation threshold.
         (c) **Responsiveness, conduction, and refractoriness.** In therapeutic doses, bretylium does not affect either responsiveness or conduction in cardiac tissue. Bretylium prolongs the duration of action potentials and the ERP of atrial and ventricular muscle and the A-V node.
      (2) **Electrocardiographic effects.** Bretylium decreases the sinus rate and increases the P–R and Q–T intervals.
   d. **Route of administration**
      (1) Bretylium tosylate is for short-term use only and is administered with patients in the supine position.
      (2) For **intravenous use,** the drug usually is diluted and infused over 10–20 minutes.
      (3) For immediately life-threatening arrhythmias, undiluted bretylium can be injected intravenously every 15–30 minutes.
      (4) For **intramuscular use,** undiluted bretylium is used.
   e. **Therapeutic uses.** Bretylium is reserved for life-threatening ventricular arrhythmias that are refractory to other therapy. Its use is confined to intensive care units.
   f. **Adverse effects**
      (1) Intravenous bretylium causes orthostatic hypotension and some degree of supine hypotension.
      (2) Nausea and vomiting can occur with rapid intravenous administration.

2. **Amiodarone** is an iodinated benzofuran derivative.
   a. **Pharmacokinetics.** Amiodarone is highly lipid-soluble; its half-life is 20–100 days.
   b. **Pharmacologic effects on the heart**
      (1) Amiodarone increases both the APD and the ERP in ventricular and atrial muscle.
      (2) It increases the P–R, QRS, and Q–T intervals.
      (3) It decreases S-A node automaticity.
      (4) It induces α- and β-adrenergic blockade by noncompetitive antagonism; therefore, it causes both systemic and coronary vasodilation.
   c. **Therapeutic use.** Amiodarone suppresses premature ventricular contractions and ventricular tachycardia. Its use is reserved for the treatment of life-threatening ventricular arrhythmias refractory to other treatment.
   d. **Adverse effects**
      (1) Pulmonary fibrosis, which is usually reversible
      (2) Cardiac effects, including sinus bradycardia, A-V block, and paradoxical ventricular arrhythmias (torsades de pointes)
      (3) Photosensitivity
      (4) Corneal microdeposits and blurred vision

    (5) Hyper- or hypothyroidism [amiodarone interferes with conversion of thyroxine (T_4) to triiodothyronine (T_3)]

    (6) Neurologic effects, such as ataxia, dizziness, tremor, peripheral neuropathy, and proximal myopathy

    (7) Anorexia, nausea, and vomiting

    (8) Increases in serum levels of digitalis, diltiazem, quinidine, and procainamide

G. Class IV antiarrhythmic agents: calcium (Ca^{2+})-channel blockers

    1. Verapamil, a Ca^{2+}-channel blocker (see III C), is considered the drug of choice for supraventricular tachycardia treated by the intravenous route.

      a. Pharmacologic effects on the heart and therapeutic uses

        (1) Verapamil significantly depresses A-V nodal conduction.

          (a) It is, therefore, very effective in paroxysmal supraventricular tachycardia.

          (b) It is also used to reduce the ventricular response in atrial fibrillation or flutter.

        (2) It is less useful than other agents for ventricular arrhythmias.

      b. Adverse effects

        (1) Because of its effects on the A-V node, verapamil should not be used in patients with A-V nodal dysfunction.

        (2) Verapamil can depress myocardial contractility; therefore, care should be exercised when administering it to patients with CHF.

        (3) Verapamil is contraindicated in patients with atrial fibrillation who have Wolff-Parkinson-White syndrome.

    2. Other Ca^{2+}-channel blockers are not at present approved for use as antiarrhythmic agents (see II A 3 d).

III. DRUGS USED IN THE TREATMENT OF ANGINA AND OTHER VASODILATORS. The nitrates, the β-adrenergic antagonists, and the Ca^{2+}-channel blockers are drugs that are useful in treating the pain resulting from ischemic heart disease. They provide symptomatic treatment of angina pectoris but do not affect the course of the disorder. Several vasodilators that are not used in the treatment of angina are also briefly discussed in this section.

A. Nitrates

    1. Chemistry

      a. The term **nitrates** will be used in this chapter to encompass both **nitrites** (esters of nitrous acid) and **nitrates** (polyol esters of nitric acid).

      b. Glyceryl trinitrate (**nitroglycerin**) is the prototype of this group.

      c. Nitroglycerin and **amyl nitrite** are volatile liquids at room temperature. Other nitrates (**isosorbide dinitrate, pentaerythritol tetranitrate, erythrityl tetranitrate**) are solids.

    2. Mechanism of action

      a. The nitrates relax all smooth muscle, including vascular smooth muscle. The proposed biochemical action involves the formation of free radical nitric oxide (NO), which stimulates guanylate cyclase. The resultant guanosine 3′, 5′-monophosphate (cyclic GMP) activates a protein kinase, which mediates dephosphorylation of myosin. The formation of endothelial-derived relaxation factor (EDRF) is also a contributory action.

      b. They reduce venous tone, thereby increasing venous capacitance and decreasing venous return to the heart.

      c. They decrease peripheral arteriolar resistance.

    3. Pharmacokinetics

      a. The nitrates are readily absorbed through the buccal mucous membranes, the skin, the gastrointestinal tract, and the lungs.

        (1) Sublingual administration produces rapid onset (2–5 minutes) and short duration of action (less than 30 minutes) and, thus, provides the best treatment for acute attacks of angina.

        (2) Oral preparations, which often come in a sustained-release form, can provide more prolonged prophylaxis against angina than sublingual forms.

      b. The nitrates are broken down in the liver by a glutathione-dependent organic nitrate reductase and are excreted in the form of various nitrites and nitrates.

4. Pharmacologic effects

a. Effects on the heart

(1) The major effect of the nitrates on the heart is to reduce myocardial oxygen require-ments relative to myocardial oxygen delivery.

(a) The arterial dilation produced by nitrates causes a reduction in the mean systemic arterial pressure, which reduces the afterload of the heart and, thus, diminishes the oxygen requirements of the heart.

(b) The venous dilation produced by nitrates results in increased peripheral pooling of blood, which decreases ventricular end-diastolic pressure and volume (decreased preload). This reduction in ventricular pressure and size results in a decreased my-ocardial wall tension and, therefore, in decreased oxygen requirements.

(c) In addition, the decrease in left ventricular end-diastolic pressure reduces tissue pressure around subendocardial vessels, favoring the redistribution of coronary blood flow to this area.

(2) Nitrates are believed to dilate the large epicardial and collateral coronary arteries se-lectively, an action that favors the distribution of blood to ischemic areas. (They do *not* increase the total coronary blood flow in patients with atherosclerosis.)

b. Extracardiac effects

(1) Vasodilation of cerebral vessels produced by nitrates results in increased intracerebral pressure and sometimes in headache.

(2) The nitrates dilate vessels in the skin, resulting in flushing.

(3) They relax bronchial and biliary tract smooth muscle with the latter action resulting in a reduction of biliary pressure.

5. Route of administration

a. Nitroglycerin (glyceryl trinitrate) is usually given sublingually. However, for long-lasting effects, nitroglycerin may be administered either orally or topically (**transdermally**) via ointment or patch.

(1) Transdermal nitroglycerin patches become ineffective if they are left in place for 24 hours and reapplied daily, even if the dosage is increased.

(2) Nitroglycerin patches delivering 10 mg or more remain effective if removed for 12 hours daily.

b. Nitroglycerin may also be given intravenously in medical emergencies.

c. Nitroglycerin tablets quickly lose potency when stored in contact with cotton, paper, or plastic and should be kept in a dark glass container.

6. Therapeutic uses

a. The primary use of nitrates is to treat acute attacks of angina pectoris and, in anticipation of attacks, to prevent their occurrence.

b. Paroxysmal nocturnal dyspnea can be relieved with nitroglycerin by improving left ven-tricular pressure and reducing pulmonary pressure.

7. Adverse effects

a. Headache is a common early side effect of nitrates that usually decreases after the first few days of treatment (i.e., patients usually develop a tolerance to headache).

(1) Temporarily discontinuing the drugs for a few days causes a recurrence of suscepti-bility to headache (as well as to the direct vascular effect of the drugs) when the nitrates are readministered.

(2) Decreasing the dose of nitrates is sometimes beneficial for headache.

b. Dizziness, weakness, and cerebral ischemia associated with postural hypotension occa-sionally occur.

c. Nitrite ions, when present in large amounts, can oxidize enough hemoglobin to methe-moglobin to result in hypoxia.

d. Death can occur with acute nitrate poisoning from circulatory collapse or respiratory failure.

8. Tolerance. When nitrates are appropriately administered intermittently, tolerance does not oc-cur (see III A 5 a).

B. Propranolol

1. Mechanism of action

a. The β-adrenergic blocking action of propranolol (see Chapter 2 III B 1) decreases sympa-thetic stimulation of the heart and, thus, reduces the heart rate, especially during exercise,

and decreases myocardial contractility. These effects in turn decrease the oxygen requirements of the myocardium, both during exercise and at rest.
  b. Propranolol may also decrease arterial pressure.

2. **Route of administration.** Propranolol is usually administered orally for the treatment of angina.

3. **Therapeutic uses**
  a. Propranolol is used prophylactically to decrease the severity and frequency of anginal attacks.
  b. Propranolol can be administered concomitantly with nitroglycerin, in which case it reduces the amount of nitroglycerin needed to control angina. While no data conclusively
show a synergistic effect of these drugs, the two drugs tend to counteract each other's non-
therapeutic effects; for example, the ability of nitroglycerin to reduce ventricular end-
diastolic pressure mitigates the tendency of propranolol to increase end-diastolic pressure.
  c. Propranolol should not be used for Prinzmetal's (variant) angina, which is caused by coronary vasospasm.

4. **Adverse effects**
  a. As noted in II E 1 e, propranolol can worsen congestive heart failure and can precipitate
bronchospasm in patients with bronchial asthma.
  b. Bradycardia and hypotension can occur.
  c. Renal plasma flow and glomerular filtration rate may be reduced.

C. Ca^{2+}-channel blockers

1. **Classification. Verapamil, nifedipine, diltiazem,** and **nicardipine** belong to the Ca^{2+}-channel
blocker, or Ca^{2+} antagonist, class of antianginal drugs.
  a. These drugs selectively inhibit Ca^{2+} influx into heart muscle (i.e., they block the slow in-
ward channel for Ca^{2+}) and inhibit Ca^{2+} influx into vascular smooth muscle.
  b. They do not change the serum Ca^{2+} concentration.

2. **Pharmacokinetics**
  a. Verapamil, diltiazem, nifedipine, and nicardipine are rapidly and almost fully absorbed
after oral administration.
  b. Peak blood levels of nifedipine occur in about 30 minutes; peak levels of diltiazem occur
in about 1 hour, and peak levels of verapamil occur in 1–2 hours. The steady-state terminal
plasma half-life of nicardipine is 8–9 hours.
  c. All four drugs are highly bound by serum proteins.
  d. Verapamil undergoes extensive first-pass biotransformation in the liver. All four drugs are
excreted as metabolites in the urine.

3. **Pharmacologic effects**
  a. **Cardiovascular effects.** By their inhibition of Ca^{2+} influx into myocardial and vascular
smooth muscle cells, Ca^{2+}-channel blockers have diverse effects on the cardiovascular
system.
    (1) They dilate the main coronary arteries and coronary arterioles, and by inhibiting cor-
onary artery spasm, they increase myocardial oxygen delivery in patients with Prinzmetal's angina.
    (2) The drugs dilate peripheral arterioles and reduce the total peripheral vascular resis-
tance, thereby reducing the oxygen requirements of the myocardium.
    (3) The more precise mechanism of action of the Ca^{2+}-channel blockers as antianginal
agents remains to be determined.
    (4) The drugs slow A-V and S-A node conduction and prolong the ERP within the A-V
node in isolated heart tissue; verapamil and diltiazem seem to have a greater effect
than nifedipine on these parameters in clinical situations.
    (5) Nifedipine reduces cardiac preload and may actually increase the heart rate.
    (6) Nicardipine may be more vasoselective than other Ca^{2+}-channel blockers.
    (7) These agents have also been shown to antagonize the aggregation of thrombocytes
and, thus, to inhibit the release of thromboxane A_2 (TXA_2).
  b. **Extracardiac effects.** Verapamil produces nonspecific sympathetic antagonism and has a
local anesthetic effect.

4. **Route of administration.** Ca^{2+}-channel blockers may be given orally; for use in medical emergencies, verapamil is also available in intravenous form.

5. **Therapeutic uses**
   a. **Use in angina.** Ca^{2+}-channel blockers are useful in the treatment of both Prinzmetal's (variant) angina and classic exertional angina. Nifedipine appears to be the most effective for Prinzmetal's angina.
   b. **Other uses**
      (1) Verapamil, diltiazem, and nicardipine have been approved for use in hypertension.
      (2) Verapamil is used to treat certain cardiac arrhythmias (see II G).
      (3) The Ca^{2+}-channel blockers are being studied for their value in migraine.

6. **Adverse effects**
   a. The Ca^{2+}-channel blockers, perhaps especially when used in combination with β-adrenergic blocking agents, can produce or aggravate the following:
      (1) Hypotension
      (2) A-V block
      (3) Congestive heart failure
      (4) Asystole
   b. Most of their adverse effects are mild; dizziness and peripheral edema are among the more common.
   c. Treatment with verapamil increases serum levels of digitalis during the first week of therapy and, thus, can cause digitalis toxicity.
   d. Nicardipine can produce a negative effect on cardiac contractility when administered intravenously to patients with congestive heart failure.

D. Other vasodilators

1. **Nylidrin**
   a. Nylidrin is an **adrenergic vasodilator**. It acts primarily on the vascular bed of skeletal muscle by β-receptor stimulation.
   b. Because it is a cardiac stimulant, nylidrin is **contraindicated** in progressive angina pectoris, acute myocardial infarction, and paroxysmal tachycardia.
   c. The efficacy of nylidrin in increasing the blood supply in vasospastic disorders has not been proven.

2. **Dipyridamole**
   a. By inhibiting the uptake of adenosine into erythrocytes and other tissues, dipyridamole allows metabolically released adenosine, which is a coronary vasodilator, to accumulate in the plasma. The drug decreases coronary vascular resistance and increases coronary blood flow and coronary sinus oxygen saturation. (Dipyridamole also inhibits in vitro platelet aggregation and can be used to prevent the formation of thromboemboli in patients with prosthetic cardiac valves.)
   b. Dipyridamole has not been proven to be superior to placebo treatment for angina; it does not prevent the appearance of electrocardiographic signs of myocardial ischemia during exercise tolerance tests.

IV. DRUGS USED IN THE TREATMENT OF HYPERTENSION

A. General considerations

1. Because the etiology of essential hypertension is still unknown, drug therapy for this condition is empiric and often rather nonspecific.

2. Traditionally, the first choice for the **initial treatment of chronic hypertension** has been a thiazide-type diuretic or a β-adrenergic receptor blocker. More recently some physicians prefer to start therapy with an ACE inhibitor or a Ca^{2+}-channel blocker. If the first agent is ineffective or poorly tolerated, another agent is substituted. If more than one agent is needed, a diuretic is added.

3. In **hypertensive emergencies,** parenteral therapy is indicated, usually with nitroprusside or diazoxide; intravenous labetalol or sublingual nifedipine are also suitable. Oral therapy should be started as soon as possible because parenteral therapy is not suitable for long-term management of hypertension.

B. Diuretic agents (see Chapter 6) are useful antihypertensive drugs when employed alone, as well as when used in combination therapy, where they potentiate the action of other hypotensive drugs. Although the exact mechanism of their antihypertensive action is unknown, it is believed to result from their ability to produce a negative Na^+ balance.

1. The **thiazides** are the most frequently used diuretics. Their early hypotensive effect is related to a reduction in blood volume; their long-term effect is related to a reduction in peripheral vascular resistance.

2. **Furosemide, ethacrynic acid,** and **bumetanide** produce greater diuresis than the thiazides, but they have a weaker antihypertensive effect and can cause severe electrolyte imbalance. Because they retain their effectiveness in the presence of impaired renal function, they are useful in cases where renal function is so impaired that the thiazides can no longer promote sodium excretion.

3. **Spironolactone, triamterene,** and **amiloride** have modest hypotensive and diuretic effects and are useful in combination with a thiazide diuretic, whose effects they potentiate and where they minimize K^+ loss. Spironolactone is useful in treating patients whose hypertension is due to mineralocorticoid excess (see Chapter 6 IX).

C. β-Adrenergic blocking agents have become increasingly important as antihypertensive agents. They are discussed in Chapter 2 III B.

1. These agents are useful both alone and in combination antihypertensive therapy.

2. Their mechanism of action in hypertension is not known, but several consequences of β-adrenergic blockade probably play a role. For example:
   a. The β-blockers reduce cardiac output.
   b. They also inhibit renin secretion.

3. **Sympathetic selectivity.** The various β-blockers all appear to be equally effective for the treatment of hypertension. However, they vary in their selectivity for adrenoreceptors (see Chapter 2 III B).
   a. Propranolol, timolol, nadolol, pindolol, penbutolol, and carteolol are nonselective, while metoprolol, acebutolol, and atenolol (in low doses) are cardioselective (i.e., they have a greater effect on $β_1$ adrenoreceptors).
   b. Pindolol, acebutolol, penbutolol, and carteolol also possess intrinsic sympathomimetic activity. They decrease blood pressure with less of a decrease in cardiac output or heart rate at rest. They are also unlikely to cause serum lipid abnormalities.
   c. Labetalol is a nonselective β blocker but possesses intrinsic sympathomimetic activity and blocks vascular postsynaptic α-adrenergic receptors.

4. **Adverse effects** (see Chapter 2 III B)
   a. The β-adrenergic receptor antagonists can exacerbate congestive heart failure, asthma, and chronic obstructive pulmonary disease.
   b. They can mask symptoms of hypoglycemia in individuals with diabetes mellitus.
   c. They can increase serum triglycerides and decrease high-density lipoprotein cholesterol (exceptions are β blockers with intrinsic sympathomimetic activity).
   d. Labetalol, when used chronically, causes more frequent orthostatic hypotension and sexual dysfunction than do other β blockers.

D. Ca^{2+}-channel blockers (see III C) are rapidly becoming important antihypertensive agents by virtue of their vasodilating effects. Verapamil and nicardipine have been approved for this therapeutic use.

1. Diltiazem, verapamil, and nicardipine increase vasodilation and decrease peripheral resistance.

2. Verapamil and diltiazem cause little change in heart rate, while nicardipine produces an initial increase, which is reflex-mediated.

3. Diltiazem and verapamil depress A-V conduction and should not be used with β blockers.

4. Diuretics may enhance the efficacy of Ca^{2+}-channel blockers.

E. Arteriolar vasodilators

1. **General considerations.** This group of antihypertensive drugs directly relaxes arteriolar smooth muscle and, thus, decreases peripheral vascular resistance and arterial blood pressure.
   a. However, the beneficial effect of these drugs on peripheral vascular resistance can be partially negated by the increased reflex sympathetic activity they produce, which can result in increased heart rate, stroke volume, and cardiac output.
   b. These drugs also can increase plasma renin activity as a result of increased reflex sympathetic discharge, causing a pressor effect.
   c. Finally, this group of drugs often causes salt and water retention and, thus, expansion of the extracellular fluid and plasma volume.
   d. Therefore, arteriolar vasodilators should be used in conjunction with diuretic and β-adrenergic blocking therapy.

2. **Hydralazine.** This phthalazine derivative has a greater effect on arterioles than on veins (which minimizes the incidence of postural hypotension). It may reduce diastolic more than systolic blood pressure.
   a. **Pharmacokinetics**
      (1) Hydralazine is well absorbed orally.
      (2) It is subject to extensive first-pass hepatic metabolism after oral administration.
      (3) It is extensively metabolized by several pathways, including acetylation, the rate of which is subject to genetic variation among individuals.
      (4) Some 85% is bound to plasma.
      (5) Its duration of effect ranges from 2–6 hours.
      (6) Tolerance develops after 24 months of therapy.
   b. **Route of administration.** Hydralazine can be given orally or intramuscularly.
   c. **Therapeutic uses**
      (1) Hydralazine is used to treat moderate to severe hypertension.
      (2) It has also been used in the treatment of acute and chronic congestive heart failure.
      (3) For long-term treatment, hydralazine is administered orally.
         (a) Oral hydralazine is combined with a β blocker to prevent tachycardia and increased renin secretion due to reflex sympathetic stimulation.
         (b) Oral hydralazine is combined with a diuretic agent to prevent salt and water retention.
   d. **Adverse effects**
      (1) Headache, anorexia, nausea, dizziness, and sweating occur frequently but tend to diminish as hydralazine is administered over a period of time.
      (2) Hydralazine can worsen coronary artery disease because of the myocardial stimulation it produces.
      (3) Hydralazine can cause a reversible lupus-like syndrome, especially when more than 400 mg/day are administered to slow acetylators of the drug (usually Caucasians).

3. **Minoxidil**
   a. **Pharmacokinetics**
      (1) Minoxidil is at least 90% absorbed following oral administration.
      (2) Approximately 90% of the drug is excreted as metabolites in the urine.
      (3) Although the plasma half-life averages around 4 hours, the duration of action may be significantly longer, since it is affected by hepatic blood flow and function.
   b. **Pharmacologic effects**
      (1) Minoxidil, a piperidinopyrimidine derivative, directly relaxes arteriolar smooth muscle.
      (2) It decreases peripheral vascular resistance more than hydralazine does.
      (3) It decreases renal vascular resistance while preserving renal blood flow and the glomerular filtration rate.
   c. **Route of administration.** Minoxidil is administered orally in single or divided doses.
   d. **Therapeutic uses**
      (1) Minoxidil is indicated for the treatment of severe hypertension that does not respond adequately to more conventional antihypertensive therapy.
      (2) It may be particularly useful for severe hypertension coupled with renal functional impairment.
      (3) Like hydralazine, minoxidil should be used in combination with a β-adrenergic blocking agent and a diuretic to avert increased sympathetic activity and salt and water retention.

e. Adverse effects
(1) Like hydralazine, minoxidil can produce side effects related to increased reflex sympathetic stimulation and to salt and water retention.
(2) Pericardial effusion and tamponade can occur, especially in patients with inadequate renal function.
(3) Hirsutism occurs for unknown reasons; it is not associated with virilism or other endocrine abnormalities.

4. Diazoxide is chemically similar to the thiazide diuretics, but it causes salt and water retention rather than diuresis.

a. Pharmacokinetics
(1) Diazoxide is used as an antihypertensive drug in intravenous form only.
(2) It has a rapid onset of action (3–5 minutes), and a given amount injected quickly produces a greater antihypertensive effect than the same amount injected slowly.
(3) The drug is extensively bound to serum proteins.
(4) The plasma half-life averages 28 hours, but the antihypertensive effects usually last only 4–12 hours.

b. Pharmacologic effects
(1) Diazoxide exerts its vasodilator effect principally on arterioles and has little effect on capacitance vessels.
(2) It causes a fall in both systolic and diastolic pressure, accompanied by an increase in both heart rate and cardiac output.
(3) The drug relaxes other smooth muscle in addition to vascular muscle.
(4) It inhibits the release of insulin.

c. Route of administration. Diazoxide is given by rapid injection into a peripheral vein. Administration is started with a bolus dose, which can be repeated at 5–15-minute intervals until the desired effect on blood pressure is attained.

d. Therapeutic uses. Intravenous diazoxide is one of two major drugs used for hypertensive emergencies (see IV F 1 c). (Diazoxide is also used orally to treat hypoglycemia that is caused by hyperinsulinemia.)

e. Adverse effects
(1) Diazoxide can cause severe hypotension.
(2) Its reflex sympathetic stimulation can cause angina and worsen myocardial ischemia.
(3) Diazoxide inhibits the release of insulin from the pancreas and can produce hyperglycemia.
(4) It can produce edema due to significant retention of salt and water.

F. Arterial and venous vasodilators. These drugs reduce both arterial resistance and venous tone and markedly decrease arterial blood pressure.

1. Sodium nitroprusside
a. Pharmacokinetics
(1) Onset of action occurs within 1 minute of intravenous administration, and effects cease within 5 minutes of stopping an infusion.
(2) The drug is rapidly inactivated by hepatic enzymes, first to cyanide and then to thiocyanate.

b. Pharmacologic effects
(1) Nitroprusside acts directly on arterial and venous smooth muscle but has little effect on other smooth muscle.
(2) It decreases blood pressure in both the supine and upright positions.
(3) The increased venous capacitance that it produces results in decreased cardiac preload and, thus, decreases myocardial oxygen demand for a given output.
(4) Nitroprusside causes a slight increase in heart rate and decrease in cardiac output except when heart failure is present; in the latter case, the heart rate may decrease and the cardiac output increase.
(5) Renal blood flow is maintained with nitroprusside, and renin secretion is increased.

c. Route of administration
(1) Na^+ nitroprusside is administered only as an intravenous infusion with sterile 5% dextrose in water. Once prepared, the solution must be protected from light and used within 4 hours.
(2) Blood pressure must be monitored continuously while the drug is being given.

d. Therapeutic uses

(1) Nitroprusside, like diazoxide, is used for short-term, rapid reduction of blood pressure in hypertensive emergencies. It is preferable to diazoxide for treating hypertensive emergencies in patients with coronary insufficiency or pulmonary edema because, in contrast to diazoxide, it reduces cardiac preload (by increasing venous capacitance) and, thus, myocardial oxygen demand.

(2) Nitroprusside can also be used to produce controlled hypotension to minimize bleeding during surgery.

(3) Nitroprusside can improve left ventricular function (lower ventricular filling pressure) in patients with acute myocardial infarction and has beneficial hemodynamic effects in the treatment of acute congestive heart failure.

e. Adverse effects

(1) Hypotension, nausea, diaphoresis, headache, restlessness, palpitations, and retrosternal pain can occur secondary to excessive, rapid vasodilation.

(2) The rate of conversion of nitroprusside from its metabolite cyanide to thiocyanate is dependent on the availability of sulfur (usually as thiosulfate). Rarely, when high doses of nitroprusside are administered for a prolonged period and sulfur stores are low, cyanide toxicity can occur.

(3) Because thiocyanate is cleared slowly by the kidneys, it can accumulate during prolonged nitroprusside therapy, especially in patients with poor renal function. A plasma thiocyanate concentration of greater than 10 mg/dl can cause weakness, nausea, muscle spasms, and psychosis, as well as hypothyroidism due to interference with iodine transport.

(4) A case of methemoglobinemia following prolonged infusion of nitroprusside has been reported.

2. Prazosin. This quinazoline derivative is a selective postsynaptic α_1-adrenergic receptor blocking agent that causes vasodilation of both the arteries and veins.

a. Pharmacokinetics

(1) Prazosin is highly bound to plasma protein.

(2) Its plasma concentration peaks in about 3 hours. Plasma half-life is usually 2–3 hours but can be prolonged by congestive heart failure.

(3) Prazosin is extensively metabolized, may undergo significant first-pass metabolism, has a bioavailability of about 60%, and is probably excreted in the feces and bile.

b. Pharmacologic effects

(1) Prazosin reduces peripheral vascular resistance and lowers arterial blood pressure in both supine and erect patients.

(2) Unlike nonselective α-adrenergic blockers, it does not usually produce reflex tachycardia.

(3) It does not increase plasma renin activity.

(4) Prazosin seems to produce minimal changes in cardiac output, renal blood flow, and glomerular filtration rate.

(5) Fluid retention occurs during long-term therapy.

c. Route of administration. Prazosin is given orally, two or three times daily.

d. Therapeutic uses

(1) Prazosin is used to treat mild to moderate hypertension. It may be more effective in conjunction with a diuretic or an α-adrenergic blocking agent than when used alone.

(2) It is also used in the treatment of acute congestive heart failure.

e. Adverse effects

(1) Dizziness, headache, drowsiness, and palpitations can occur but often disappear with continued therapy and rarely cause discontinuation of the drug.

(2) The initial dose of prazosin, especially if larger than 1 mg can induce postural hypotension and syncope, probably due to decreased venous return to the heart. It is, therefore, best to give the initial dose at bedtime.

(3) Tests for antinuclear factor may become positive with prazosin therapy.

3. Terazosin. This α_1-adrenergic receptor blocker has a longer half-life (12 hours) and longer duration of action (24 hours) than does prazosin but is otherwise similar to prazosin.

G. Centrally acting sympatholytic agents. Clonidine and methyldopa act centrally on the vasomotor centers of the brain and are predominantly **α-receptor agonists**.

1. Clonidine. This imidazoline derivative is thought to stimulate α-adrenergic receptors (probably presynaptic α_2 receptors) in the vasomotor centers of the brain, resulting in decreased sympathetic outflow to the peripheral vessels.

   a. Pharmacokinetics

   (1) The antihypertensive effects of clonidine develop within 30–60 minutes of oral administration, peak in 2–4 hours, and last for approximately 8 hours.

   (2) The drug and its metabolites are excreted primarily in the urine.

   b. Pharmacologic effects

   (1) Intravenous injection of clonidine causes an initial increase in both systolic and diastolic pressure; oral administration does not normally produce this hypertensive effect. The initial rise in blood pressure is caused by direct stimulation of peripheral α-adrenergic receptors, producing transient vasoconstriction. Clonidine also causes peripheral α-adrenergic blockade, and thus, it is a partial agonist.

   (2) The increase in blood pressure following intravenous injection is transient and is soon followed by a fall in blood pressure, resulting from a decrease in cardiac output and heart rate, usually not accompanied by a significant change in peripheral resistance. During long-term oral clonidine therapy, cardiac output tends to return to control values, and peripheral vascular resistance and heart rate are decreased.

   (3) Vagal discharge is increased by clonidine in association with increased baroreceptor reflex sensitivity.

   (4) Clonidine does not block the homeostatic control mechanisms of the peripheral autonomic system.

   (5) It decreases plasma renin activity, primarily through a centrally mediated decrease in sympathetic stimulation of the juxtaglomerular cells of the kidney.

   (6) Renal vascular resistance decreases, while renal blood flow remains essentially unchanged.

   c. Route of administration

   (1) Clonidine is given orally. It is often administered in two unequal doses with the larger one given at bedtime to minimize problems resulting from its sedative effects.

   (2) Clonidine is also available as a transdermal patch, which is applied once weekly.

   d. Therapeutic uses

   (1) Clonidine can be used to treat mild hypertension or moderate to severe hypertension.

   (2) It can be used as a single agent or in combination with other antihypertensive agents.

   (3) It cannot be administered to patients taking tricyclic antidepressants because these drugs block its hypotensive effect.

   e. Adverse effects

   (1) Dry mouth, drowsiness, and sedation are the most frequent problems and may require discontinuation of clonidine.

   (2) Rebound hypertensive crises can result from abrupt cessation of clonidine tablets or patches when the drug is used as a single agent.

   (3) Fluid retention often occurs, requiring concurrent diuretic therapy.

   (4) Clonidine can cause or worsen depression.

2. Methyldopa

   a. Mechanism of action

   (1) Methyldopa is an effective inhibitor of dopa decarboxylase and was initially thought to act as an antihypertensive agent by decreasing stores of norepinephrine in the sympathetic nervous system. However, as is now apparent, its primary mode of action is via a central effect.

   (2) Methyldopa is metabolized by decarboxylation and β-hydroxylation in adrenergic neurons of the CNS. The metabolite, α-methylnorepinephrine, stimulates α-adrenergic receptors in the brain, inhibiting sympathetic outflow. This effect on the CNS is believed to be the principal mechanism by which methyldopa exerts its antihypertensive effect.

   (3) Methyldopa reduces renal vascular resistance, possibly as a result of an α-methylnorepinephrine being a weaker vasoconstrictor than norepinephrine in renal beds, and is thought to exert other direct actions on peripheral adrenergic neurons that contribute to its antihypertensive effect.

b. **Pharmacokinetics**
(1) Methyldopa is poorly absorbed (<25%) following oral administration and may be subject to first-pass intestinal metabolism.
(2) Its peak effect is exerted 4–6 hours after administration, and its effect may last up to 24 hours.
(3) Methyldopa is excreted largely by the kidneys.

c. **Pharmacologic effects**
(1) Methyldopa decreases blood pressure and peripheral arteriolar resistance.
(2) It has little effect on cardiac output, renal blood flow, or glomerular filtration rate.
(3) It does not abolish sympathetic reflexes.

d. **Route of administration.** Methyldopa is given orally or by slow intravenous infusion.

e. **Therapeutic uses.** Methyldopa is used orally to treat mild or moderate to severe hypertension, usually in combination with a diuretic. Adverse effects limit its usefulness.

f. **Adverse effects**
(1) Sedation is common, and although it may decrease with continued administration of methyldopa, mental acuity may remain decreased.
(2) Methyldopa can produce "drug fever" that mimics sepsis, with chills and high fever. Febrile episodes may be accompanied by alterations in liver function, which on rare occasions terminate in hepatic necrosis.
(3) A positive direct Coombs' test develops in as many as 25% of patients taking methyldopa for more than 6 months. Hemolytic anemia, usually reversible on discontinuation of the drug, occurs in a small percentage of these patients.
(4) Edema caused by salt and water retention can develop if a diuretic is not administered.
(5) Rebound hypertension can follow the sudden withdrawal of methyldopa but occurs less frequently than with clonidine.
(6) Orthostatic hypotension occurs more frequently than with clonidine but less frequently than with guanethidine.
(7) Lactation can occur in either sex, and impotence can occur in some men.
(8) Gastrointestinal disturbances can occur but usually are mild.

H. **Agents that block postganglionic adrenergic neurons** (see Chapter 2 III C). This group of drugs selectively inhibits sympathetic neuron function through interference with chemical mediation at ganglionic nerve endings; one or more mechanisms may be involved.

1. **Reserpine**
a. **Mechanism of action**
(1) Reserpine, a rauwolfia alkaloid, depletes catecholamine and serotonin stores in the peripheral and central nervous systems and causes impaired sympathetic nerve discharge (see Chapter 2 III C 1).
(a) It interferes with intracellular storage of catecholamines by inhibiting the binding of norepinephrine to neurosecretory vesicles at the vesicle membrane, both centrally and peripherally. Norepinephrine that diffuses from the storage site is degraded intracellularly by monoamine oxidase (MAO).
(b) Reserpine decreases the synthesis of norepinephrine and increases its turnover rate.
(2) Reserpine also exerts a direct vasodilating effect on vascular smooth muscle when administered intra-arterially and may have several other actions.

b. **Pharmacokinetics**
(1) With oral administration, reserpine usually takes several days to several weeks to reach a maximum effect.
(2) A likely possibility for the breakdown of reserpine involves hydrolysis of the ester linkage and demethylation.
(3) Reserpine is concentrated in tissues with a high lipid content.

c. **Pharmacologic effects**
(1) Reserpine decreases blood pressure, usually decreases heart rate and cardiac output, and may decrease peripheral vascular resistance.
(2) In usual therapeutic doses, reserpine only partially inhibits cardiovascular reflexes.
(3) Reserpine exerts central actions that produce sedation.

d. **Route of administration.** Reserpine is usually given orally but is also available for parenteral administration.

 e. Therapeutic uses. Reserpine is used principally in low oral doses in combination with other antihypertensive agents (e.g., a thiazide diuretic and vasodilator) to control moderate hypertension.

 f. Adverse effects

  (1) Reserpine regularly causes sedation and can cause episodes of severe depression, which are probably due to a reduction of biogenic amine levels in subcortical areas of the brain. Reserpine, therefore, should not be administered to patients prone to depression.

  (2) Because reserpine decreases sympathetic activity, unopposed parasympathetic activity can result in bradycardia, nasal congestion, and increased gastrointestinal activity. It is contraindicated for patients with active peptic ulcers.

  (3) Some studies have suggested that reserpine increases the incidence of breast cancer; however, recent data do not support this.

2. Guanethidine

 a. Mechanism of action

  (1) Guanethidine acts presynaptically to inhibit the release of neurotransmitter from peripheral adrenergic neurons, thus reducing the response to sympathetic nerve activation. Acutely, it produces sympathetic blockade before any appreciable decrease in norepinephrine stores has occurred; with chronic administration, it impairs the release of neurotransmitter from peripheral adrenergic neurons. (See Chapter 2 III C 2 for further discussion.)

   (a) For guanethidine to exert an antihypertensive effect, it must be taken up and stored in adrenergic nerve terminals in a manner similar to norepinephrine uptake.

   (b) Agents that prevent this uptake, such as cocaine and tricyclic antidepressants, inhibit the therapeutic effect of guanethidine.

  (2) Unlike reserpine, guanethidine can inhibit the pressor action of indirect-acting amines such as tyramine.

  (3) As with reserpine, the norepinephrine released by guanethidine is deaminated intraneuronally by MAO but to a lesser degree than with reserpine.

  (4) Although guanethidine displaces norepinephrine from storage granules and is subsequently released as a "false" neurotransmitter in response to stimulation of sympathetic nerves, this does not seem to be a primary mechanism of action.

  (5) The drug does not cross the blood–brain barrier like reserpine, and thus, it does not affect serotonin and norepinephrine stores in the CNS.

  (6) It is believed to decrease plasma renin activity.

 b. Pharmacokinetics

  (1) Absorption of guanethidine following oral administration varies from patient to patient and is low (3%–30%).

  (2) The drug has a long duration of action.

  (3) Guanethidine is thought to be metabolized by hepatic enzymes and is excreted with its metabolites in the urine.

 c. Pharmacologic effects

  (1) Initially, guanethidine displaces and releases enough unchanged norepinephrine to cause mild, transient hypertension and cardiac stimulation.

  (2) Hypotension and bradycardia follow. Because guanethidine depresses vasoconstrictor reflexes, blood pressure is reduced significantly more when the patient is erect than when lying down. Venous return and cardiac output are decreased.

  (3) Guanethidine has a direct inhibitory effect on skeletal muscle contraction.

  (4) It increases the sensitivity of tissues to catecholamines.

 d. Route of administration. Guanethidine is given orally. The dose can be increased at intervals of not less than 5 days until either the desired effect is attained or untoward effects develop.

 e. Therapeutic uses. Guanethidine is used in the treatment of moderate to severe hypertension, usually in combination with a thiazide diuretic or a diuretic and a vasodilator.

 f. Adverse effects

  (1) Significant orthostatic hypotension and syncope frequently occur, especially during exercise, when patients first arise in the morning, during hot weather, and when patients ingest alcohol.

  (2) Salt and water retention occur but can be prevented or treated with a mild diuretic.

(3) Gastrointestinal hyperactivity occurs, probably as a result of the parasympathetic predominance that follows sympathetic blockade.

(4) Muscular aching and weakness can occur.

3. Guanadrel (see Chapter 2 III C 3) is similar to guanethidine but has a much shorter duration of action.

I. Drugs that interfere with the renin–angiotensin system (see Chapter 8 V C). The kidneys synthesize renin, which acts on a plasma globulin substrate to produce angiotensin I. This, in turn, is converted (by a peptidyl dipeptidase) to angiotensin II, a potent vasoconstrictor. Drugs in this group exert an antihypertensive effect by interfering with either the formation or the utilization of angiotensin II.

1. Captopril, enalapril, and lisinopril (see Chapter 8 V C 2)

  a. Chemistry

    (1) Enalapril is a prodrug that is hydrolyzed in the liver to the active compound enalaprilate. It differs structurally from captopril in lacking a sulfhydryl group.

    (2) Lisinopril is the lysine analog of enalaprilate.

  b. Mechanism of action

    (1) Captopril, enalapril, and lisinopril are specific competitive inhibitors of peptidyl dipeptidase (an ACE), the enzyme that converts angiotensin I to angiotensin II. They are, therefore, often termed **ACE inhibitors**.

      (a) Angiotensin II is a potent direct vasoconstrictor. Thus, captopril, enalapril, and lisinopril inhibit vasoconstriction.

      (b) Angiotensin II stimulates the secretion of aldosterone, which promotes salt and water retention. Thus, captopril, enalapril, and lisinopril inhibit salt and water retention and slightly increase serum K^+ levels.

    (2) Because peptidyl dipeptidase is necessary to catalyze the degradation of bradykinin, the ACE inhibitors may increase the concentration of bradykinin, which is a potent vasodilator.

    (3) The ACE inhibitors also exert an antihypertensive effect in low-renin hypertension; the mechanism of action in this case is not explained.

  c. Pharmacokinetics

    (1) **Captopril** is rapidly absorbed following oral administration and reaches peak blood levels within an hour. Approximately 95% of a dose is eliminated by the kidneys within 24 hours.

    (2) **Enalapril** is more potent than captopril, and its duration of action is more than 24 hours, twice as long as that of captopril. Due to its hepatic conversion and activation, enalapril does not reach clinically active levels for 2–4 hours, but it has a half-life of 11 hours.

    (3) **Lisinopril** is absorbed more slowly than enalapril and has a slower onset of action.

  d. Pharmacologic effects. The cardiovascular effects of captopril and enalapril include a reduction in total peripheral resistance and mean arterial blood pressure, and either no change or an increase in cardiac output.

  e. Route of administration

    (1) **Captopril** is given orally, 1 hour before meals. The initial dose can be increased at 1- to 2-week intervals.

    (2) **Enalapril** is given orally once or twice a day.

    (3) Lisinopril is given orally once a day.

  f. Therapeutic uses

    (1) **ACE inhibitors** are increasingly used for the treatment of mild to moderate hypertension because they are without the side effects associated with adrenergic blockers.

      (a) ACE inhibitors are effective for low-renin, as well as high-renin, hypertension.

      (b) They are effective when used alone but are often administered with a thiazide diuretic, in which case the antihypertensive effects appear to be additive. An ACE inhibitor can also be given with a β blocker, but in this case, the antihypertensive effect appears to be less than additive.

    (2) ACE inhibitors also relieve chronic congestive heart failure by reducing both preload and afterload.

    (3) These agents may be less effective than a diuretic for hypertension in black patients.

  g. Adverse effects
    (1) Proteinuria can occur, especially in patients with compromised renal function. Monitoring of urinary protein levels is recommended.
    (2) ACE inhibitors are contraindicated in patients with bilateral renal artery stenosis because acute renal failure may ensue.
    (3) Hypotension has followed the first dose of ACE inhibitors in Na^+-depleted patients.
    (4) Neutropenia can occur, and in patients who have impaired renal function or serious autoimmune disease (e.g., systemic lupus erythematosus), captopril should be used with caution. Neutropenia is rare with enalapril or lisinopril.
    (5) Approximately 10% of patients treated with captopril develop reversible skin rashes, alterations in taste, proteinuria, and leukopenia. The incidence is lower (1.5%) with enalapril and lisinopril because they lack a sulfhydryl group.
    (6) Headache, dizziness, and fatigue are the most common side effects associated with enalapril.
    (7) Cough and bronchospasm can occur.
    (8) Hyperkalemia has been reported.
  2. Drugs that block receptors for angiotensin (see Chapter 8 V C 1). **Saralasin,** an angiotensin II analog, exemplifies the drugs that interfere with the renin–angiotensin system by this mechanism.
    a. These drugs can be given only by intravenous infusion.
    b. They are primarily used diagnostically to detect a renal cause of hypertension.

V. DRUGS USED IN THE TREATMENT OF CORONARY ARTERY THROMBOSIS (see Chapter 7 IV C). More than 80% of patients with acute transmural myocardial infarction demonstrate thrombotic coronary artery occlusion within 6 hours of symptoms. **Streptokinase, urokinase, and tissue-type plasminogen activator (t-PA)** are available for intravenous administration in the treatment of coronary artery thrombosis associated with myocardial infarction.

A. Mechanism of action

  1. Streptokinase, urokinase, and t-PA all facilitate the conversion of plasminogen to plasmin. Plasmin is fibrinolytic.

  2. Because t-PA is more selective than the kinases, it has a high affinity for fibrin and induces the degradation of plasminogen to plasmin only in the presence of fibrin. Theoretically, it should be less likely to have systemic effects on clotting.

B. Pharmacokinetics. The plasma half-life of t-PA is 5 minutes, compared to 16 minutes for urokinase and 23 minutes for streptokinase.

C. Therapeutic uses

  1. Clinical studies comparing t-PA to streptokinase indicate the following:
    a. Both t-PA and streptokinase have comparable efficacy in the reduction of mortality and improvement of left ventricular function.
    b. Streptokinase appears most effective when given less than 3 hours after the onset of symptoms.

  2. Route of administration. Thrombolytic therapy is begun as soon as possible after the onset of symptoms of myocardial infarction.
    a. Streptokinase is given by intravenous or intracoronary infusion.
    b. Urokinase is infused into the occluded coronary artery.
    c. t-PA is given by intravenous administration only.

D. Adverse effects and contraindications

  1. Serious bleeding can occur; most importantly gastrointestinal and intracranial hemorrhage are possible.

  2. Streptokinase can cause anaphylaxis.

  3. With any thrombolytic agent, cardiac arrhythmias can occur upon reperfusion of the occluded vessels.

4. Contraindications to the use of thrombolytic agents include internal bleeding, cerebral vascular accident, recent intracranial or intraspinal trauma, or surgery, known bleeding diathesis, or severe uncontrolled hypertension.

5. Any condition in which bleeding would be a significant hazard is a relative contraindication and calls for a careful risk–benefit analysis before using thrombolytic therapy.

VI. DRUGS USED IN THE TREATMENT OF HYPERLIPIDEMIA

A. General considerations

1. **Classes of lipoproteins and transport pathways**
   a. **Exogenous pathways**
      (1) **Chylomicrons** are formed from dietary triglycerides and cholesterol.
      (2) In adipose tissue and muscle, the enzyme **lipoprotein lipase** removes the triglycerides, leaving **chylomicron remnants** containing intact cholesterol esters.
      (3) When chylomicron remnants reach the liver, they are taken up by hepatocytes and then cleaved, releasing **free cholesterol**.
      (4) The cholesterol can be:
         (a) Stored in hepatocytes as cholesterol esters
         (b) Released in bile as cholesterol or as bile acids
         (c) Used to form membranes or endogenous lipoproteins
   b. **Endogenous pathways**
      (1) **Very low-density lipoprotein (VLDL)** is formed in the liver from triglycerides and cholesterol, generally as a result of high caloric intake.
      (2) VLDL is released into the plasma, where lipoprotein lipase cleaves the triglycerides from VLDL.
      (3) The hydrolysis of VLDL produces **intermediate-density lipoprotein (IDL)**. The metabolic fate of IDL is twofold:
         (a) Some IDL particles are taken up by the liver via endocytosis and then cleaved to produce free cholesterol. This receptor-mediated action is via the **low-density lipoprotein (LDL) receptor**.
         (b) Some IDL particles remain in the circulation, where triglycerides are removed so that IDL is eventually metabolized to LDL.
      (4) **LDL** is involved in the transport of endogenous cholesterol ester to the liver or to extrahepatic tissues. LDL constitutes 60%–70% of plasma cholesterol levels. Metabolic demand for cholesterol (for synthesis of bile acids, steroids, or membranes) is met by increased synthesis of LDL receptors, which promote endocytosis and release of free cholesterol.
      (5) **High-density lipoprotein (HDL)** is involved in the transport of cholesterol from peripheral cells back to the liver. HDL absorbs free cholesterol released during cell turnover. This cholesterol is esterified by the enzyme **lecithin:cholesterol acyltransferase (LCAT),** and the cholesterol esters are transferred to VLDL or IDL particles.
   c. **Nonspecific pathways**
      (1) When plasma lipoprotein concentrations are high, macrophages and other scavenger cells take part in lipoprotein degradation.
      (2) This leads to cholesterol deposits in macrophages or arterial walls **(atheromas)** and of tendons and skin **(xanthomas)**.

2. **Hyperlipoproteinemias**
   a. **Causes**
      (1) **Primary hyperlipoproteinemias** may be single-gene congenital defects or polygenic (multifactorial).
      (2) **Secondary hyperlipoproteinemia** may occur in diabetes, hypothyroidism, alcoholism, biliary cirrhosis, or renal disease, or in women taking oral contraceptives.
   b. **Use of drug therapy**
      (1) In persons with hyperlipoproteinemia, lowering the serum lipid concentration reduces the risk of atherosclerosis and its consequences. Specifically, a reduction in plasma LDL can reduce the risk of coronary heart disease.
      (2) Some types of hypertriglyceridemia can cause life-threatening pancreatitis. Reduction of serum lipids has been demonstrated to be beneficial.

(3) Drug therapy is usually tried after dietary fat restriction, reduction of atherosclerosis risk factors, and moderate exercise programs have failed to lower serum lipids to an acceptable level.

(4) Bile acid sequestrants, niacin, β-hydroxy-β-methylglutaryl coenzyme A (HMG CoA) reductase inhibitors, and fibric acid derivatives demonstrably lower the risk of coronary artery disease; only niacin has been shown to reduce overall mortality.

B. Antihyperlipidemic agents (Table 5-6)

1. Cholestyramine, colestipol: bile acid sequestrants
  a. Mechanism of action and pharmacologic effects
   (1) Cholestyramine and colestipol are resins that bind bile acids in the intestine, forming insoluble complexes, which are then excreted in the feces.
   (2) The loss of bile acids leads to an increased conversion of cholesterol into bile acids.
   (3) There is also a compensatory increase in hepatic LDL receptors.
   (4) The net effect is a reduction in serum LDL and cholesterol levels.
  b. Therapeutic uses
   (1) The earliest use of bile acid sequestrants was to control pruritus in patients with cholestasis and elevated plasma bile acids.
   (2) These agents are now also used to reduce elevated LDL levels.
   (3) Patients with heterozygous familial hypercholesterolemia or polygenic hypercholesterolemia can be expected to respond.
   (4) The bile acid sequestrants are not effective for treating patients with elevated chylomicrons, VLDL, or IDL; in addition, these agents elevate triglyceride levels.
  c. Adverse effects
   (1) Since bile acid sequestrants are not absorbed, they have no adverse systemic effects.
   (2) The most common untoward effects are gastrointestinal discomfort and constipation.
   (3) The resins may cause or aggravate steatorrhea and may impede absorption of fat-soluble vitamins.
   (4) These agents may bind other drugs (e.g., chlorothiazide, anticoagulants, digitalis glycosides), impeding their absorption.

Table 5-6. Antihyperlipidemic Agents

		Therapeutic Uses	
Drug	**Effects**	**Lipoprotein State**	**Clinical Condition**
HMG CoA reductase inhibitors (lovastatin, prevastatin, mevastatin)	↓LDL	High LDL	Hypercholesterolemias with risk of myocardial infarction; diabetes- and nephrosis-related hypercholesterolemias
Fibric acid derivatives (clofibrate, gemfibrozil)	↓ ↑LDL ↓VLDL ↑HDL	Low HDL, high VLDL, high IDL (clofibrate); also high LDL (gemfibrozil)	Familial type III hyperlipoproteinemia (both derivatives); hypertriglyceridemia with or without hypercholesterolemia, type V hyperlipoproteinemia (gemfibrozil)
Bile acid sequestrants (cholestyramine, colestipol)	↓LDL ↑HDL	High LDL	Heterozygous familial and polygenic hypercholesterolemias
Probucol	↓LDL ↓HDL	High LDL	Hypercholesterolemia (given with other lipid-lowering agents)
Niacin (nicotinic acid)	↓LDL ↓VLDL ↑HDL	Low HDL; high VLDL; high LDL	All hyperlipoproteinemias except lipoprotein lipase deficiency

Arrows indicate changes: ↑ = increased; ↓ = decreased.

2. Lovastatin pravastatin, and mevastatin: HMG CoA reductase inhibitors

a. Mechanism of action and pharmacologic effects

(1) 3-HMG CoA reductase is the rate-limiting enzyme in cholesterol biosynthesis.

(2) Drugs that inhibit HMG CoA reductase are highly effective in lowering serum LDL-cholesterol levels.

(a) HMG CoA reductase inhibitors block the hepatic synthesis of cholesterol.

(b) This block leads to a compensatory reduction of serum LDL.

(c) There is also a compensatory increase in synthesis of HMG CoA reductase so that inhibition of cholesterol synthesis is not complete.

(3) These drugs reduce serum levels of LDL, LDL-cholesterol, VLDL-cholesterol, and triglycerides. They elevate HDL-cholesterol.

(a) The decrease in LDL appears to result from an increase in hepatic LDL receptors, which causes an increase in receptor-mediated clearance of LDL and IDL.

(b) Lovastatin does not decrease LDL levels in homozygous LDL-receptor–negative hypercholesterolemia, since these patients lack LDL receptors; this finding supports the presumed mechanism.

b. Therapeutic uses

(1) Lovastatin is indicated for patients with hypercholesterolemia who are at high risk of myocardial infarction.

(2) It is specifically indicated for types IIa and IIb hyperlipoproteinemia in which IDL and total cholesterol are elevated.

(3) Lovastatin is also useful in secondary hyperlipoproteinemia due to diabetes mellitus or nephrotic syndrome.

(4) The drug may be useful in patients with combined elevated cholesterol and triglycerides.

c. Adverse effects

(1) Serum hepatic transaminases are elevated in 2% of patients receiving lovastatin, and muscle creatine phosphokinase (CPK) levels are elevated in 11%.

(2) Gastrointestinal reactions include flatulence and diarrhea.

(3) Periodic slit-lamp examinations are suggested before and during therapy, because ocular opacities have been noted in dogs.

(4) Lovastatin therapy, when combined with another lipid-lowering drug or with cyclosporine, can cause myopathies, sometimes progressing to rhabdomyolysis and renal failure.

(5) Teratogenicity occurs in animals.

3. Niacin (nicotinic acid)

a. Mechanism of action and pharmacologic effects

(1) In large doses, niacin reduces serum triglycerides by lowering VLDL, usually within 1–4 days.

(2) The reduction of VLDL in turn reduces IDL and LDL.

(3) Niacin usually produces a mild to moderate increase in HDL.

(4) The VLDL-reducing action of niacin is independent of its vitamin activity. The mechanism may involve:

(a) Inhibition of lipolysis in adipocytes

(b) Inhibition of hepatic triglyceride esterification

(c) Increased activity of lipoprotein lipase

(5) Niacin does not significantly affect either total body production or biliary excretion of cholesterol.

b. Therapeutic uses

(1) Niacin is helpful in controlling a wide range of hyperlipidemias.

(2) It is particularly useful for type V hyperlipoproteinemia, characterized by severe hypertriglyceridemia and elevated chylomicrons.

(3) It is not useful in familial lipoprotein lipase deficiency.

c. Adverse effects. These can be minimized by taking the drug with meals and increasing the dosage gradually.

(1) Niacin produces prostaglandin-mediated intense flushing and itching.

(2) Gastrointestinal distress is common, and peptic ulceration has occurred.

(3) Hepatic dysfunction can occur with high-dose regimens.

(4) Glucose intolerance and hyperuricemia can occur.

4. Clofibrate, gemfibrozil: fibric acid derivatives

a. Mechanism of action and pharmacologic effects

(1) **Effects on serum lipids**

(a) The fibric acid derivatives lower serum VLDL levels, thus reducing serum triglycerides.

(b) With **clofibrate,** the net effect on serum cholesterol in most patients is minimal. However, serum cholesterol is significantly reduced in patients with familial type III hyperlipoproteinemia.

(c) Clofibrate has no effect on chylomicron levels or on HDL levels.

(d) **Gemfibrozil** lowers plasma VLDL-cholesterol levels, lowers LDL-cholesterol to a lesser degree, and raises HDL-cholesterol.

(2) **Mechanism of action.** This is not yet fully established.

(a) Fibric acid derivatives increase the activity of lipoprotein lipase, the enzyme that degrades chylomicrons and VLDL.

(b) Other proposed mechanisms include:

(i) Decreased hepatic synthesis and release of VLDL

(ii) Reduced VLDL–HDL lipid exchange, causing increased HDL-cholesterol levels

(iii) Increased hepatic clearance of VLDL and IDL, causing lower LDL-cholesterol levels

b. Therapeutic uses

(1) Fibric acid derivatives are indicated for patients with familial type III hyperlipoproteinemia, in which VLDL and IDL levels are increased.

(2) Gemfibrozil is the first-choice drug for hypertriglyceridemia, whether or not accompanied by hypercholesterolemia.

(3) Gemfibrozil is also useful in type V hyperlipoproteinemia in which both chylomicron and triglyceride levels are increased.

(4) Neither clofibrate nor gemfibrozil is useful in type I hyperlipoproteinemia with elevated chylomicrons or triglycerides but normal VLDL levels.

c. Adverse effects

(1) These agents are generally well tolerated. The most common unwanted effects are mild gastrointestinal reactions.

(2) Some patients may show a paradoxic increase in LDL-cholesterol.

(3) Myositis with elevated CPK and serum glutamic oxaloacetic transaminase (SGOT) levels can occur.

(4) The fibric acid derivatives increase the incidence of cholelithiasis and cholecystitis.

(5) Cardiac arrhythmias have been reported with clofibrate.

(6) Clofibrate displaces warfarin from albumin, potentiating its anticoagulant effects.

5. Probucol: lipophilic antioxidant

a. Mechanism of action and pharmacologic effects

(1) **Effect on serum lipids**

(a) Probucol reduces total serum cholesterol; it lowers HDL-cholesterol more than LDL-cholesterol.

(b) Probucol has little or no effect on VLDL or triglycerides.

(c) The mechanism of action is unclear but appears to involve:

(i) Synthesis of cholesterol-poor HDL

(ii) Inhibition of early stages of cholesterol synthesis

(iii) An increased rate of LDL degradation

(2) **Effect on cholesterol deposits**

(a) Probucol has been found to induce marked regression of xanthomas and, in rabbits, a marked reduction in atheromatous deposits.

(b) The mechanism is believed to involve the antioxidant effects of probucol, inhibiting the oxidation of LDL, thereby preventing its uptake by macrophages.

(c) Insufficient data as yet prevent clinical application of these findings.

    b. Therapeutic uses. Probucol is generally combined with another type of lipid-lowering drug for the treatment of general hypercholesterolemia.

    c. Adverse effects

       (1) Gastrointestinal reactions are the most common untoward effects.

       (2) Prolongation of the Q–T interval has been reported.

       (3) Probucol is stored in body tissue for up to 6 months. Since its safety has not been established in pregnancy, women should discontinue and practice contraception for at least 6 months before pregnancy is attempted.

STUDY QUESTIONS

Directions: Each of the numbered items or incomplete statements in this section is followed by answers or by completions of the statement. Select the **one** lettered answer or completion that is **best** in each case.

1. All of the following statements about digitalis glycosides are true EXCEPT

(A) the active moiety of the glycoside molecule is chemically similar to the adrenocorticosteroid molecule
(B) the most important property of the cardiac glycosides is their positive inotropic effect
(C) cardiac glycosides affect cardiac conductivity
(D) cardiac glycosides cause Na^+ retention
(E) intoxication due to depletion of K^+ stores is a common problem with the cardiac glycosides

2. Actions of digoxin on the heart include all of the following EXCEPT

(A) increased force of systolic contraction
(B) prolonged A-V nodal conduction time
(C) a decrease in ventricular size of the failing heart
(D) a positive chronotropic effect in the failing heart
(E) an increase in the effective refractory period of the atria

3. Digitalis glycosides are used with all of the following conditions EXCEPT

(A) atrial fibrillation
(B) high-output cardiac failure
(C) paroxysmal atrial tachycardia
(D) atrial flutter

4. All of the following measures can be used in the treatment of digoxin-induced arrhythmias EXCEPT

(A) stopping digoxin administration
(B) electrical conversion
(C) phenytoin administration
(D) lidocaine administration
(E) digoxin-specific antibody fragment

5. Which of the following antiarrhythmic agents is incorrectly matched by class?

(A) Mexiletine—class IB
(B) Encainide—class IC
(C) Esmolol—class IV
(D) Propranolol—class II
(E) Verapamil—class IV

6. A 67-year-old man with a history of recurrent ventricular tachycardia presents with joint and muscle pain, fatigue (which proves to be due to hemolytic anemia), and a skin rash. He is taking several "heart pills." A likely cause of his signs and symptoms is

(A) digoxin
(B) procainamide
(C) disopyramide
(D) minoxidil
(E) reserpine

7. When used intravenously, lidocaine has all of the following effects EXCEPT

(A) it suppresses premature ventricular contractions
(B) it reverses atrial arrhythmias
(C) it decreases Na^+ conductance in automatic cells
(D) it has no effect on sinus nodal pacemaker discharge
(E) it is rapidly metabolized by the hepatic microsomal enzyme system

8. The antiarrhythmic agent tocainide has all of the following properties EXCEPT

(A) it can be used for ventricular arrhythmias
(B) it can be given orally
(C) it is also a local anesthetic
(D) it lengthens the action potential
(E) it is a class IB antiarrhythmic agent

1-D	4-B	7-B
2-D	5-C	8-D
3-B	6-B	

9. All of the following statements regarding nitroglycerin are true EXCEPT

(A) tablets should be stored in a dark glass container
(B) headache is a common early side effect
(C) transdermal administration is effective when administered daily for 24 hours
(D) it can be given intravenously in medical emergencies
(E) the nitrates are broken down in the liver by a glutathione-dependent organic reductase

10. A 48-year-old woman who is being treated with propranolol for essential hypertension experiences a worsening of her COPD. Acceptable alternate therapy could include all of the following EXCEPT

(A) diltiazem
(B) verapamil
(C) nicardipine
(D) nadolol
(E) thiazide diuretic

11. Correct statements about the adverse effects of antihypertensive agents include all of the following EXCEPT

(A) hydralazine can induce a lupus-like syndrome
(B) diazoxide inhibits the release of insulin from the pancreas
(C) clonidine can cause fluid retention that often requires concurrent diuretic therapy
(D) reserpine augments sympathetic effects due to decreased parasympathetic activity
(E) captopril can cause cough and bronchospasm

12. A 47-year-old man has been treated for essential hypertension for 6 months. The patient's hypertension is under control; however, he now complains of impotence, vertigo, and difficulty in doing mental work. Laboratory results reveal a positive Coombs' test. Which antihypertensive agent is capable of causing these effects?

(A) Captopril
(B) Hydralazine
(C) Lisinopril
(D) Methyldopa
(E) Prazosin

13. A patient presents to the emergency room with substernal chest pain that has lasted 1 hour. Within the next hour, the diagnosis of an acute transmural myocardial infarction is made. All of the following statements regarding the use of a thrombolytic agent in this situation are true EXCEPT

(A) t-PA would facilitate the conversion of plasminogen to plasmin
(B) t-PA has a shorter half-life than streptokinase
(C) t-PA administration is more likely to benefit this patient's chances of survival than streptokinase
(D) streptokinase appears more effective when given less than 3 hours after the onset of symptoms
(E) all thrombolytic agents can cause cardiac arrhythmias upon reperfusion

14. Which antihyperlipidemic agent would reduce circulating cholesterol levels by binding to cholesterol in the gastrointestinal tract?

(A) Cholestyramine
(B) Clofibrate
(C) Gemfibrozil
(D) Lovastatin
(E) Nicotinic acid

15. All of the following lipid-reducing agents are correctly matched with their pharmacologic mechanism of action EXCEPT

(A) cholestyramine—bile acid sequestrant
(B) probucol—enhanced LDL clearance by non-receptor mechanisms
(C) clofibrate—coenzyme A reductase inhibitor
(D) gemfibrozil—increases the activity of lipoprotein lipase
(E) lovastatin—inhibits the early stage of cholesterol biosynthesis

9-C   12-D   15-C
10-D   13-C
11-D   14-A

Directions: Each item below contains four suggested answers of which **one or more** is correct. Choose the answer

A   if **1, 2, and 3** are correct
B   if **1 and 3** are correct
C   if **2 and 4** are correct
D   if **4** is correct
E   if **1, 2, 3, and 4** are correct

16. True statements about the use of diuretics in the management of hypertension include which of the following?

(1) The thiazides are the diuretics used most frequently for this purpose
(2) Diuretics are only useful in mild hypertension
(3) Triamterene is used in combination with a thiazide diuretic
(4) Furosemide is a more effective antihypertensive than chlorothiazide

17. Pairs of compounds with opposing effects on blood glucose concentrations include

(1) tolbutamide and diazoxide
(2) insulin and cortisol
(3) insulin and glucagon
(4) glucagon and isoproterenol

18. True statements about the antihypertensive agents enalapril and captopril include which of the following?

(1) Both enalapril and captopril inhibit peptidyl dipeptidase
(2) Both agents are angiotensin II antagonists
(3) Both agents reduce blood pressure in hypertensive patients with normal renin levels
(4) Both agents reduce blood pressure in normotensive individuals

16-B
17-A
18-B

ANSWERS AND EXPLANATIONS

1. The answer is D *[I B 1 a (1), 3 a, b (3), c (4), 6 c; Table 5-2]*
Cardiac glycosides promote the excretion of salt and water. This diuretic effect results from the improvement in myocardial contractility and decreased sympathetic activity, which cause an increase in renal blood flow. The other statements in the question are correct.

2. The answer is D *[I B 3 b (4)]*
Digoxin will produce increased force of systolic contraction, prolonged A-V nodal conduction time, a decrease in ventricular size of the failing heart, and an increase in the effective refractory period of the atria. It tends to slow the heart rate, especially in the failing heart (a negative chronotropic effect). By improving cardiac output, digoxin produces a decrease in sympathetic activity.

3. The answer is B *[I B 4]*
Cardiac glycosides are contraindicated in cardiac tamponade, high-output congestive heart failure, constrictive pericarditis, and idiopathic hypertrophic subaortic stenosis with outlet obstruction. In all of these conditions, a high-pressure system is involved, and a positive inotropic effect in such circumstances would be undesirable. Cardiac glycosides are very useful in supraventricular arrhythmia, such as atrial fibrillation, atrial flutter, and paroxysmal atrial tachycardia. It is of greatest value for treating low-output cardiac failure.

4. The answer is B *[I B 7 a, d, e, j, k]*
The use of phenytoin and lidocaine for various digoxin-induced arrhythmias is considered appropriate therapy. Digoxin and K^+-depleting diuretics should be discontinued. Electrical conversion can be hazardous because it can precipitate ventricular fibrillation. Digoxin-specific antibody fragment is available for life-threatening digoxin overdosage.

5. The answer is C *[III A 3 a–d]*
Esmolol, like propranolol, is a class II antiarrhythmic agent. These agents act by β-adrenergic blockade. Class I agents (e.g., mexiletine, encainide) depress phase 0 of the action potential by blocking Na^+ channels. Class III agents (e.g., amiodarone, bretylium) prolong repolarization, and phase 2 is lengthened. Class IV agents (e.g., verapamil, diltiazem) are Ca^{2+} antagonists.

6. The answer is B *[II B 2 f (4)]*
Procainamide is capable of producing a syndrome that resembles systemic lupus erythematosus, the signs and symptoms of which could be this patient's presenting problems. These untoward effects are caused by hypersensitivity to procainamide and are reversible with time once the drug is discontinued.

7. The answer is B *[II C 1 b, c]*
Lidocaine is an effective antiarrhythmic agent and is the drug of choice for premature ventricular contractions, although it is ineffective in reversing atrial arrhythmias. It decreases Na^+ but not K^+ conductance in automatic cells. It does not effect sinus nodal pacemaker discharge. Lidocaine is rapidly metabolized by the hepatic microsomal enzyme system.

8. The answer is D *[II C 3 a–d]*
Tocainide is a lidocaine analog and a class IB antiarrhythmic agent. It closely resembles lidocaine in its effects, but unlike lidocaine, it can be used orally for arrhythmias. Tocainide is used to suppress ventricular arrhythmias; it is also a local anesthetic. In arrhythmias, tocainide shortens, not lengthens, the action potential; it also shortens the ERP.

9. The answer is C *[III A 3 b, 4 b (1), 5 a–c]*
Transdermal nitroglycerin patches become ineffective if they are left in place for 24 hours and reapplied daily, even if the dosage is increased. Nitroglycerin patches delivering 10 mg or more remain effective if removed for 12 hours daily. It can be given intravenously in medical emergencies. Nitroglycerin tablets should be stored in a dark glass container so that they do not lose potency. Headache is a common early side effect, resulting from vasodilation of cerebral vessels produced by nitrates. Nitrates are broken down in the liver by a glutathione-dependent organic nitrate reductase.

10. The answer is D *[IV A 2, C 4 a, D]*
Diltiazem, verapamil, and nicardipine are all Ca^{2+}-channel blocking agents and do not worsen COPD.

Nadolol, which is similar to propranolol, is a nonselective β blocker and could exacerbate COPD. The use of a thiazide diuretic would be an acceptable alternative to propranolol.

11. The answer is D *[IV E 2 d (3), 4 e (3), G 1 e (3), H 1 f (2)]*
All of the agents in the question are correctly matched with an adverse effect except reserpine. Reserpine augments parasympathetic effects due to decreased sympathetic activity; this may result in bradycardia, increased gastrointestinal activity, and miosis.

12. The answer is D *[IV G 2 f]*
An antihypertensive agent capable of producing the adverse effects described in the question is methyldopa. In addition, methyldopa can cause sedation, extrapyramidal signs, postural hypotension, and hepatic dysfunction; rebound hypertension can occur with sudden withdrawal of methyldopa therapy.

13. The answer is C *[V A–C]*
Both t-PA and streptokinase appear to reduce mortality equally when administered after the diagnosis of an acute transmural myocardial infarction. However, streptokinase appears to be most effective when given less than 3 hours after the onset of symptoms. t-PA facilitates the conversion of plasminogen to plasmin and has a shorter half-life than streptokinase. All thrombolytic agents can cause cardiac arrhythmias upon reperfusion.

14. The answer is A *[VI B 1, 3, 4]*
Cholestyramine is a resin that binds bile acid in the intestine, thereby preventing its reabsorption. The reduction in bile acid leads to an increase in 7-α-hydroxylase, which in turn leads to an increased hepatic conversion of cholesterol into bile acids. Nicotinic acid and clofibrate alter the metabolism, not the transport, of cholesterol. Nicotinic acid depresses the synthesis of VLDL, which indirectly depresses LDL levels. Clofibrate and gemfibrozil reduce VLDL but may raise serum LDL. Lovastatin is a coenzyme A reductase inhibitor, which competitively inhibits the early stage of cholesterol biosynthesis.

15. The answer is C *[VI B 1 a, 2 a, 4 a, 5 a]*
Clofibrate, like gemfibrozil, are fibric acid derivatives that possibly increase the activity of lipoprotein lipase, the enzyme that degrades chylomicrons and VLDL. Lovastatin and pravastatin are 3-hydroxy-3-methylglutaryl coenzyme A reductase inhibitors. They competitively inhibit the early stage of cholesterol biosynthesis. Cholestyramine is a resin that binds bile acids in the intestines, which are then excreted in the feces. Probucol reduces total serum cholesterol by increasing the rate of degradation of LDL and inhibition of the early stages of cholesterol synthesis.

16. The answer is B (1, 3) *[IV B 1–3]*
Thiazides are the diuretics used most frequently in the management of hypertension and are used for mild, moderate, and severe hypertension. If a thiazide is ineffective alone in the treatment of mild hypertension, it is usually combined with another type of antihypertensive agent, such as a β-adrenergic blocking agent. Triamterene and spironolactone have only modest hypotensive effects, but they potentiate the effects of the thiazides and minimize the K^+ loss that thiazides can cause. Furosemide and ethacrynic acid produce greater diuresis than the thiazides, but they have a weaker antihypertensive effect.

17. The answer is A (1, 2, 3) *[IV E 4 b (4); Ch 2 II B; Ch 10 III G; IV; V B]*
The oral hypoglycemic agent tolbutamide decreases blood glucose concentrations, while the antihypertensive agent diazoxide increases them. Insulin decreases blood glucose concentrations, while cortisol, glucagon, and isoproterenol all increase blood glucose concentrations.

18. The answer is B (1, 3) *[IV I 1; Ch 8 V C 2]*
Both enalapril and captopril are ACE inhibitors; that is, they block the enzyme peptidyl dipeptidase, preventing the conversion of angiotensin I to angiotensin II. They are not angiotensin II antagonists. ACE inhibitors serve as indirect vasodilators by reducing the level of angiotensin II, a vasoconstrictor, and also by increasing the level of bradykinin, a vasodilator, because bradykinin is degraded by peptidyl dipeptidase. ACE inhibitors reduce blood pressure in hypertensive patients with high, normal, or low plasma renin levels; the reason is not yet known. ACE inhibitors do not affect blood pressure in normal persons who are in Na^+ balance.

I. GENERAL CONSIDERATIONS. Diuretics are drugs that promote a net loss of sodium ions (Na^+) and water from the body, the net result being an increase in urine flow. Some drugs can increase urine flow by **nonrenal mechanisms** (e.g., by increasing cardiac output in a patient with congestive heart failure), but these drugs are not generally regarded as diuretics.

A. **Classification.** Diuretics can be classified by structure and mechanism of action into eight groups listed below. Agents in the first four groups are seldom or no longer used but are discussed because their mode of action or their role in the history of diuretics is important.

1. Xanthine diuretics

2. Mercurial diuretics

3. Carbonic anhydrase inhibitors

4. Acidifying salts

5. Thiazide diuretics

6. High-ceiling (loop) diuretics

7. Osmotic diuretics

8. Potassium (K^+)-sparing diuretics

B. **Sites of action.** Although an individual diuretic can act on several areas of the nephron, the major sites of action for the diuretics may be summarized as follows:

1. Those acting on the **proximal tubule**:
   a. Osmotic diuretics
   b. Xanthine diuretics
   c. Carbonic anhydrase inhibitors
   d. Acidifying salts

2. Those acting on the **ascending limb of the loop of Henle**:
   a. High-ceiling (loop) diuretics
   b. Thiazide diuretics
   c. Mercurial diuretics

3. Those acting on the **distal tubule**: K^+-sparing diuretics

C. **Therapeutic uses**

1. Diuretics are frequently employed for the clinical management of disorders involving abnormal fluid distribution, such as edema, or for hypertension. They are also used to reduce the toxicity of ingested or administered substances. For example, mannitol, an osmotic diuretic, reduces the renal toxicity of the antitumor agent cisplatin, and acetazolamide, a carbonic anhydrase inhibitor, is used to alkalinize the urine and increase salicylate elimination.

2. The efficacy of the different classes of diuretics varies significantly, with the xanthine diuretics being the least effective and the "high-ceiling," or "loop," diuretics being the most effective. The establishment of a net negative Na^+ balance, particularly with the less efficacious diuretics, can also depend upon limiting the Na^+ intake.

D. Adverse effects

1. Prolonged use of some diuretics (e.g., mercurials, carbonic anhydrase inhibitors) results in refractoriness or a reduction in efficacy. These agents are "self-limiting" and not frequently used.

2. Reduction in serum K^+ levels (**hypokalemia**) is one of the most important adverse effects of many, but not all, diuretics.

3. A summary of the adverse effects of important diuretics is presented in Table 6-1.

II. XANTHINE DIURETICS

A. Mechanism of action

1. By increasing cardiac output, these drugs increase renal plasma flow, promoting a higher glomerular filtration rate.

2. They also appear to inhibit Na^+ reabsorption in the proximal convoluted tubule.

B. Therapeutic uses. Xanthines are rarely used as diuretics, but the diuretic action may be seen with xanthines used as bronchodilators (e.g., aminophylline) or in caffeine products (e.g., tea, coffee, soda).

C. Adverse effects. Xanthine diuretics may cause:

1. Central nervous system (CNS) stimulation

2. Gastrointestinal upset, including vomiting and consequent dehydration

3. Cardiovascular toxicity, including palpitations, hypotension, and circulatory collapse

III. MERCURIAL DIURETICS

A. Mechanism of action

1. The major effect of organomercurials is to inhibit active chloride (Cl^-) transport in the ascending limb of the loop of Henle.

2. In an **acidic environment,** the mercuric ion (Hg^{2+}) dissociates and binds to sulfhydryl enzymes, inactivating them.
   a. As a result, reabsorption of Na^+ is diminished and the excretion of Na^+ and Cl^- is increased.
   b. More Cl^- than Na^+ is lost; thus, to maintain electrical neutrality, cations such as hydrogen (H^+) and to a lesser degree K^+ are also lost.
   c. Because excess Cl^- is excreted, bicarbonate (HCO_3^-) remains to maintain balanced anions, and the resulting metabolic picture is a **hypochloremic alkalosis.**

3. In an **alkaline environment,** Hg^{2+} does not dissociate from the mercurial diuretics to take an active form; thus, patients become **refractory** to the mercurials in about a week. However, an

Table 6-1. Adverse Effects of Diuretics

Diuretic	Hyperglycemia	Hyperuricemia	Hypokalemia	Ototoxicity	Calcium Excretion
Thiazide	+	+	+	−	↓
Ethacrynic acid	+	+	+	+	↑
Furosemide	+	+	+	+	↑
Bumetanide	+	+	+	+	↑*
Mercurials	−	−	−	−	−*
Acetazolamide	−	−	+	−	−*
Indapamide	+	+	+	−	↓

+ = side effect; − = no side effect; ↑ = increase; ↓ = decrease.
*No effect.

acidifying agent, such as ammonium chloride (NH_4Cl), can be combined with mercurials to create a metabolic acidosis, offsetting the metabolic alkalosis and combating refractoriness.

B. Route of administration. Mercurial diuretics are poorly absorbed by the oral route and, thus, are given parenterally. **Mercaptomerin** is administered daily, intramuscularly or subcutaneously. The major excretory product is a cysteine complex of the intact organic mercurial molecule.

C. Therapeutic uses. The mercurials are now seldom used because they must be given parenterally and because of their adverse effects. Since the mercurial diuretics do not disrupt K^+ balance as much as many of the other diuretics, they occasionally are used for congestive heart failure, cirrhosis, and portal obstruction.

D. Adverse effects include:

1. Systemic mercury poisoning

2. Cardiac toxicity (ventricular fibrillation can follow rapid intravenous administration, possibly because of the mercurial's binding to sulfhydryl enzymes in cardiac muscle)

3. Hypersensitivity reactions

4. Aggravation of acute nephritis or renal insufficiency

IV. CARBONIC ANHYDRASE INHIBITORS

A. Mechanism of action

1. These agents inhibit the carbonic anhydrase enzyme predominantly at the proximal convoluted tubules, causing a reduction in hydrogen ions for Na^+–H^+ exchange. Carbon dioxide (CO_2) reabsorption from the glomerular filtrate is suppressed, and HCO_3^- excretion is increased.

2. Due to decreased Na^+ reabsorption, the Na^+–K^+ exchange in the distal convoluted tubule increases, causing a loss of K^+ in the urine.

3. To maintain ionic balance, Cl^- is retained by the kidney, resulting in a hyperchloremic acidosis.

4. Increased urinary amounts of Na^+, K^+, and HCO_3^- result in an alkaline urine.

5. The resulting metabolic acidosis eventually induces a refractory state or a decreased diuresis.

B. Route of administration

1. As a diuretic, **acetazolamide** is given orally once daily or every other day.

2. For use in glaucoma, it is given orally 2–4 times daily.

C. Therapeutic uses

1. Carbonic anhydrase inhibitors are weak diuretics and have largely been replaced by the thiazide diuretics. Historically, however, they are very important.

2. They are still used with moderate success for the following purposes:
   a. In **glaucoma,** for reducing the rate of aqueous humor formation
   b. In **petit mal epilepsy,** where they act as an anticonvulsant and decrease the rate of spinal fluid formation (the mechanism of action of this therapeutic effect is unclear)
   c. To **alkalinize the urine**:
      (1) In the treatment of salicylate or barbiturate poisoning
      (2) In combination with HCO_3^- to maintain electrolyte balance

D. Adverse effects with carbonic anhydrase inhibitors are few.

1. They are aromatic sulfonamides, which can cause blood dyscrasias and allergic skin reactions, but these are rare.

2. Drowsiness and paresthesias can occur with large doses but are reversible.

3. They inhibit iodide uptake by the thyroid but are not therapeutic as agents used to treat goiters.

V. ACIDIFYING SALTS

A. Mechanism of action

1. Acidifying salts such as NH_4Cl lower the pH in the extracellular fluid and urine.
   a. The ammonium (NH_4) in NH_4Cl is metabolized by the liver to urea, resulting in the net formation of H^+.
   b. H^+ then is buffered by HCO_3^-, and CO_2 is formed.
   c. Cl^- from the NH_4Cl replaces HCO_3^-, and this leads to acidosis.
   d. An excess of Cl^- also occurs in the tubular lumen and takes Na^+ along with it to maintain electrical neutrality.
   e. The glutaminase system becomes activated, producing ammonia (NH_3).
   f. The kidney secretes H^+ in exchange for Na^+, and Cl^- is excreted in combination with NH_4^+.

2. Ultimately, the amount of NH_4Cl ingested is equal to the amount excreted by the kidney, and a refractory state is produced.

B. Route of administration. NH_4Cl is administered as enteric-coated tablets given orally 4–6 times a day for 2 days.

C. Therapeutic uses

1. As a primary diuretic, NH_4Cl is effective only 1–2 days, and thus, it is seldom used.

2. The drug has been used to augment the effect of mercurial and high-ceiling diuretics by maintaining an available source of Cl^- in the blood to compensate for diuretic-induced alkalosis.

D. Adverse effects include:

1. Gastric irritation

2. Uncompensated acidosis that occurs when renal function is impaired

3. Exacerbation of hepatic failure

VI. THIAZIDE DIURETICS (BENZOTHIADIAZIDES)

A. Mechanism of action

1. The thiazide diuretics vary widely in their potency of carbonic anhydrase inhibition (Figure 6-1). Structurally, these drugs have a sulfonamyl group, which accounts for their inhibition of carbonic anhydrase activity. Their primary mechanism of action does not, however, rely on inhibition of carbonic anhydrase.

2. They inhibit Cl^- reabsorption, particularly in the distal portion of the ascending limb of Henle's loop and the very early portion of the distal tubule.

3. There is increased renal excretion of Na^+, Cl^-, HCO_3^-, and K^+.

4. Refractoriness does not occur.

5. The initial hypotensive effect of the thiazide diuretics is a result of a reduction in blood volume, and a continued hypotensive effect occurs because of direct relaxation of arteriolar smooth muscle.

6. Certain other sulfonamide diuretics—indapamide, chlorthalidone, quinethazone, and metolazone—are pharmacologically similar to the thiazides.

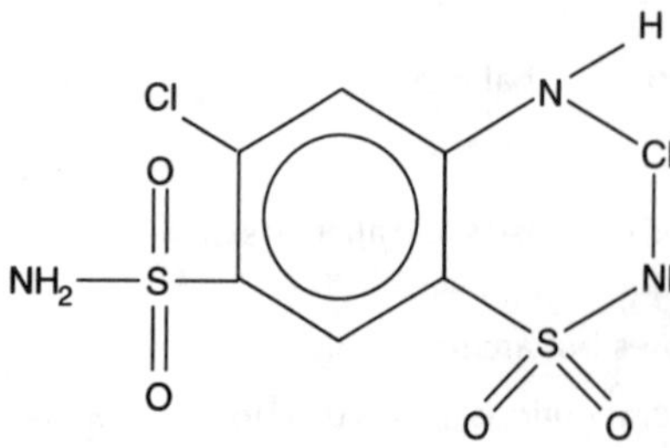

Figure 6-1. Hydrochlorothiazide.

B. Route of administration. There are many analogs, but the two most important prototypes are:

1. **Chlorothiazide,** given orally 1–2 times a day

2. **Hydrochlorothiazide,** given orally 1–2 times a day

C. Therapeutic uses

1. Thiazide diuretics are used to treat chronic edema, usually associated with cardiac decompensation. A diuretic response occurs in 2–3 hours and lasts for about a day.

2. Thiazides are used in the treatment of essential hypertension.

3. They sometimes are effective in the treatment of nephrosis.

4. They are occasionally used for the palliation of nephrogenic and pituitary [antidiuretic hormone (ADH)-sensitive] diabetes insipidus. By decreasing the urinary volume through their natriuretic action, these drugs may enhance the action of ADH.

5. They are used in the management of hypercalciuria.

D. Adverse effects

1. Electrolyte abnormalities such as **hypokalemia** can occur.
   a. Thus, K^+ supplementation is recommended.
   b. Particular caution is needed when a thiazide is administered in combination with a digitalis preparation for the treatment of congestive heart failure. If digitalis is administered in the presence of hypokalemia, digitalis intoxication and serious cardiac arrhythmias can result.

2. **Hyperuricemia** may result from an inhibition of renal tubular secretion of uric acid. Since thiazides are excreted by glomerular filtration and tubular secretion, the thiazides compete with uric acid for tubular secretion.

3. **Hyperglycemia** can occur, aggravating preexisting diabetes mellitus. Thiazides may interfere with the conversion of proinsulin to insulin.

4. Thiazide diuretics may **reduce urinary calcium excretion**.
   a. **Hypercalcemia** and **hypophosphatemia** have occurred in a few patients on prolonged thiazide therapy.
   b. Suppression of parathyroid hormone and reduction in intestinal calcium absorption may occur.

5. Thiazide diuretics occasionally may **aggravate renal or hepatic insufficiency**.

6. Lassitude, weakness, and vertigo can occur with large doses.

7. Recently, **thiazide-induced pancreatitis** has been reported.

8. Recently, several reports have implicated thiazides in **elevating lipid** and lipoprotein changes that could enhance **atherogenesis**.

E. Sulfonamide diuretics

1. The nature of their heterocyclic ring makes them chemically different from the thiazides.

2. Pharmacologically, they are similar to the thiazides though their duration of action is sufficiently long (24 hours) to allow once a day oral administration.

3. Preparations include:
   a. Chlorthalidone (Figure 6-2)
   b. Quinethazone
   c. Metolazone
   d. Indapamide

VII. HIGH-CEILING (LOOP) DIURETICS

A. Mechanism of action

1. These diuretics inhibit electrolyte reabsorption in the thick ascending limb of the loop of Henle.

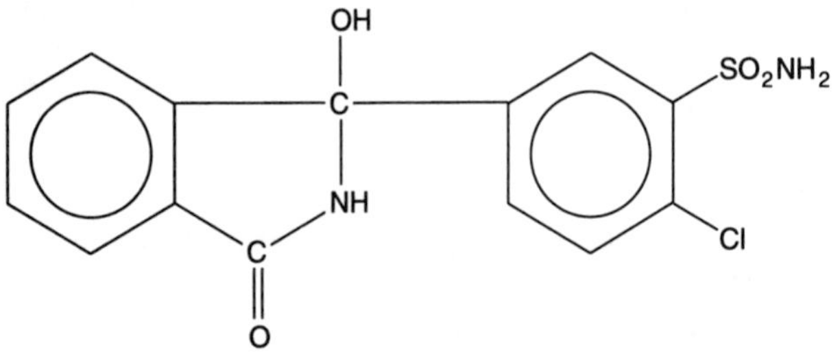

Figure 6-2. Chlorthalidone.

2. Cl^- excretion is greater than Na^+ excretion.

3. These diuretics increase renal blood flow without increasing the glomerular filtration rate.

4. Large doses promote uric acid excretion.

5. Hypochloremic alkalosis can occur, but it does not produce a refractory state.

6. Furosemide, a structural derivative of the thiazides (Figure 6-3), and **bumetanide** are weak inhibitors of carbonic anhydrase, probably as a result of the diuretics' substituted sulfonamide side chain.

7. Ethacrynic acid lacks a sulfonamyl group and does not inhibit carbonic anhydrase.

B. Route of administration

1. Furosemide and **bumetanide** are usually administered orally in a single dose once or twice daily. Both also can be administered intramuscularly or (more frequently) intravenously.

2. Ethacrynic acid is administered orally or intravenously once or twice daily. One of the main differences between furosemide and ethacrynic acid is that the former has a broader dose–response curve.

C. Therapeutic uses

1. The high-ceiling diuretics are the most efficacious oral diuretic agents available.

2. They are useful for the treatment of acute episodes of pulmonary edema.

3. They are also effective for edema associated with congestive heart failure, cirrhosis, and renal disease.

4. Because of its potent edema-reducing ability, furosemide has been used to treat elevated intracranial pressure.

D. Adverse effects

1. Fluid and electrolyte imbalances are the most commonly seen adverse effects. The high-ceiling diuretics frequently are administered to patients on digitalis so hypokalemia may be a particular problem.

2. Hyperuricemia results because these diuretics are actively secreted by the renal and biliary secretory systems, and thus, they block (by competition) renal uric acid secretion. While hyperuricemia is relatively common, it is benign.

3. Transient deafness is a risk if a potentially ototoxic drug (e.g., an aminoglycoside antibiotic) is administered concomitantly. In such circumstances, another class of diuretic should be employed.

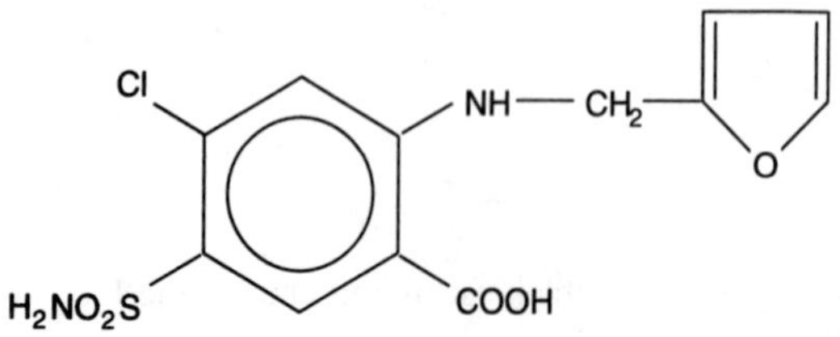

Figure 6-3. Furosemide.

4. Transient granulocytopenia and thrombocytopenia have occurred.

5. Severe muscle pain and tenderness have been reported in patients with renal failure taking a loop diuretic.

VIII. OSMOTIC DIURETICS

A. Mechanism of action

1. Osmotic diuretics are filtered at the glomerulus but are poorly reabsorbed due to their molecular size.

2. The presence of these unresorbed solutes in the proximal tubule causes decreased reabsorption of Na^+ and water, resulting in a large volume of urine.

3. Mannitol causes an increase in renal medullary blood flow via a prostaglandin-mediated mechanism.

4. Osmotic diuretics do not markedly influence Na^+ and Cl^- excretion.

B. Route of administration

1. **Mannitol** is a six-carbon sugar alcohol that is administered intravenously because it is not absorbed well from the gastrointestinal tract. It is not metabolized.

2. **Urea** is the least used osmotic diuretic. It can be given orally but because of its bitter taste is generally administered intravenously.

3. **Isosorbide** is used orally for ophthalmologic emergencies such as acute angle-closure glaucoma.

C. Therapeutic uses

1. The osmotic diuretics are used to reduce cerebrospinal fluid pressure.

2. They will transiently reduce intraocular fluid pressure.

3. They have also served as an adjunct in the prevention or treatment of oliguria and anuria.

4. The osmotic diuretics, especially mannitol, are employed prophylactically for acute renal failure in situations such as cardiovascular operations, treatment with nephrotoxic anticancer agents, severe traumatic injury, and management of hemolytic transfusion reactions.

D. Adverse effects

1. Because they do not penetrate cells and their mode of excretion is by glomerular filtration, osmotic diuretics increase blood volume, which can cause decompensation in patients with congestive heart failure.

2. When osmotic diuretics are used for the treatment of renal failure or cirrhotic disease, hyperosmolality and hyponatremia can occur.

IX. POTASSIUM (K^+)-SPARING DIURETICS

A. Triamterene and amiloride

1. **Mechanism of action**
   a. Triamterene (Figure 6-4) and amiloride (Figure 6-5) inhibit active Na^+ reabsorption.
      (1) The increased excretion of Na^+ and Cl^- disrupts normal Na^+ transport and produces a net change in the electrogenic force across tubular membranes.
      (2) This reduces the net driving force for K^+ secretion.
   b. Triamterene and amiloride cause a moderate increase in Na^+, Cl^- and HCO_3^- excretion.
   c. Their action is independent of aldosterone.

2. **Route of administration**
   a. **Triamterene** is administered orally twice daily.
   b. **Amiloride** is administered orally once daily.

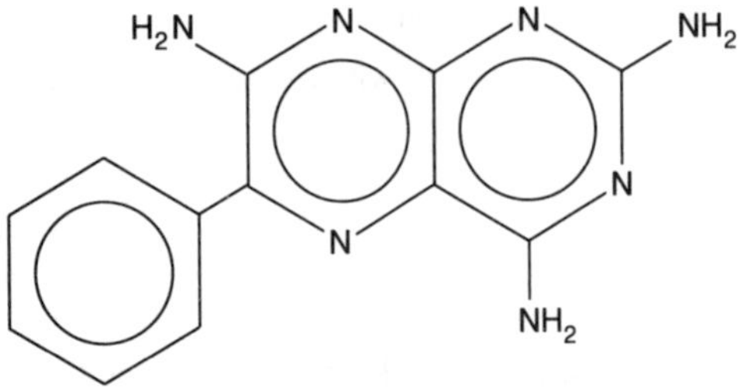

Figure 6-4. Triamterene.

3. Therapeutic uses. Triamterene or amiloride is used in combination with other diuretic agents for the treatment of hypertension; this combined therapy augments the natriuretic effect while diminishing kaliuresis.

4. Adverse effects

    a. Hyperkalemia can occur; thus, K^+-sparing diuretics are not given in combination with one another and are contraindicated in hyperkalemic patients. Hyperkalemia is especially likely in diabetics or in those with impaired renal function.

    b. Reversible azotemia is relatively common.

    c. Gastrointestinal disturbances, including nausea and vomiting, occur on occasion.

    d. Leg cramps may occur.

    e. Dizziness has been reported.

    f. Triamterene causes a slight increase in serum acid and, thus, should be used with caution in patients with gout.

B. Spironolactone

  1. Mechanism of action

    a. Spironolactone is a competitive antagonist of the mineralocorticoid, aldosterone.

    b. It interferes with the aldosterone-mediated Na^+–K^+ exchange, increasing Na^+ loss at the distal tubular site while decreasing K^+ loss.

    c. It is most effective when circulating aldosterone levels are high.

  2. Route of administration. Spironolactone is usually given orally four times a day.

  3. Therapeutic uses

    a. Spironolactone is often used as an adjunct to other diuretics to reduce the loss of K^+ in the management of refractory edema, such as that associated with Laënnec's cirrhosis.

    b. It also is used when adrenal gland tumors result in increased aldosterone levels.

    c. It can be used for edema due to congestive heart failure, although other diuretic agents are more effective.

  4. Adverse effects

    a. Hyperkalemia can occur or be exacerbated, especially in patients with impaired renal function. Spironolactone is **contraindicated** in patients with acute renal insufficiency or hyperkalemia and is not given in combination with another K^+-sparing diuretic.

    b. Gastrointestinal disturbances include diarrhea.

    c. Androgenic side effects include menstrual irregularities and hirsutism.

    d. CNS disturbances include lethargy and mental confusion.

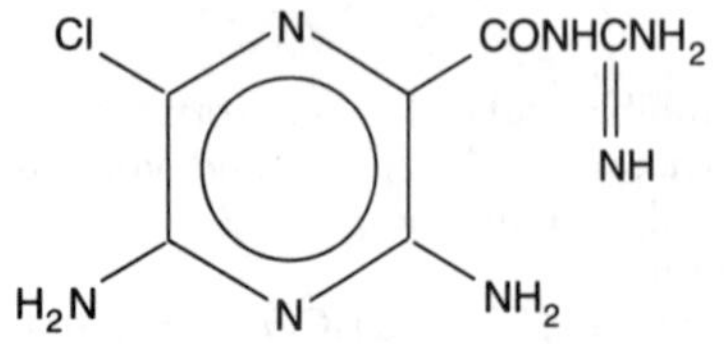

Figure 6-5. Amiloride.

STUDY QUESTIONS

Directions: Each of the numbered items or incomplete statements in this section is followed by answers or by completions of the statement. Select the **one** lettered answer or completion that is **best** in each case.

1. Properties of triamterene include all of the following EXCEPT

(A) it acts primarily in the distal nephron
(B) it inhibits the secretion of K^+
(C) it produces reversible azotemia relatively commonly
(D) it is weakly uricosuric
(E) it is a weak competitive antagonist of aldosterone

2. All of the following statements about xanthine diuretics are true EXCEPT

(A) they promote a high glomerular filtration rate by increasing cardiac output
(B) they are less effective than newer diuretics
(C) they can produce CNS stimulation
(D) they rarely produce cardiovascular toxicity
(E) they are closely related to substances in tea and coffee

3. All of the following statements about mercurial diuretics are true EXCEPT

(A) their mercuric ion dissociates in an acidic environment
(B) they can induce a hypochloremic alkalosis
(C) they rarely produce a refractory state
(D) they must be given parenterally
(E) rapid intravenous administration can result in ventricular fibrillation

4. A patient with a history of glaucoma, epilepsy, and edema would be a candidate for treatment with which of the following diuretics?

(A) Ethacrynic acid
(B) Chlorothiazide
(C) Furosemide
(D) Acetazolamide
(E) Spironolactone

5. The thiazide diuretics have a useful therapeutic effect in all of the following conditions EXCEPT

(A) chronic edema associated with cardiac decompensation
(B) ADH-secreting pulmonary tumors
(C) hypercalciuria
(D) hypertension
(E) nephrosis

Questions 6 and 7

A 70-year-old woman with a history of congestive heart failure, for which she takes digoxin and a diuretic agent, is seen because of an arrhythmia. Electrolyte determination reveals a serum potassium level of 2.8 mEq/L.

6. Diuretics capable of producing this patient's hypokalemia include all of the following EXCEPT

(A) bumetanide
(B) ethacrynic acid
(C) hydrochlorothiazide
(D) furosemide
(E) amiloride

7. Immediate therapy for this patient should include

(A) high doses of spironolactone
(B) insulin and glucose administration
(C) high doses of amiloride
(D) K^+ supplementation
(E) high doses of triamterene

8. Adverse effects resulting from the administration of furosemide include all of the following EXCEPT

(A) hypercalcemia
(B) hyperuricemia
(C) hypokalemia
(D) ototoxicity
(E) alkalosis

1-E	4-D	7-D
2-D	5-B	8-A
3-C	6-E	

9. Furosemide is useful for the treatment of all of the following conditions EXCEPT

(A) congestive heart failure

(B) acute pulmonary edema

(C) hypocalcemia

(D) edema resulting from hepatic or renal disease

(E) hypertensive crisis

10. The potential for digitalis-induced cardiac arrhythmias is increased by each of the following diuretics EXCEPT

(A) ethacrynic acid

(B) chlorothiazide

(C) spironolactone

(D) furosemide

(E) mercaptomerin

Directions: Each item below contains four suggested answers of which **one or more** is correct. Choose the answer

A if **1, 2, and 3** are correct

B if **1 and 3** are correct

C if **2 and 4** are correct

D if **4** is correct

E if **1, 2, 3, and 4** are correct

11. At present, the most commonly used diuretics belong to which of the following classes?

(1) Mercurials

(2) Thiazides

(3) Carbonic anhydrase inhibitors

(4) High-ceiling diuretics

12. A 22-year-old woman who sustains a severe head injury in an automobile accident is found to have elevated intracranial pressure. Proper therapy for this patient would include the use of which of the following diuretic agents?

(1) Urea

(2) Furosemide

(3) Mannitol

(4) Spironolactone

Directions: The group of items in this section consists of lettered options followed by a set of numbered items. For each item, select the **one** lettered option that is most closely associated with it. Each lettered option may be selected once, more than once, or not at all.

Questions 13–16

For each of the following diuretic agents, choose the anatomic site in the renal nephron where the principal action of the agent occurs.

(A) Glomerulus

(B) Proximal tubule

(C) Ascending limb of the loop of Henle

(D) Distal tubule

(E) Collecting duct

13. Acetazolamide

14. Spironolactone

15. Furosemide

16. Chlorothiazide

ANSWERS AND EXPLANATIONS

1. The answer is E *[I B 3; IX A]*
A K$^+$-sparing diuretic, triamterene acts primarily in the distal nephron. The increased excretion of Na$^+$ and Cl$^-$ induced by triamterene disrupts normal Na$^+$ transport and causes a net change in electrogenic forces across the tubular membranes. This reduces the net driving force for K$^+$ secretion, resulting in decreased excretion of K$^+$. Triamterene also causes a slight increase in uric acid excretion. Triamterene is not a competitive antagonist of aldosterone. Unlike spironolactone, triamterene acts independently of aldosterone.

2. The answer is D *[II A 1, B, C; Ch 5 I D 4 c (2)]*
Cardiovascular toxicity can occur with xanthine diuretics. The cardiovascular toxicity can include palpitations, hypotension, and circulatory collapse. Being phosphodiesterase inhibitors, the xanthine diuretics increase cyclic adenosine 3′,5′-monophosphate (cyclic AMP) levels, which can cause an increase in cardiac output. If toxicity ensues, the above cardiovascular effects can occur.

3. The answer is C *[III A, D 2]*
With the use of mercurial diuretics, refractoriness does occur. Mercurial diuretics can produce a clinical metabolic picture of hypochloremic alkalosis. In an alkalotic environment, the mercuric ion will not dissociate from the drug into its active form; the result is that a refractory state soon develops, requiring use of an acidifying agent (e.g., NH$_4$Cl) to reverse the alkalosis. Ventricular fibrillation is probably the result of binding to cardiac sulfhydryl enzymes.

4. The answer is D *[IV C]*
The carbonic anhydrase inhibitor, acetazolamide, although a weak diuretic, is useful in the treatment of glaucoma and petit mal epilepsy. The high-ceiling diuretics, namely ethacrynic acid and furosemide, the thiazide diuretic, chlorothiazide, and the K$^+$-sparing diuretic, spironolactone, are not effective agents in the treatment of glaucoma or epilepsy, although they are more effective as diuretics.

5. The answer is B *[VI C]*
The thiazide diuretics are not useful in treating pulmonary tumors that secrete ADH. By decreasing the urinary volume (due to their natriuretic action), thiazide diuretics may enhance the action of ADH and have been used for the palliative treatment of diabetes insipidus.

6. The answer is E *[VI D 1; VII D 1; IX A 4 a]*
Hypokalemia is a potential complication of furosemide, ethacrynic acid, bumetanide, and hydrochlorothiazide therapy. If a patient is concurrently receiving digoxin therapy, aggravated toxicity of this cardiac glycoside can become a major therapeutic problem. Correction of the hypokalemia is essential. Amiloride is a potassium-sparing diuretic.

7. The answer is D *[VI D 1; IX; Ch 5 I B 7 b]*
Spironolactone, triamterene, and amiloride are used as adjunct diuretics for preventing hypokalemia, but they are not used for the treatment of hypokalemia once it occurs. Insulin and glucose are used for the treatment of hyperkalemia. Immediate K$^+$ supplementation with oral preparations is indicated.

8. The answer is A *[VII A 5, D; Table 6-1]*
Furosemide administration does not produce hypercalcemia. In fact, furosemide lowers plasma Ca^{2+} concentrations by increasing the renal excretion of Ca^{2+}. Hyperuricemia results because furosemide is actively secreted by the renal and biliary secretory systems. Transient deafness has occurred, particularly when another potentially ototoxic drug was given concomitantly. Electrolyte imbalance, especially hypokalemia, can be a particular problem if furosemide is administered with digitalis. Alkalosis can occur but is not refractory.

9. The answer is C *[VII C]*
The therapeutic uses of furosemide are many, including the treatment of both acute and chronic edema from such conditions as cirrhosis, renal disease, acute pulmonary edema, and congestive heart failure. Because of its efficacy in reducing edema, furosemide has also been used to treat elevated intracranial pressure (e.g., from hypertensive crisis). Furosemide is not used for the treatment of hypocalcemia; however, it is useful in treating hypercalcemia, in which it increases the renal excretion of Ca^{2+}.

10. The answer is C *[IX B]*
Reduction in serum K$^+$ levels (hypokalemia) is a common adverse effect of most diuretics. Hypokalemia greatly increases the potential for digitalis-induced cardiac arrhythmias. The K$^+$-sparing diuretics, such as spironolactone, do not produce hypokalemia and, thus, do not add to the toxic potential of digitalis.

11. The answer is C (2, 4) *[I A]*

Diuretic agents are used most commonly for the treatment of edematous states or hypertension. Both the mercurial diuretics and the carbonic anhydrase inhibitors have been replaced by more effective, more convenient, or less toxic diuretics, such as the thiazides and the high-ceiling, or loop, diuretics. The mercurials are effective diuretics, but they must be given parenterally. Carbonic anhydrase inhibitors are given orally and are considered weak diuretics. Moreover, a refractory state soon develops with both of these agents.

12. The answer is A (1, 2, 3) *[VII C 4; VIII C]*

Cerebral edema resulting in increased intracranial pressure is helped by diuretic therapy. Mannitol and urea are osmotic diuretics that reduce cerebrospinal fluid pressure. Furosemide, due to its potent edema-reducing ability, has also been used in the treatment of elevated intracranial pressure.

13–16. The answers are: 13-B *[IV A 1]*, 14-D *[IX B 1 b]*, 15-C *[VII A 1]*, 16-C *[VI A 2]*

Although acetazolamide acts on both the proximal and distal convoluted tubules, its effects on the proximal tubules are quantitatively most important for its diuretic actions. Spironolactone, a K^+-sparing diuretic, acts as a competitive antagonist of aldosterone. The receptor for aldosterone is located in the distal convoluted tubule, and thus, this is the site of action for spironolactone. Furosemide is a high-ceiling diuretic and, like ethacrynic acid, it inhibits reabsorption in the ascending limb of the loop of Henle. Chlorothiazide is one of a variety of thiazide diuretics. The thiazides, like the high-ceiling diuretics, act primarily on the ascending limb of the loop of Henle. The thiazides inhibit chlorine reabsorption and cause increased renal excretion of Na^+, Cl^-, HCO_3^-, and K^+.

Drugs Affecting Hematopoiesis and Hemostasis

I. DRUGS FOR IRON-DEFICIENCY ANEMIA

A. Physiology

1. The major portion of iron in body stores is found in **hemoglobin**.
   a. Molecular oxygen is bound reversibly by the iron in hemoglobin.
   b. The ferric state of iron (Fe^{3+}) in **methemoglobin** is less able to carry oxygen than the ferrous form (Fe^{2+}) in hemoglobin.

2. Inorganic iron in the ferrous form is most readily absorbed from the gastrointestinal tract.
   a. Men require a nutritional input of about 0.5–1 mg iron per day.
   b. Menstruating women require up to 2 mg per day.
   c. Pregnant women (especially in the last two trimesters) require 5–6 mg per day.

3. About 1 mg of iron is lost per day in the feces, sweat, and desquamated skin.
   a. Menstruating women can lose up to 30 mg of iron per menstrual period.
   b. Pregnant women can lose up to 500 mg per full-term pregnancy.

4. About 1 g of iron is stored as **ferritin** and **hemosiderin** in the bone marrow, liver, and spleen. This stored iron is available for the synthesis of hemoglobin should blood be lost from the body.

5. Internal exchange of iron is mediated by a plasma transport protein, **transferrin**. Transferrin receptors on cell membranes mediate endocytosis of the transferrin–iron complex.

B. Pathophysiology of iron-deficiency anemia

1. **Symptoms.** Depletion of body iron can be associated with fatigability, anorexia, headache, and a characteristic hypochromic, microcytic anemia.

2. **Laboratory findings.** A low plasma iron level in iron-deficiency anemia is associated with an elevated total iron-binding capacity of plasma transferrin so that the ratio of serum iron to iron-binding capacity is less than 10%:

$$\frac{\text{Serum iron level}}{\text{Total iron-binding capacity}} < 10\%$$

In other words, the serum iron carrier, transferrin, is less than 10% saturated with iron. This ratio in normal individuals is 35% ± 15%.

3. **Diagnosis.** A definitive diagnosis of iron-deficiency anemia is made by confirming reduced bone marrow iron stores.

4. **Complications.** Severe iron deficiency can cause Plummer-Vinson syndrome, which is associated with dysphagia, hypopharyngeal webs, gastritis, and hypochlorhydria.

5. **Etiology.** Iron-deficiency anemia is often caused by significant blood loss. Underlying disorders should be sought where appropriate.

C. Oral iron

1. **Preparations and therapeutic uses.** The different ferrous salt forms used in oral iron preparations have about the same bioavailability and are absorbed about three-fold better than ferric salt forms.

      a. Ferrous sulfate, containing about 20% elemental iron, is the drug of first choice for iron-deficiency anemia.

      b. Ferrous fumarate contains 33% elemental iron. It is principally used in multivitamin–mineral mixtures.

      c. Ferrous choline citrate and **ferrous gluconate** both contain 12% elemental iron.

  2. Adverse effects are related to the amount of soluble iron in the upper gastrointestinal tract.

      a. Nausea, heartburn, diarrhea, and constipation can all occur.

      b. Hemochromatosis is rare and is usually the result of an underlying disorder that augments the absorption of iron.

D. Parenteral iron is used in patients unable to take iron orally and in patients with malabsorption syndromes.

  1. Preparations. Iron dextran is the preparation used parenterally.

      a. Iron dextran is a complex of ferric hydroxide and low-molecular-weight dextran.

      b. Each milliliter of iron dextran preparation contains 50 mg of elemental iron.

      c. Reticuloendothelial cells phagocytize the iron dextran, splitting off the iron from the dextran molecule.

      d. Iron dextran delivered intramuscularly may become fixed (up to 50%) locally.

      e. Due to serious local reactions, the intravenous route is preferred. A test dose is first given over a 5-minute period to test for anaphylaxis.

  2. Adverse effects

      a. If given intramuscularly, iron dextran may cause local discomfort, discoloration, and potentially malignant skin changes. This route is, therefore, inappropriate unless the intravenous route is inaccessible.

      b. Headache, fever, arthralgias, and lymphadenopathy can occur.

      c. Anaphylactic reactions, although rare, can be fatal.

II. DRUGS FOR MEGALOBLASTIC ANEMIAS

A. Etiology of megaloblastic anemia

  1. Megaloblastic anemia is almost always caused by deficiencies of vitamin B_{12} or folic acid; however, nitrous oxide can also mimic the symptoms of vitamin B_{12} deficiency. These vitamins are essential in DNA synthesis, and thus, the high cell turnover in hematopoiesis is dramatically affected by deficiencies.

  2. The most helpful diagnostic tests are serum folate and vitamin B_{12} levels, the Schilling test for urinary vitamin B_{12} excretion, and analysis of gastric function.

  3. A characteristic morphologic feature is the abnormal macrocytic red blood cell.

B. Folic acid

  1. Daily requirements

      a. Folic acid is found in a wide variety of foods with its highest content being found in yeast, liver, and green vegetables.

      b. The minimum daily adult dietary requirement is 50 μg, although pregnant or lactating women may need 100–200 μg per day.

  2. Physiology

      a. Folic acid is completely absorbed in the proximal third of the small intestine.

      b. Folates present in food are in the reduced polyglutamate form. The mucosa of the duodenum and the upper jejunum contains dihydrofolate reductase, which methylates the reduced folate.

      c. Once absorbed, folate is transported to tissues where it is stored within cells as polyglutamates.

      d. Supplies are maintained by food intake and by the enterohepatic cycle.

      e. The urine is the major route of excretion for folates and their cleavage products.

      f. Folic acid is a precursor of several coenzymes, and several derivatives of tetrahydrofolic acid are important in single carbon atom transfers, such as the synthesis of thymidylate from deoxyuridylate.

3. Folate deficiency

  a. Folate deficiency can result from:

   (1) Inadequate dietary supply

   (2) Disease involving the small intestine

   (3) Defects in the folate enterohepatic cycle (e.g., hepatic toxicity from alcoholism)

   (4) A low concentration of folate-binding proteins in plasma

   (5) Certain drugs (e.g., methotrexate, trimethoprim, anticoagulants, contraceptives)

   (6) Normal pregnancy, which produces an increased requirement for folate

  b. Folate deficiency can result in megaloblastic anemia.

   (1) The onset is more rapid than with a vitamin B_{12} deficiency.

   (2) There is *no* neurologic abnormality associated with folate deficiency.

4. Therapeutic uses

  a. The major therapeutic use for folic acid is in the therapy of folic acid deficiency.

  b. Leucovorin calcium injection (folinic acid) is used to circumvent the action of dihydrofolate reductase inhibitors, such as methotrexate. It is not used as a treatment for ordinary folate deficiency.

5. Preparations and administration

  a. Folic acid can be given orally (or parenterally) and will usually cure an uncomplicated megaloblastic anemia resulting from folate deficiency.

  b. Folic acid injection contains the sodium salt and is principally used in acute illness. It is given by intramuscular, intravenous, or deep subcutaneous injection.

6. Adverse effects

  a. The oral form is nontoxic at therapeutic doses.

  b. Large amounts may counteract the antiepileptic action of phenobarbital, phenytoin, and primidone.

  c. There have been rare allergic reactions to parenteral administration.

C. Vitamin B_{12}

1. Physiology

  a. Vitamin B_{12} (cyanocobalamin) is a cobalt-containing compound that is synthesized by the bacterial flora in the colon. However, it cannot be absorbed there, and humans must obtain the vitamin from the dietary intake of meat and vegetables that possess B_{12}-forming bacteria.

  b. **Intrinsic factor,** a glycoprotein produced by the gastric parietal cells, is necessary for the gastrointestinal absorption of vitamin B_{12}.

   (1) Gastric acid releases the vitamin from proteins, allowing it to become complexed to intrinsic factor.

   (2) The vitamin B_{12}–intrinsic factor complex binds to ileal mucosal cell receptors, whence it is transported into the circulation.

  c. Once in the circulation, vitamin B_{12} is transported to the tissues by a plasma β-globulin, transcobalamin II.

  d. The liver preferentially stores vitamin B_{12}. A portion of the stored vitamin is secreted into the bile each day and is normally reabsorbed in the ileum.

  e. Vitamin B_{12} is essential for cell growth and for maintenance of normal myelin. It is also important for the normal metabolic functions of folate.

2. Vitamin B_{12} deficiency

  a. Vitamin B_{12} deficiency can result from:

   (1) Inadequate secretion of intrinsic factor

   (2) Intestinal disorders, including ileal disease, gastric atrophy, or surgery

   (3) An insufficient dietary supply, although this is rarely the case

   (4) Congenital absence of transcobalamin II

   (5) Interference with the reabsorption of vitamin B_{12} excreted in the bile

  b. Vitamin B_{12} deficiency can result in:

   (1) Megaloblastic anemia; although this is most common, all blood cell lines can be affected, resulting in pancytopenia

   (2) Demyelination and cell death, which can produce irreversible damage to the central nervous system (CNS)

3. Therapeutic uses
   a. The most common therapeutic use for vitamin B_{12} is the treatment of pernicious anemia (addisonian anemia). This condition is usually caused by atrophy of the gastric mucosa with achlorhydria and failure to secrete intrinsic factor.
   b. Lifetime maintenance therapy with vitamin B_{12} is required.

4. Preparations and administration
   a. If the patient lacks intrinsic factor or has ileal disease, vitamin B_{12} must be administered parenterally. Cyanocobalamin injection, a bright red solution, is administered by the intramuscular or deep subcutaneous route but never intravenously.
   b. Oral combinations of vitamin B_{12} with intrinsic factor usually produce unreliable absorption, and therefore, this approach is not recommended.

5. Adverse effects from vitamin B_{12} administration are rare.

III. ERYTHROPOIETIN FOR ANEMIA ASSOCIATED WITH CHRONIC RENAL FAILURE

A. Physiology

1. Erythropoietin is a glycoprotein hormone produced by the kidneys and released in response to tissue hypoxemia. It is a primary regulator of erythropoiesis.

2. Erythropoietin stimulates the proliferation of immature erythroid progenitor cells. These cells give rise to marrow normoblasts, the immediate precursors of reticulocytes and mature red blood cells.

3. Erythropoietin has been produced by recombinant DNA technology as a 165 amino acid glycoprotein. It contains the identical amino acid sequence of isolated natural erythropoietin.

B. Pharmacokinetics

1. Erythropoietin is administered parenterally (intravenously or subcutaneously) because it is broken down in the gastrointestinal tract.

2. The $t_{1/2}$ ranges from 5–13 hours when administered intravenously to patients in chronic renal failure.

3. The pharmacokinetics of erythropoietin are not affected by dialysis.

C. Therapeutic uses

1. Erythropoietin is indicated for the treatment of anemia associated with chronic renal failure, including patients on and off dialysis.

2. It elevates or maintains red blood cell levels, decreasing the need for transfusions.

3. It is not intended for patients needing immediate correction of severe anemia.

4. Recent data suggest that erythropoietin may also be useful for treating anemia in patients with acquired immune deficiency syndrome (AIDS) treated with zidovudine.

D. Adverse effects

1. Hypertension may occur.

2. Seizures may occur, especially during the first 90 days of treatment.

3. High doses of heparin may be needed for adequate anticoagulation during hemodialysis.

4. Antibodies to erythropoietin have not been detected.

IV. ANTICOAGULANTS FOR HEMOSTASIS

A. Heparin

1. Pharmacokinetics
   a. Heparin is a highly negatively charged mucopolysaccharide that is prepared commercially from bovine lung and porcine intestinal mucosa. Because of its highly negative charge and large molecular size, it is administered parenterally.

    b. It displays dose-dependent half-life kinetics, although the half-life may be prolonged in cirrhotic patients or patients with renal dysfunction.

    c. Heparin is metabolized in the liver by heparinase. The inactive products are excreted in the urine.

2. Pharmacologic effects

    a. Heparin prolongs the clotting time of blood, both in vivo and in vitro.

    b. Heparin prevents fibrin formation in the process of coagulation.

        (1) It increases the activity of antithrombin III.

        (2) Antithrombin III then inhibits the conversion of prothrombin to thrombin by thromboplastin.

        (3) Antithrombin III also directly inactivates thrombin.

    c. Injected heparin causes the release of tissue-bound lipoprotein lipase, which hydrolyzes the triglycerides of chylomicrons and low-density lipoproteins bound to capillary endothelial cells. This produces a clearing effect on postprandial turbid lipemic plasma.

    d. Heparin suppresses the rate of aldosterone secretion and increases the concentration of free thyroxine.

    e. Heparin slows wound healing and probably also depresses cell-mediated immunity.

3. Therapeutic uses

    a. Since heparin and oral anticoagulants reduce the rate of fibrin formation, they are primarily used in the prophylaxis of venous thrombosis. Venous (red) thrombi consist of a fibrin network enmeshed with red blood cells and platelets.

    b. The anticoagulants are generally ineffective in the treatment of arterial (white) thrombi, made up of adhering platelets. Arterial thrombi are treated with the antithrombotics and thrombolytics (see IV C).

4. Preparations and administration

    a. The prophylactic treatment of venous thrombotic disease usually involves continuous infusion of heparin, as well as intravenous bolus administration.

    b. In the preoperative use of heparin to prevent postoperative venous thrombosis and embolism, a low dose is given by subcutaneous injection. This is followed by additional intermittent subcutaneous injections.

    c. Heparin therapy is monitored by the **partial thromboplastin time (PTT)**.

        (1) The test is done at any time during continuous infusion therapy; if the heparin is given intermittently, the PTT is measured prior to an injection.

        (2) During therapy, the PTT should be twice the control value.

        (3) Once the PTT is stable, daily monitoring is performed.

    d. Intramuscular injections are contraindicated because they can cause painful hematomas.

5. Adverse effects and contraindications

    a. Hypersensitivity reactions can occur. A test dose should be given to patients with a prior allergic history.

    b. Hemorrhage due to excessive blockade of fibrin formation and interference with normal hemostasis accounts for the primary toxicity of heparin. Bleeding should be reduced by careful control of dosage.

    c. Osteoporosis may complicate prolonged heparin therapy.

    d. Transient alopecia can occur.

    e. Transient thrombocytopenia can occur in up to 25% of patients receiving heparin therapy, resulting from heparin-induced platelet aggregation; severe cases result from the formation of heparin-dependent antiplatelet antibodies.

    f. Heparin is **contraindicated** in patients who are hypersensitive to the drug. Bacterial endocarditis, active tuberculosis, recent head trauma, neurosurgery, and recent major surgery are also contraindications to the use of heparin or other anticoagulants.

6. Reversal of anticoagulant effects

    a. Often, discontinuation of heparin therapy is sufficient to correct excessive anticoagulant effects.

    b. If rapid reversal is indicated, the strongly basic **protamine sulfate** is given by slow intravenous injection. About 1–1.5 mg of protamine sulfate usually antagonizes 100 units of heparin.

B. Oral anticoagulants. Warfarin sodium is the drug of choice and is considered the prototype of the **coumarin-derived anticoagulants**.

1. **Pharmacokinetics**
   a. Racemic warfarin (i.e., the mixture of the dextro- and levo-forms) is well absorbed orally and reaches peak plasma concentrations in 1 hour.
   b. It is 99% bound to plasma albumin, which prevents its diffusion into red blood cells, cerebrospinal fluid, urine, and breast milk.
   c. It is metabolized in the liver, undergoes enterohepatic circulation, and then is excreted in the urine and feces.

2. **Pharmacologic effects**
   a. The coumarin-derived anticoagulants interfere with vitamin K–dependent synthesis of active coagulation factors II (prothrombin), VII, IX, and X.
   b. The oral anticoagulants are effective only in vivo. Their therapeutic effect is dependent on the half-lives of factors II, VII, IX, and X, and thus 8–12 hours are required for action.

3. **Preparations and administration**
   a. For warfarin sodium and warfarin potassium, the maintenance dose is determined by **one-stage prothrombin activity,** which should be about 1½–2½ times the control value. For most adults, this dosage is 5 mg/day. Once the prothrombin activity is stable, bimonthly checks are sufficient.
   b. Warfarin sodium is available in injectable form, but parenteral administration is seldom needed.

4. **Factors affecting activity**
   a. Conditions that **increase** the response to anticoagulants include:
      (1) Anything that can cause vitamin K deficiency, such as disease of the small bowel
      (2) Hypermetabolic states, such as hyperthyroidism
      (3) Debilitating states, such as congestive heart failure
      (4) Age: the older the patient, the greater the response to these anticoagulants
   b. Impaired hepatic synthesis of clotting factors can lead to an increased hypoprothrombinemic response to oral anticoagulants during hepatic disease or in alcoholic individuals. Excessively reduced levels of prothrombin will result in hemorrhage.
   c. During pregnancy, vitamin K–dependent factors are increased, resulting in a **decreased** responsiveness to oral anticoagulants. Since heparin does not cross the placenta, it is considered safe for the fetus.
   d. Table 7-1 lists the drugs that increase or decrease the response to oral anticoagulants.

Table 7-1. Drug Interactions with Oral Anticoagulants

Drugs	Effect on Response to Anticoagulant	Mechanism
Acetylsalicylic acid	↑	↓ ADP release by platelets, impairing platelet aggregation
Barbiturates, glutethimide	↓	Induce drug microsomal metabolizing system
Cholestyramine	↓	↓ hypoprothrombinemia; ↑ plasma clearance of drug
Cimetidine	↑	Unknown
Clofibrate	↑	↓ platelet adhesiveness and ↑ turnover of vitamin K–dependent factors
Disulfiram, metronidazole, trimethoprim–sulfamethoxazole	↑	↑ hypoprothrombinemia by prolonging levowarfarin half-life
Phenobarbital	↓	↑ biotransformation of coumarin
Phenylbutazone, oxyphenbutazone	↑	Impair platelet aggregation; displace warfarin from albumin
Rifampin	↓	↓ blood concentration of drug

Note: ↑ = increased; ↓ = decreased.

5. Therapeutic uses
   a. These agents are widely used in the secondary prophylactic treatment of venous thrombosis and pulmonary embolism to prevent the recurrence or extension of venous thrombus formation.
   b. Since oral anticoagulants have no effect on platelets, they are not used in the treatment of thrombotic disease in the arterial system.

6. Adverse effects
   a. Major bleeding occurs in 2% of patients while minor bleeding occurs in 5%.
   b. Warfarin necrosis is a painful erythematous patch on the skin, which can progress to gangrene. This condition usually occurs within 3–10 days of starting warfarin therapy, most frequently in women. Thrombi occur in the vasculature of affected tissue.
   c. A "purple toe" syndrome can occur 3–8 weeks after starting warfarin therapy. It is caused by cholesterol emboli from atheromatous plaques, following bleeding into the plaques.
   d. Warfarin is contraindicated in pregnancy but not for the nursing mother since it is not excreted in milk.
   e. Subdural or intracerebral hematoma is 10-fold higher in long-term patients over 50 years of age.

7. Reversal of anticoagulant effects
   a. Following discontinuation of oral anticoagulants, the one-stage prothrombin time (PT) gradually returns to normal. Oral administration of **vitamin K₁ (phytonadione)** will enhance recovery.
   b. For severe hemorrhage, phytonadione is given intravenously. The one-stage prothrombin activity will return to normal within 6–12 hours, whatever the amount of coumarin anticoagulant ingested. The phytonadione is administered slowly to avoid precipitating a hypotensive episode. Fresh frozen plasma or coagulation-factor concentrate may be needed when bleeding is severe.

C. Antithrombotic and thrombolytic drugs. Antithrombotic agents are those that prevent or reduce the formation of arterial platelet thrombi. The antithrombotic actions of **aspirin** and **sulfinpyrazone** are discussed in Chapter 9 II A 3 h and IV C 4, respectively, and those of **dipyridamole** in Chapter 5 III D 2. Thrombolytic drugs are used in acute, extensive thromboembolic disease, acting via the conversion of endogenous plasminogen to plasmin, a protease. The newly formed plasmin hydrolyzes fibrin in hemostatic plugs and degrades fibrinogen and factors V and VII.

1. General considerations
   a. Thrombotic coronary artery occlusion occurs in more than 80% of patients with acute transmural myocardial infarction.
   b. Urokinase, streptokinase, anistreplase (eminase), and recombinant tissue plasminogen activator (t-PA) promote the conversion of plasminogen to plasmin, which is fibrinolytic.
   c. The use of thrombolytic agents is contraindicated in the presence of recent stroke, craniotomy, head trauma, or brain tumor.

2. Preparations
   a. Streptokinase is a purified preparation of a bacterial protein elaborated by group C β-hemolytic streptococci.
      (1) Pharmacokinetics
         (a) Streptokinase produces an activator complex that converts plasminogen to plasmin. The $t_{1/2}$ of the activator complex is 80 minutes.
         (b) The mechanism of elimination is unknown. The complex is inactivated in part by antistreptococcal antibodies.
         (c) A loading dose of 25 mg (250,000) must be given to overcome plasma antibodies.
      (2) Pharmacologic effects
         (a) Streptokinase decreases fibrinogen levels for 24–36 hours.
         (b) Plasma and blood viscosity and red blood cell aggregation is decreased.
         (c) Intravenous administration reduces blood pressure, total peripheral resistance, and cardiac afterload.
      (3) Therapeutic uses
         (a) The primary use is for the management of acute myocardial infarction due to intracoronary thrombi. Fibrinolytics may be administered intravenously or by the intracoronary route.

    (b) Reduction in acute mortality is 20%–30% and is time-dependent with the greatest recovery rate among patients treated within 1 hour of onset of chest pain.
    (c) Left ventricular ejection fraction also improves in 3%–6% of patients.
    (d) It is also used for lysis of pulmonary emboli, deep venous thrombosis, and acute arterial thrombi and emboli not originating from the left side of the heart.
    (e) It can be used to clear occluded arteriovenous cannulae.
   (4) Adverse effects
    (a) Systemic bleeding, particularly intracranial hemorrhage, occurs in 1% of patients. Gastrointestinal bleeding occurs in 5%–10% of patients.
    (b) Hypotension may occur.
    (c) Allergic reactions, ranging from minor bronchospasm to anaphylactic reactions, are fairly common.
    (d) Reperfusion atrial or ventricular dysrhythmias may occur.
 b. Anistreplase (eminase) is a plasminogen activator approved for the intravenous treatment of coronary thrombosis. Anistreplase is an acylated inactive complex of streptokinase and human lys-plasminogen.
  (1) Pharmacokinetics. Anistreplase has a $t_{1/2}$ of 90 minutes. Slow hydrolysis of the acyl group accounts for its long half-life. It does not require a prolonged infusion.
  (2) Pharmacologic effects
   (a) After injection, the acyl group slowly hydrolyzes, producing an activator that converts plasminogen to plasmin, initiating fibrinolysis.
   (b) It breaks down circulating fibrinogen similar to streptokinase and urokinase.
   (c) Reduction in mortality and improvement in left ventricular ejection fraction is similar to that of streptokinase.
  (3) Therapeutic uses. Management of acute myocardial infarction consists of the intravenous administration of anistreplase to lyse intracoronary thrombi. Intravenous administration is more convenient because it does not require prolonged infusion.
  (4) Adverse effects
   (a) Bolus injections may produce systemic bleeding and hematoma formation at the catheter entry site (30%), intracranial hemorrhage (< 21%), and gastrointestinal bleeding (5%–10%).
   (b) Hypotension, allergic reactions, and reperfusion dysrhythmias have been reported.
 c. Tissue plasminogen activator (t-PA) is a commercial formulation of a naturally occurring thrombolytic enzyme.
  (1) Pharmacokinetics. t-PA is rapidly metabolized in the liver and excreted in the urine. The $t_{1/2}$ is only 5 minutes. After 10 minutes, 80% of the dose is cleared from the blood.
  (2) Pharmacologic effects
   (a) t-PA selectively promotes the conversion of plasminogen to plasmin in the presence of fibrin.
   (b) t-PA binds to fibrin and activates bound plasminogen several hundredfold more rapidly than circulating plasminogen.
   (c) Heparin is generally given with t-PA to maintain patency of catheters and prevent reocclusion of coronary arteries.
   (d) Reduction in mortality and improvement in left ventricular ejection fraction is similar to streptokinase.
  (3) Therapeutic uses
   (a) Management of acute myocardial infarction due to intracoronary thrombi is the primary use of t-PA.
   (b) As with other thrombolytics, treatment should be initiated as soon as possible after the onset of symptoms.
  (4) Adverse effects
   (a) Bleeding complications include:
    (i) Hematomas at the catheterization site (40%)
    (ii) Intracranial hemorrhage (1%)
    (iii) Gastrointestinal bleeding (5%–10%)
   (b) Serious allergic reactions have *not* been reported.
   (c) Reperfusion dysrhythmias have been reported.
 d. Urokinase is an enzyme produced by the kidney and found in the urine.
  (1) Pharmacokinetics. Urokinase is administered intravenously and is cleared rapidly by the liver. The $t_{1/2}$ is 20 minutes.

(2) Pharmacologic effects
   (a) Urokinase converts endogenous plasminogen to the enzyme plasmin.
   (b) Plasmin degrades fibrin clots, fibrinogen, and other plasma proteins.
(3) Therapeutic uses
   (a) Acute massive pulmonary emboli
   (b) Restoration of patency to intravenous catheters
   (c) Acute thrombi obstructing coronary arteries (It has not been demonstrated that intracoronary administration during transmural myocardial infarction results in myocardial salvage or improved mortality.)
(4) Adverse effects
   (a) Systemic bleeding, similar to streptokinase, is due to poor plasminogen selectivity.
   (b) Allergic reactions are usually mild and rare.
   (c) Fever occurs in 2%–3% of treated patients.

D. Other drugs affecting blood flow

1. Pentoxifylline, a methylxanthine derivative, is used for the treatment of intermittent claudication due to occlusive arterial disease.
   a. Mechanism of action
      (1) Pentoxifylline is thought to increase the flexibility of erythrocytes, thereby easing their passage through the capillary microcirculation.
      (2) Serum fibrinogen is also reduced, and platelet aggregation is inhibited.
   b. Pentoxifylline is metabolized by the liver and is excreted by the kidney within 24 hours after an oral dose.
   c. Adverse effects include minor nausea, dizziness, and headache.

2. Danazol, a synthetic androgen, has been found to increase serum concentrations of clotting factors VIII and IX, but long-term use in the treatment of hemophilias A and B has not proved efficacious. However, danazol has been associated with a rise in platelet count in patients with idiopathic thrombocytopenic purpura and with a rise in serum α_1-antitrypsin activity in those with α_1-antitrypsin deficiency.

STUDY QUESTIONS

Directions: Each of the numbered items or incomplete statements in this section is followed by answers or by completions of the statement. Select the **one** lettered answer or completion that is **best** in each case.

1. All of the following statements about iron-deficiency anemia are true EXCEPT

(A) menstruating females require about twice as much dietary iron as men do
(B) iron deficiency can lead to the Plummer-Vinson syndrome
(C) ferrous sulfate is the drug of first choice for iron-deficiency anemia
(D) ferrous sulfate contains more than 90% elemental iron
(E) diarrhea or constipation can occur with ferrous sulfate use

2. Correct statements about folic acid include all of the following EXCEPT

(A) it is completely absorbed in the proximal third of the small intestine
(B) the urine is the major route of excretion
(C) deficiency can be a result of inadequate dietary intake
(D) a deficiency of folic acid is usually associated with neurologic complications
(E) it is the precursor of several coenzymes

3. Folate deficiency can result from all of the following EXCEPT

(A) inadequate secretion of intrinsic factor
(B) inadequate dietary supply
(C) disease involving the small intestine
(D) low concentration of folate-binding proteins in plasma
(E) defects in the folate enterohepatic cycle

4. Vitamin B_{12} has all of the following characteristics EXCEPT

(A) it is a cobalt-containing compound
(B) it is synthesized by the bacterial flora in the colon
(C) it is preferentially stored in the bone marrow
(D) it is obtained from the dietary intake of animal products
(E) it is required for myelin maintenance

5. Vitamin B_{12} deficiency can result from all of the following EXCEPT

(A) an insufficient dietary supply
(B) inadequate secretion of intrinsic factor
(C) ileal disease
(D) excessive transcobalamin II
(E) interference with the reabsorption of vitamin B_{12} excreted in the bile

6. A patient with chronic renal failure is given erythropoietin. Adverse effects that need monitoring include all of the following EXCEPT

(A) hypertension
(B) seizures
(C) antibody production of erythropoietin
(D) increased doses of heparin for adequate anticoagulation

7. Which of the following drug and drug effect pairs is INCORRECTLY matched?

(A) Urokinase—converts plasminogen to plasmin
(B) Heparin—prevents fibrin formation
(C) Heparin—antagonized by zinc sulfate
(D) Warfarin sodium—interferes with vitamin K–dependent reactions
(E) Warfarin sodium—warfarin necrosis

8. Heparin administration would be contraindicated in all of the following situations EXCEPT

(A) active tuberculosis
(B) bacterial endocarditis
(C) certain types of surgery
(D) diffuse intravascular coagulopathy
(E) known hypersensitivity

9. The therapeutic effect of sodium warfarin is dependent on the half-lives of all of the following coagulation factors EXCEPT

(A) II
(B) V
(C) VII
(D) IX
(E) X

1-D	4-C	7-C
2-D	5-D	8-D
3-A	6-C	9-B

10. All of the following drugs, if given concomitantly with warfarin, would probably require a reduction in warfarin dosage EXCEPT

(A) aspirin
(B) barbiturates
(C) cimetidine
(D) disulfiram
(E) phenylbutazone

11. A useful thrombolytic agent that leads to plasmin activation is

(A) vitamin K
(B) heparin
(C) streptokinase
(D) aminocaproic acid
(E) aspirin

Directions: Each item below contains four suggested answers of which **one or more** is correct. Choose the answer

A	if **1, 2, and 3** are correct
B	if **1 and 3** are correct
C	if **2 and 4** are correct
D	if **4** is correct
E	if **1, 2, 3, and 4** are correct

12. True statements about folic acid include which of the following?

(1) It is a cobalt-containing compound
(2) It can be given orally or parenterally
(3) It often causes allergic reactions
(4) It can reduce the effects of antiseizure agents

13. Correct statements concerning vitamin B_{12} deficiency include which of the following?

(1) It is capable of producing demyelination and irreversible neurologic damage
(2) It is associated with a defect in folate-binding proteins
(3) It is one of two major causes of megaloblastic anemia
(4) It is treated by leucovorin administration

14. The response to a dose of an anticoagulant is often changed by concomitant administration of other drugs, which affect the dose–response by different mechanisms. Which of the following drugs and mechanisms are CORRECTLY matched?

(1) Phenylbutazone—impairs platelet aggregation
(2) Phenobarbital—induces drug microsomal metabolism system
(3) Acetylsalicylic acid—impairs platelet aggregation
(4) Glutethimide—inhibits drug microsomal metabolizing system

15. In which of the following pairs is the anticoagulant drug correctly matched with its characteristic?

(1) Heparin—is a strongly positively charged molecule
(2) Warfarin sodium—overdose is treated with vitamin K
(3) Warfarin sodium—overdose results in a shortened prothrombin time (PT)
(4) Heparin—prevents the conversion of prothrombin to thrombin

16. Correct statements about the anticoagulant heparin include which of the following?

(1) It is effective in vivo and in vitro
(2) It is antagonized by vitamin K
(3) It prolongs the partial thromboplastin time (PTT)
(4) Approximately 25% is orally absorbed

17. Substances that help to prevent or reduce arterial thrombi include which of the following?

(1) Warfarin
(2) Urokinase
(3) Heparin
(4) Aspirin

10-B	13-B	16-B
11-C	14-A	17-C
12-C	15-C	

18. In which of the following pairs is the anticoagulant drug correctly matched with its characteristic?

(1) Heparin—overdose doubles the PTT
(2) Warfarin—overdose is treated with vitamin K
(3) Warfarin—overdose results in a shortened PT
(4) Heparin—overdose is treated with protamine sulfate

Directions: The group of items in this section consists of lettered options followed by a set of numbered items. For each item, select the **one** lettered option that is most closely associated with it. Each lettered option may be selected once, more than once, or not at all.

Questions 19–21

Match each thrombolytic agent with the statement that most aptly describes it.

(A) Streptokinase
(B) Tissue plasminogen activator (t-PA)
(C) Urokinase
(D) Anistreplase

19. Slow hydrolysis of the acyl group, accounting for the longer half-life

20. Least likely agent to cause serious allergic reactions

21. Enzyme produced by the kidney

18-C   21-C
19-D
20-B

ANSWERS AND EXPLANATIONS

1. The answer is D *[I A 2, B 4, C 1 a, 2]*
Ferrous sulfate contains about 20% elemental iron. All of the other statements are true. Men require about 0.5–1 mg of iron daily, while menstruating females require up to 2 mg/day. The Plummer-Vinson syndrome is associated with severe iron deficiency and is characterized by dysphagia, hypopharyngeal webs, gastritis, and hypochlorhydria. Diarrhea or constipation, nausea, and heartburn can all occur with oral iron preparations.

2. The answer is D *[II B 2, 3]*
Folate deficiency can result in megaloblastic anemia. There is *no* neurologic abnormality associated with folate deficiency. This is in contrast to vitamin B_{12} deficiency, which produces both effects. The remaining statements listed in the question are true.

3. The answer is A *[II B 3 a (1)–(4)]*
Folate deficiency can result from an inadequate dietary supply or disease, which would affect its absorption in the small intestine. Low concentrations of folate–binding proteins in plasma can result in folate deficiency. Hepatic toxicity from alcoholism can result in defects in the folate enterohepatic cycle. Inadequate secretion of intrinsic factor can result in vitamin B_{12} deficiency.

4. The answer is C *[II C 1 a, d, e]*
Vitamin B_{12} is a cobalt-containing compound that is synthesized by the bacterial flora in the colon. However, because it cannot be absorbed there, humans must obtain vitamin B_{12} from the dietary intake of animal products, some legumes, or vitamin supplements. The liver, not the bone marrow, preferentially stores vitamin B_{12}. A portion of the stored vitamin is secreted into the bile each day and is absorbed in the ileum. Vitamin B_{12} is essential for cell growth and for the maintenance of normal myelin. It is also important for the normal metabolic functions of folate.

5. The answer is D *[II C 2 a]*
Because vitamin B_{12} is available in many dietary animal products, some legumes, and many vitamin supplements and because only minute amounts are required, vitamin B_{12} deficiency is highly unlikely to occur, except in strict vegetarians or in individuals with reabsorption defects, including those with ileal disease or with inadequate secretion of intrinsic factor. Congenital absence of transcobalamin II, the plasma β-globulin that transports vitamin B_{12}, can also result in vitamin B_{12} deficiency.

6. The answer is C *[III D 1–4]*
A patient with chronic renal failure who has been given erythropoietin should be monitored for hypertension, seizures, and the need for increased doses of heparin for adequate anticoagulation. Antibodies to erythropoietin have not been detected.

7. The answer is C *[IV A 2 b, 6 b, B 2 a, 6 b, C 2 d]*
The antidote for heparin is protamine sulfate. It is strongly basic, and 1–1.5 mg of protamine sulfate will antagonize 100 units of heparin. All of the other drugs listed in the question are correctly matched with their effects.

8. The answer is D *[IV A 5 f]*
Hypersensitivity reactions to heparin can occur, and patients with a known hypersensitivity should not be given the drug. Bacterial endocarditis, active tuberculosis, and certain types of surgery are also contraindications to heparin use. Heparin is an acceptable form of therapy for diffuse intravascular coagulation.

9. The answer is B *[IV B 2 b]*
Sodium warfarin is the prototype of the coumarin-derived anticoagulants. The therapeutic effect of this class of anticoagulants is dependent on the half-lives of factors II, VII, IX, and X, and thus, 8–12 hours are required for action. Factor V is unaffected.

10. The answer is B *[IV B 3; Table 7-1]*
Disulfiram, aspirin, phenylbutazone, and cimetidine increase the response to warfarin and other oral anticoagulants, and thus, their use would probably require a reduction in warfarin dosage. Disulfiram affects warfarin activity by prolonging the half-life of levowarfarin, and this effect increases hypoprothrombinemia. Aspirin and phenylbutazone both impair platelet aggregation. Cimetidine binds to cytochrome P-450, thereby diminishing the activity of the hepatic microsomal mixed-function oxidases. Barbiturates and glutethimide have the reverse effects on anticoagulation. These drugs reduce the response to warfarin and, thus, would probably require an increase in warfarin dosage because they induce the hepatic enzyme system that increases drug metabolism.

11. The answer is C *[IV C 2 a (1) (a)]*
Vitamin K is required for the synthesis of several coagulation factors; the coumarin-derived anticoagulants act by interfering with this function. Heparin is an anticoagulant, not a thrombolytic agent; it acts by inhibiting the conversion of prothrombin to thrombin. Aminocaproic acid antagonizes the effects of thrombolytic drugs. Aspirin inhibits platelet aggregation, thereby preventing thrombus formation, presumably through its effects on platelet cyclooxygenase. The value of aspirin as an antithrombotic agent is still under study. Thus, streptokinase is the only drug of those in the question that produces thrombolysis by plasmin activation.

12. The answer is C (2, 4) *[II B 5, 6]*
The vitamin B_{12} molecule, not folic acid, contains cobalt. Folic acid is usually given orally to correct a folate deficiency but can be given parenterally when a prompt response is important. Allergic reactions are rare. Large amounts of folic acid may counteract the antiseizure effects of phenytoin, phenobarbital, and primidone.

13. The answer is B (1, 3) *[II C]*
Vitamin B_{12} is essential for the maintenance of myelin and for normal cell growth. Neurologic abnormalities are associated with vitamin B_{12} deficiency. A deficiency of either folate or vitamin B_{12}, or of both, accounts for 95% of megaloblastic anemias. Folate-binding proteins are important for folic acid transport but are not involved in vitamin B_{12} transport. Leucovorin (folinic acid) is an antidote for the antimetabolite methotrexate but is not used to treat vitamin B_{12} deficiency, nor is it usually used for ordinary folate deficiency.

14. The answer is A (1, 2, 3) *[IV; Table 7-1]*
Both phenylbutazone and aspirin affect platelet aggregation; phenylbutazone is also capable of displacing warfarin from albumin, which increases the warfarin blood level. These two drugs, therefore, *increase* the response to oral anticoagulants, which can cause severe hemorrhage. Glutethimide, like phenobarbital and other barbiturates, induces the drug microsomal metabolizing system. This *decreases* the response to oral anticoagulants, so that higher doses are required to produce the desired anticoagulant effect.

15. The answer is C (2, 4) *[IV A 1, 2, B 3 a, 7]*
Heparin is a negatively charged mucopolysaccharide, which does interfere with the conversion of prothrombin to thrombin. An overdose of warfarin sodium is effectively treated with vitamin K; however, an overdose will result in a lengthened prothrombin time (PT).

16. The answer is B (1, 3) *[IV A 1 a, 2 a, 4 c, 6 b]*
Heparin is effective in vivo and in vitro. It is antagonized by protamine sulfate, not by vitamin K. The partial thromboplastin time (PTT) is the only laboratory test that is used to monitor the action of heparin; during therapy, the PTT should be twice the control value. Due to its large molecular size and polarity, heparin is only administered parenterally.

17. The answer is C (2, 4) *[IV A 3 b, B 5 b, C 1, 2; Ch 9 II A 3 h]*
Heparin and warfarin are anticoagulants and, thus, are ineffective in the treatment of arterial (white cell) thrombi, which are made up of adhering platelets. Heparin reduces the rate of fibrin formation and, thus, is primarily used in the prophylaxis of venous thrombosis, which consists of a fibrin network of red cells and platelets. Warfarin is used in the secondary prophylactic treatment of venous thrombosis and pulmonary embolism. Aspirin and urokinase are both antithrombotic drugs, that is, agents that prevent or reduce the formation of platelet thrombi in the arterial system.

18. The answer is C (2, 4) *[IV A 4 c, 6, B 3 a, 7]*
The PTT is the laboratory test that is used to monitor the action of heparin. During therapy, the PTT should be twice the control value. With an overdose, therefore, the PTT would be more than doubled. For rapid reversal of heparin's anticoagulant effects, protamine sulfate is given. An overdose of warfarin sodium is effectively treated with vitamin K; however, an overdose will result in a lengthened, not shortened, PT.

19–21. The answers are: 19-D *[IV C 2 b (1)]*, **20-B** *[IV C 2 c (4)]*, **21-C** *[IV C 2 d]*
Anistreplase is a plasminogen activator, which is an acylated inactive complex of streptokinase and human lys-plasminogen. Slow hydrolysis of the acyl group accounts for its long half-life.

Tissue plasminogen activator (t-PA) is a formulation of naturally occurring thrombolytic enzyme where no serious allergic reactions have been reported. Streptokinase and anistreplase have the greatest chance of causing an allergic reaction.

Urokinase is an enzyme produced by the kidney and found in the urine. It converts endogenous plasminogen to the enzyme plasmin.

8
Autacoids and Their Antagonists

I. INTRODUCTION

A. Definitions

1. Autacoids are circulating or locally acting hormone-like substances, which originate from diffuse tissues.

2. Autacoid antagonists inhibit the synthesis or the receptor interactions of certain autacoids.

B. Physiologic roles

1. The two main functions of the autacoids are to modulate local circulation and to influence the process of inflammation.

2. Many autacoids have other physiologic and pathologic functions, which are not readily understood.

3. Some autacoid antagonists have therapeutic value.

C. Major classes. Autacoids can be divided into three categories on the basis of their structure:

1. Decarboxylated amino acids: Histamine, serotonin

2. Polypeptides: Angiotensins, kinins, vasoactive intestinal polypeptide, substance P

3. Eicosanoids: Prostaglandins, leukotrienes, thromboxanes

II. DECARBOXYLATED AMINO ACIDS

A. Histamine (Figure 8-1)

1. Chemistry

    a. Biosynthesis. Histamine is derived chiefly from dietary histidine, which is decarboxylated by *l*-histidine decarboxylase.

    b. Metabolism. In humans, histamine is metabolized primarily by methylation to form 1-methylhistamine, which can undergo oxidation by monoamine oxidase (MAO) to form 1-methylimidazole acetic acid.

    c. Storage sites. Histamine is stored in almost all mammalian tissues, although its concentration varies greatly.

        (1) The **principal sites of storage** are the **lungs, skin,** and **intestinal mucosa**.

            (a) Histamine that is stored in the **mucosal cells of the stomach** can be released by mechanical stimuli, such as food and vagal stimulation. The released gastric histamine regulates intestinal contraction and gastric secretion.

            (b) In **skin and lung tissue,** histamine is thought to be important in tissue growth and repair as well as in allergic responses.

            (c) In the central nervous system (CNS), a high concentration of histamine can be found in the **hypothalamus,** where it is thought to be released as a neurotransmitter.

        (2) Histamine is stored chiefly in **mast cells**. Although some nonmast cells can store the autacoid, in most such cells, histamine is synthesized but not stored.

2. Receptor classification. Two classes of receptors mediate the action of histamine.

    a. H$_1$ receptors are responsible for the contraction of bronchial and intestinal smooth muscle, vasodilation, increased capillary permeability, and pruritus.

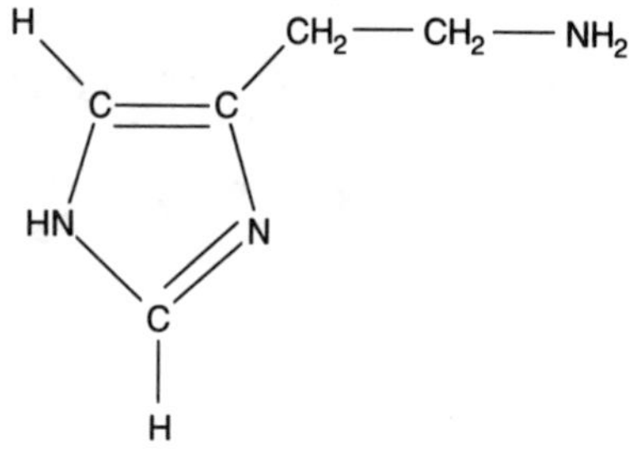

Figure 8-1. Histamine.

(1) The prototypic agonist is 2-methylhistamine.

(2) Prototypic antagonists include pyrilamine, chlorpheniramine, and diphenhydramine.

b. **H_2 receptors** principally regulate gastric acid secretion but can also cause vasodilation and inhibit neutrophil activation and T-cell cytotoxicity.

(1) Prototypic agonists include 4-methylhistamine and impromidine.

(2) Prototypic antagonists include cimetidine and ranitidine.

3. Mechanism of action

a. **Release.** Histamine can be released from storage cells by either chemical or physical insults. The mechanism is thought to involve a high intracellular calcium (Ca^{2+}) concentration.

(1) The **primary mechanism for histamine release is immunologic** during anaphylaxis and allergic reactions. Immunoglobulin E (IgE) antibody interacts with antigen on the surface of mast cells and basophils, which leads to histamine release without cell membrane disruption (immediate hypersensitivity reaction).

(2) **Enzymes, venoms, organic bases** (e.g., morphine), and **polymers** (e.g., dextran) can liberate histamine without prior sensitization by disrupting the mast cell membrane.

(3) **Tissue injury,** such as that from trauma or burns, can cause histamine release from storage sites.

b. **Inhibition of release** can occur with high intracellular levels of adenosine 3′,5′-monophosphate (cyclic AMP).

4. Pharmacologic effects

a. **Extravascular smooth muscle**

(1) The activation of H_1 receptors in smooth muscle results in **contraction**. In bronchial smooth muscle, this is seen in bronchoconstriction and decreased lung capacity; in gastrointestinal smooth muscle, this is seen in spasmodic contractions.

(a) Activation of H_1 receptors indirectly leads to increased intracellular levels of free Ca^{2+}; the Ca^{2+}, in turn, helps to regulate contraction and secretion of histamine.

(b) Contraction by H_1 receptors produces a rise in guanosine 3′,5′-monophosphate (cyclic GMP) levels.

(2) The activation of H_2 receptors produces relaxation of smooth muscle and a rise in cyclic AMP levels.

b. **Cardiovascular system**

(1) Histamine dilates the fine vessels of the microcirculation, an effect that involves activation of both H_1 and H_2 receptors.

(a) Capillary permeability is the characteristic effect of histamine on the fine vessels and results in edema.

(b) Decreased systemic blood pressure reflects capillary and arteriolar dilation.

(c) Vasodilation is most prominent in the skin of the upper body.

(d) Unilateral cluster, or histamine, headaches result from the dilation of cranial blood vessels.

(2) Histamine produces positive inotropic and chronotropic effects, which are mediated by both H_1 and H_2 receptors.

(3) An intradermal injection of histamine results in the classic **triple response**:

(a) A **reddening** at the site of injection due to local vasodilation

(b) A **wheal,** or disk of edema, due to increased capillary permeability seen within 1–2 minutes after the histamine injection

(c) A bright crimson **flare,** or halo, surrounding the wheal, which may be as large as 5 cm and may last for 10 minutes

c. **Exocrine glands**

(1) When bound to H_2 receptors, histamine becomes a potent gastric secretagogue, causing the release of large quantities of highly acidic gastric juices, pepsin, and intrinsic factor.

(2) Histamine potentiates the release of gastric acid induced by gastrin and acetylcholine.
(3) Histamine also can stimulate pancreatic and bronchiolar secretion, as well as lacrimation and salivation.
  d. **CNS.** Although the brain contains histamine, little is known about histamine's physiologic role there. Histamine does not penetrate the blood–brain barrier.

5. **Physiologic and pathologic roles**
  a. **Gastric secretion.** Histamine is a mediator of normal gastric secretion. It stimulates gastric acid and pepsin secretion by directly affecting parietal cell H_2 receptors.
  b. **Allergic reactions and anaphylactic shock.** Histamine is one of several autacoids that participate in hypersensitivity reactions. Antigenic substances cause the release of histamine when they bind to IgE molecules located on a mast cell membrane.
  c. **Inflammation.** Histamine may be responsible for the delayed vasodilation seen in inflammatory responses.
  d. **Tissue repair and growth.** A high histamine-synthesizing capacity is found in rapidly proliferating tissues, such as liver, bone marrow, and a variety of malignancies.
  e. **Neurotransmission.** Histamine may be involved in the initiation of sensory impulses for pain and itching; also, high concentrations are found in the hypothalamus.
  f. **Regulation of the microcirculation.** Histamine plays a role through its vasoactive properties.
  g. **Immunoreactivity**
    (1) H_2-receptor activation elevates levels of intracellular cyclic AMP, blocking T-cell–mediated cytotoxicity.
    (2) H_2-receptor activation can also suppress lymphocyte proliferation and the release of cytokines.
    (3) The activation of H_1 receptors on T lymphocytes inhibits suppressor cell function.

6. **Preparations**
  a. **Histamine phosphate** is injected intravenously. It has been used as a diagnostic agent for testing gastric acid secretion, but side effects (see II A 8) have limited its use.
  b. **Betazole** is an isomer of histamine with preferential effects on gastric secretion; it is 10 times more potent as a stimulator of gastric secretion than as a vasodilator. It is used as an alternative for histamine phosphate in tests of gastric function because it does not require premedication with an H_1- or H_2-receptor blocker.
  c. **Pentagastrin** is a pentapeptide that also stimulates the secretion of gastric acid, pepsin, and intrinsic factor. The gastric secretory responses are similar to those induced by histamine or betazole. It is short-acting and has few adverse effects.
  d. **Impromidine** stimulates the activity at H_2 receptors more than 10,000 times than at H_1 receptors.

7. **Therapeutic uses**
  a. Histamine and its analogs have no well-established therapeutic uses.
  b. **They can, however, be used diagnostically.**
    (1) Histamine and its analogs can be used to distinguish between pernicious anemia and other forms of anemia. The loss of the gastric parietal cells in pernicious anemia results in an inability to secrete gastric acid in response to histamine.
    (2) More selective H_2-receptor agonists, such as impromidine, can be used in tests of gastric acid secretion, as can pentagastrin, which is also used to test for achlorhydria.

8. **Adverse effects**
  a. The cardiovascular effects include vasodilation, which produces a decrease in blood pressure, flushing, and tachycardia.
  b. Skin temperature increases, and headache and visual disturbances occur.
  c. Bronchoconstriction, dyspnea, and diarrhea are caused by smooth muscle stimulation.
  d. To reduce the effects of histamine in patients not in shock, epinephrine, rather than an antihistamine, is preferred because of its fast action.

B. Serotonin (5-hydroxytryptamine, 5-HT; Figure 8-2)

1. **Chemistry**
  a. **Biosynthesis.** This autacoid is primarily derived from dietary tryptophan, which is first hydroxylated and then decarboxylated to form 5-hydroxytryptamine (serotonin).
  b. **Metabolism, distribution, and function**
    (1) Serotonin is initially deaminated by MAO to form 5-hydroxyindoleacetaldehyde and is then rapidly oxidized to the major metabolite, 5-hydroxyindoleacetic acid.

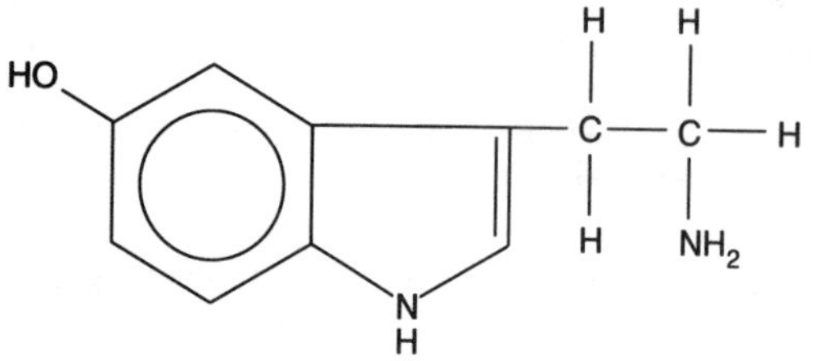

Figure 8-2. Serotonin.

    (2) Approximately 90% of the body's serotonin is found in the enterochromaffin and enterochromaffin-like cells of the gastrointestinal tract. The function of this serotonin is uncertain.

    (3) Serotonin is also found in platelets, where its function has not been established, and in the CNS, where it is believed to be involved with the regulation of temperature, sleep, aggression, pain, and mood. As a component of the pineal gland, serotonin functions as a precursor of melatonin, a hormone that may influence endocrine function.

    (4) Carcinoid tumors synthesize large quantities of serotonin.

  2. Pharmacologic effects. Serotonin, like histamine, shows wide species variations; human pharmacology is given here.

    a. Serotonin **constricts most arteries and veins,** especially in the renal and splanchnic beds, and **dilates the blood vessels** in skeletal muscle.

    b. Serotonin produces positive inotropic and chronotropic effects on the heart, but these effects may be masked by reflex responses.

    c. The effects of a serotonin injection are complex.

      (1) Initially, a brief depressor phase is seen, which is the result of a transient reflex response to serotonin and vagus nerve stimulation.

      (2) This phase is followed by an increase in blood pressure, which is due to an increase in cardiac output and a reduction in peripheral resistance.

      (3) Finally, a prolonged depressor action results from the dilation of blood vessels in skeletal muscles.

  3. Therapeutic uses. Serotonin currently has no therapeutic use.

III. POLYPEPTIDES

  A. Angiotensins

    1. Chemistry

      a. The precursor for all angiotensins is **angiotensinogen,** a plasma α-globulin.

      b. Angiotensinogen is metabolized by **renin** to form the decapeptide **angiotensin I.**

      c. Angiotensin I is hydrolyzed by a peptidyl dipeptidase called **angiotensin-converting enzyme (ACE).** This enzyme is found in large quantities on capillary endothelial cells. Its product is the pharmacologically active octapeptide **angiotensin II.**

      d. Angiotensin II is metabolized by an aminopeptidase to form a less active autacoid, **angiotensin III.**

      e. Other routes of metabolism have been observed but appear to be less important.

    2. Mechanism of action

      a. Angiotensin II acts through specific cell surface receptors located on target tissues.

      b. The precise mechanism responsible for the ultimate pharmacologic effects of angiotensin II remains unknown, but both prostaglandins and cyclic nucleotides have been implicated.

    3. Pharmacologic effects

      a. One of the major functions of the **renin–angiotensin system** is to regulate blood pressure.

      (1) **Renin,** a juxtaglomerular enzyme, controls the formation of angiotensin II.

      (2) **Angiotensin II** is one of the most potent vasoconstrictors known, being 40 times more potent than norepinephrine.

      (3) Angiotensin II produces **positive inotropic and chronotropic effects,** which are due to central and peripheral sympathetic stimulation.

      b. In addition to its centrally mediated hypertensive effect, blood-borne angiotensin II has a centrally mediated dipsogenic action.

   c. Angiotensin II also stimulates sympathetic ganglion cells and enhances ganglionic transmission. This may be mediated by increased biosynthesis of norepinephrine, decreased reuptake of norepinephrine, or increased release of the neurotransmitter.

   d. Angiotensin II stimulates the synthesis and secretion of aldosterone, but this has very little effect on blood pressure.

   e. Angiotensin II can stimulate the secretion of antidiuretic hormone (ADH) when injected intraventricularly.

  4. Therapeutic uses

   a. There are no approved clinical uses for angiotensin.

   b. Angiotensin II amide, given as an infusion, has produced a sustained pressor response, but its value in the treatment of patients in shock is controversial because the vasoconstriction that angiotensin produces can lead to decreased tissue and organ perfusion.

B. Kinins

  1. Chemistry

   a. Like angiotensin, the kinins are vasodilating polypeptides.

   b. Two enzymes called **kallikreins** catalyze the formation of the plasma kinins **bradykinin,** a nonapeptide, and **kallidin** (lysyl-bradykinin), a decapeptide, from α_2-globulin precursors called **kininogens.**

     (1) High-molecular-weight (HMW) kininogen is the precursor of **bradykinin.**

       (a) The formation of bradykinin is catalyzed by plasma kallikrein.

       (b) Plasma kallikrein is formed from prekallikrein in a reaction catalyzed by either activated Hageman factor or plasmin.

     (2) Low-molecular-weight (LMW) kininogen is the precursor of **kallidin.** The formation of kallidin is catalyzed by tissue kallikrein or by kininogens formed by complement-mediated cell lysis.

   c. Kinin synthesis and degradation show extensive **interactions** with other biochemical processes.

     (1) Hageman factor can activate prekallikrein.

     (2) Prekallikrein and HMW kininogen both activate Hageman factor.

     (3) Complement activation creates products that inhibit plasma kallikrein but promote tissue kallikrein.

     (4) Bradykinin is inactivated by ACE, the same peptidyl dipeptidase that converts angiotensin I to angiotensin II (see III A 1 c).

  2. Mechanism of action. Although the mechanism of action of kinins is not well understood, some responses may be mediated by prostaglandins resulting from the stimulation of phospholipase A_2 (see IV A 1 b).

  3. Pharmacologic effects

   a. Kinins are powerful **algesic agents;** the algetic action is mediated by a direct stimulation of nerve endings.

   b. Kinins are potent **vasodilators.** They act directly on smooth muscles of fine resistance vessels and also cause the classic triple response seen with histamine [see II A 4 b (3)].

   c. In contrast to their actions on the fine resistance vessels, plasma kinins cause **constriction** of large arteries and most large and small veins.

     (1) Kinins dilate the fetal pulmonary artery and affect the neonatal circulation by promoting closure of the ductus arteriosus and constriction of the umbilical vessels.

     (2) Kinins are capable of constricting most nonvascular smooth muscle (e.g., bronchiolar, gastrointestinal).

  4. Therapeutic uses. No therapeutic use currently exists for kinins.

C. Vasoactive intestinal polypeptide (VIP)

  1. This autacoid derives its name from the original site of isolation, but it is prevalent in both central and peripheral nerves, including those serving the pancreas.

  2. It is a potent vasodilator and a pancreatic secretagogue.

D. Substance P

  1. An undecapeptide, substance P produces vasodilation, contraction of various smooth muscles, including intestinal muscle, salivary secretion, and diuresis.

2. Substance P causes depolarization of central and peripheral nervous system neurons, an action that is believed to be responsible for many of its effects. Stimulation of the preganglionic sympathetic nerve to the adrenal medulla results in a release of substance P and acetylcholine.

3. Substance P is thought to be a neurotransmitter and, in addition, is found in enterochromaffin cells. It is secreted by enterochromaffin tumors and, thus, plays a role in the carcinoid syndrome.

IV. EICOSANOIDS

A. General considerations

1. Chemistry (Figure 8-3)

a. The eicosanoids—**prostaglandins (PGs), thromboxanes (TXs),** and **leukotrienes (LTs)**—are derived from unsaturated 20-carbon essential fatty acids, primarily **arachidonic acid,** which is a component of membrane phospholipids.

b. The release of arachidonic acid from lipid storage sites by phospholipases, most notably **phospholipase A_2,** can be initiated by a variety of physical, chemical, hormonal, and neurochemical stimuli.

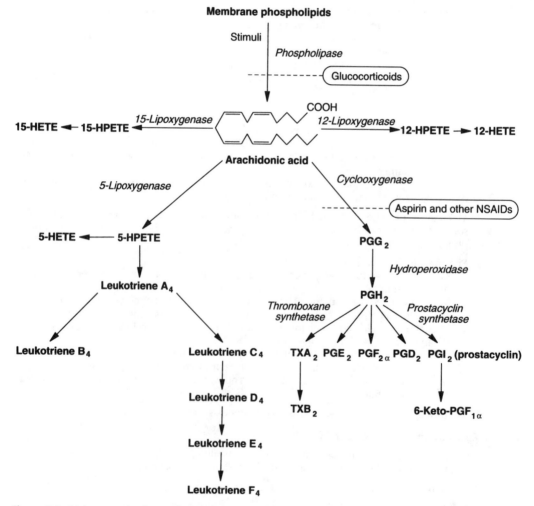

Figure 8-3. Major steps in the synthesis of eicosanoids and sites of inhibition by various agents. *HETE* and *HPETE* = hydroxy and hydroperoxy derivatives of eicosatetraenoic acid; *NSAIDs* = nonsteroidal anti-inflammatory drugs; *PG* = prostaglandin; *TX* = thromboxane. (Adapted from Zipser RD, Laffi G: Prostaglandins, thromboxanes, and leukotrienes in clinical medicine. *West J Med* 143:485–497, 1985.)

   c. Arachidonic acid metabolism follows several oxidative **pathways**.

      (1) The **cyclooxygenase** (prostaglandin synthetase) **pathway** leads to the prostaglandins and thromboxanes.

      (2) The **5-lipoxygenase pathway** leads to the leukotrienes.

      (3) Other lipoxygenase pathways lead to 12- and 15-hydroperoxy and hydroxy derivatives of eicosatetraenoic acid (12-HPETE and 12-HETE; 15-HPETE and 15-HETE).

2. Nomenclature and structure

   a. The **eicosanoids** are so named because of their 20-carbon fatty acid derivation (from the Greek *eikosi,* "twenty"). Arachidonic acid is 5,8,11,14-eicosatetraenoic acid.

   b. The **prostaglandins** are so named because early researchers identified them in seminal fluid.

   c. The **leukotrienes,** first found in **leuko**cytes, are conjugated **trienes**.

   d. The **thromboxanes** are synthesized in platelets (**thrombo**cytes) and contain an **oxane** ring rather than the cyclopentane ring of the prostaglandins.

   e. **Numeric subscripts** denote the number of double bonds in the alkyl side chain, which derives from the fatty acid precursor. **Greek-letter subscripts** refer to the type of substituent at C_9 of the cyclopentane ring.

3. The eicosanoids are ubiquitous substances. They are generally not stored but are synthesized de novo.

   a. Most are rapidly inactivated and, thus, have short-lived biologic activities.

   b. For example, 95% of PGE_2 is inactivated in the first pass through the lungs.

B. Prostaglandins (PGs)

1. Pharmacologic effects

   a. **PGG** and **PGH** cause platelet aggregation and are potent vasoconstrictors.

   b. **PGD** has mixed actions on smooth muscle, constricting interpulmonary veins and relaxing renal vasculature.

   c. **PGE** causes smooth muscle relaxation and vasodilation. It promotes edema via plasma extrusion. It inhibits platelet aggregation. It is a secretagogue for various hormones; for example, it is luteotropic (i.e., it increases luteal progesterone secretion). At low doses, PGE_2 causes uterine contractions.

   d. **PGF** causes smooth muscle contraction and vasoconstriction. It is luteolytic (i.e., it causes the corpus luteum to regress and to stop producing progesterone).

   e. **PGI** inhibits platelet aggregation, inhibits gastric and intestinal secretions, and promotes vascular and bronchial smooth muscle relaxation.

   f. Several prostaglandins serve as mediators of the inflammatory response:

      (1) Heat: PGE_1, PGE_2

      (2) Vasodilation and redness: PGE_1, PGE_2, PGD_2, PGA_2

      (3) Edema: PGE, PGI_1, PGI_2 (by potentiating bradykinin effects)

      (4) Pain: PGI_2 (hyperalgesia for 30 minutes), PGE_1, PGE_2, (hyperalgesia for 2 hours)

2. Preparations

   a. **Alprostadil** (PGE_1) is available for use in infants with congenital heart defects, to maintain a patent ductus arteriosus until definitive surgery can be performed.

   b. **Carboprost** (15-methyl $PGF_{2\alpha}$) induces second-trimester abortion. It is a more powerful uterine contractor than oxytocin. The methyl group is present to prevent oxidation.

   c. **Dinoprost** ($PGF_{2\alpha}$) **tromethamine** is used intra-amniotically to induce abortion, usually in pregnancy of longer than 15 weeks.

   d. **Dinoprostone** (PGE_2) is used in suppository form to induce abortion in pregnancies of less than 28 weeks. It is also used to induce full-term labor.

   e. **Doxaprost,** a PGE analog, may be useful for preventing bronchospasm. PGEs are more potent than isoproterenol as a bronchial relaxant, but they irritate the respiratory mucosa.

   f. **Misoprostol** (PGE_2) and numerous PG analogs (arbaprostil, enprostil, enisoprost, deprostil, rioprostil, trimoprostil) inhibit gastric acid secretion; this may be the mechanism of the gastrointestinal damage that follows exposure to nonsteroidal anti-inflammatory drugs (NSAIDs). These agents are being developed for the treatment of gastrointestinal ulceration by virtue of their cytoprotective effects on the gastric mucosa.

      (1) Misoprostol is rapidly absorbed and metabolized in the liver and excreted in the urine. It has a half-life of less than 30 minutes.

(2) When administered chronically, misoprostol can prevent gastric ulceration caused by NSAIDs.

(3) Dose-related diarrhea can occur in as many as 40% of patients taking misoprostol.

(4) Misoprostol is contraindicated during pregnancy. It causes bleeding in 40% of women and, in a lower percentage, partial or complete expulsion of the products of conception.

C. Thromboxane A_2 (TXA_2) and prostacyclin (PGI_2)

1. **Pharmacologic effects**
   a. **TXA_2** is synthesized in platelets.
      (1) It is a potent stimulator of platelet aggregation.
      (2) It is similar to angiotensin II in its vasoconstrictor effects.
      (3) It is also a bronchoconstrictor.
   b. **PGI_2** is synthesized in intact vascular endothelium.
      (1) PGI_2 is a vasodilator and bronchodilator.
      (2) It inhibits TXA_2 production and platelet aggregation by a mechanism that involves cyclic AMP.
   c. PGI_2 synthesis is believed to prevent platelet aggregation and adherence and, therefore, to help prevent thrombus formation.
   d. When a vessel wall is damaged, a hemostatic plug forms because TXA_2 is released and PGI_2 synthesis is reduced.

2. **Therapeutic uses.** PGI_2 is being studied for its ability to inhibit platelet aggregation and for its vasodilating effects. It has been used as a heparin substitute in procedures involving extracorporeal circulation, such as hemodialysis and cardiopulmonary bypass surgery.

3. **Thromboxane antagonists**
   a. **Thromboxane synthetase inhibitors** may prevent thrombus formation in thromboembolic disorders. Agents in this category include **nictindole, imidazole** and its derivatives (**dazoxiben, anagrelide, trifenagrel**), and **hydralazine**.
   b. **Dipyridamole** (see Chapter 5 III D 2) increases cyclic AMP, thereby potentiating the actions of PGI_2.
   c. **Pinane-thromboxane A_2,** a TXA_2 analog, prevents platelet aggregation and vasoconstriction. At high concentrations, it may be a TXA_2 inhibitor.
   d. The antithrombotic actions of **aspirin** and **sulfinpyrazone** are discussed in Chapter 9 II A 3 e (5) and IV C 4, respectively.

D. Leukotrienes (LTs)

1. **Chemistry** (see Figure 8-3). Leukotriene synthesis takes place chiefly in leukocytes.
   a. Signals that induce leukotriene generation include:
      (1) Anti-IgE antibody in mast cells
      (2) Phagocytosis and immune complexes in macrophages
      (3) Platelet-activating factors, released by basophils and mast cells
      (4) 12-HPETE, a platelet-derived lipoxygenase product
   b. The enzymes 5-lipoxygenase and leukotriene synthetase produce the common intermediate, **LTA_4,** which has two possible **pathways**:
      (1) To LTB_4
      (2) Via glutathione-S-transferase, to LTC_4, LTD_4, and LTE_4, the **slow-reacting substance of anaphylaxis (SRS-A)**

2. **Pharmacologic effects**
   a. **LTC_4, LTD_4, and LTE_4 (SRS-A)**
      (1) These leukotrienes are potent vasoconstrictors; their relative potency is $LTD_4 > LTC_4 > LTE_4 >>>$ histamine.
      (2) They are also potent bronchoconstrictors.
      (3) They increase the permeability of postcapillary venules.
      (4) They increase mucus secretion.
   b. **LTB_4** is chemotactic and chemokinetic: It causes leukocytes to adhere to the vascular endothelium and to extravasate.
   c. **Interactions**
      (1) LTC_4 and LTD_4 enhance the production of PGE, PGI, and TXA.
      (2) PGE and PGD enhance the chemotactic effects of LTB_4.
      (3) PGE potentiates the vascular permeability induced by LTC_4 and LTD_4.

3. Leukotriene receptor antagonists are a new class of experimental agents that may prove useful in bronchial asthma, pulmonary fibrosis, bronchitis, and bronchiectasis, renal endotoxic shock, myocardial infarction, coronary artery disease, and inflammatory diseases.

V. AUTACOID ANTAGONISTS

A. Histamine antagonists fall into **two categories,** depending on whether they block H_1 or H_2 receptors.

1. H_1-receptor antagonists are the classic **antihistamine agents**.
  a. Mechanism of action. H_1-receptor antagonists block the histamine effect on:
    (1) Bronchial smooth muscle
    (2) Intestinal smooth muscle
    (3) Small blood vessels
    (4) Sensory impulses for itching
  b. Structure and classification
    (1) H_1-receptor antagonists are substituted ethylamines (Figure 8-4).
    (2) The major classes, their substituents at X in Figure 8-4, and typical drugs of each class are shown in Table 8-1.
  c. Pharmacokinetics
    (1) H_1-receptor antagonists are rapidly and almost completely absorbed from the gastrointestinal tract, allowing effective oral administration.
    (2) The onset of action is usually within 30 minutes, and the duration of effect is between 4 and 6 hours.
    (3) Most H_1-receptor antagonists are metabolized by hydroxylation and are capable of inducing the hepatic microsomal enzyme system.
  d. Pharmacologic effects
    (1) Sedation is a common effect and may be desirable in some clinical settings. There is little correlation between antihistamine potency and degree of sedation. Alcohol consumption will greatly increase sedation.
    (2) The **anticholinergic properties** of H_1-receptor antagonists are useful in the treatment of motion sickness.
    (3) The **local anesthetic and antipruritic effects** of the H_1-receptor antagonists are due to their ability to prevent histamine-induced itching and pain in the skin and mucous membranes.
  e. Therapeutic uses
    (1) H_1-receptor antagonists are useful in the symptomatic treatment of patients with allergic conditions.
      (a) Disorders that respond include urticaria and seasonal rhinitis and conjunctivitis.
      (b) H_1 blockers are also effective for drug reactions caused by allergic phenomena.
      (c) They have an adjuvant role in systemic anaphylaxis.
    (2) H_1-receptor antagonists are ineffectual in patients with bronchial asthma.
      (a) Prophylaxis of asthma is accomplished with **cromolyn sodium,** which is neither an antihistamine nor a bronchodilator agent.
      (b) Cromolyn sodium inhibits the release of histamine and other autacoids from mast cells in the lung.
    (3) H_1-receptor antagonists are used in cough preparations.
    (4) They are used prophylactically for motion sickness and for vestibular disturbances such as Meniere's disease. The ethanolamines and piperazines are especially useful in the treatment of patients with motion sickness.
    (5) H_1 blockers are also used as somnifacients.
    (6) H_1-receptor antagonists can be used topically as well as orally for treating patients with urticaria and pruritus.
  f. Preparations
    (1) Examples of the classic antihistamine agents are given in Table 8-1.
    (2) Terfenadine is a nonsedating antihistamine.

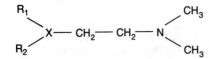

Figure 8-4. Structure of the nucleus of H_1-receptor antagonists (H_1 blockers). *X* can be nitrogen, carbon, or an ether moiety (see Table 8-1). R_1 and R_2 are cyclic structures.

Table 8-1. Classes of Antihistamine Agents (H$_1$ Blockers) and Typical Members

Class	Substituent at X*	Typical Members
Ethylenediamines	N	Tripelennamine (Pyribenzamine) Pyrilamine (Neo-Antergan)
Phenothiazines	N	Promethazine (Phenergan)
Alkylamines	C	Chlorpheniramine (Chlor-Trimeton)
Piperazines	C—N	Cyclizine (Marezine) Meclizine (Antivert, Bonine)
Ethanolamines	C—O	Diphenhydramine (Benadryl) Dimenhydrinate (Dramamine) Carbinoxamine (Clistin)
Other		Terfenadine (Seldane) Astemizole (Hismanal)

C = carbon; N = nitrogen; O = oxygen.
*See Figure 8-4.

        (a) Terfenadine is absorbed from the gastrointestinal tract, reaching maximal plasma concentration within 2 hours. Suppression of the histamine-induced wheal response lasts 12 hours.

        (b) Terfenadine is as effective as the classic agents in relieving seasonal rhinitis.

        (c) Terfenadine lacks CNS sedating and adverse anticholinergic effects.

    (3) Astemizole is a nonsedating antihistamine that is effective in the treatment of patients with chronic urticaria and seasonal allergic rhinitis.

        (a) Although rapidly absorbed from the gastrointestinal tract, absorption is decreased in the presence of food.

        (b) It dissociates very slowly from H$_1$ receptors. Astemizole and its major active metabolite have half-lives of 9 days.

        (c) Because astemizole is extremely long-acting, adverse effects could be troublesome. Serious ventricular arrhythmias have been reported with overdosage. Astemizole does not appear to be dialyzable.

  g. Adverse effects

    (1) In general, antihistamines possess a high therapeutic index. Acute toxicity is rare.

    (2) Acute poisoning due to overdosage with these agents does occur, especially in children, and the principal symptoms reflect CNS stimulation:

        (a) Hallucinations

        (b) Excitement

        (c) Ataxia

        (d) Convulsions, which precede death

    (3) With therapeutic doses, sedation is the most frequently seen adverse effect, and it can interfere with the patient's daily activities. This effect can be avoided by reducing the dose or changing the antihistaminic agent.

    (4) Other CNS effects include tinnitus, nervousness, and lassitude.

    (5) Nausea, vomiting, or other gastric distress can occur, which can be minimized by giving the agent with meals.

    (6) Atropine-like adverse effects can occur.

    (7) Allergic manifestations can occur when the drug is topically administered.

    (8) The piperazine compounds are, rarely, teratogenic.

2. H$_2$-receptor antagonists (Figure 8-5) inhibit gastric acid secretion. They have no significant action at H$_1$ receptors.

  a. Cimetidine, the prototype of the H$_2$-receptor blockers, is a substituted imidazole compound that acts as a competitive antagonist at H$_2$ receptors.

    (1) Pharmacokinetics. Cimetidine is well absorbed when administered orally, and it is rapidly excreted by the kidney. It undergoes extensive first-pass biotransformation.

    (2) Pharmacologic effects. Cimetidine inhibits all phases of physiologic secretion of gastric acid.

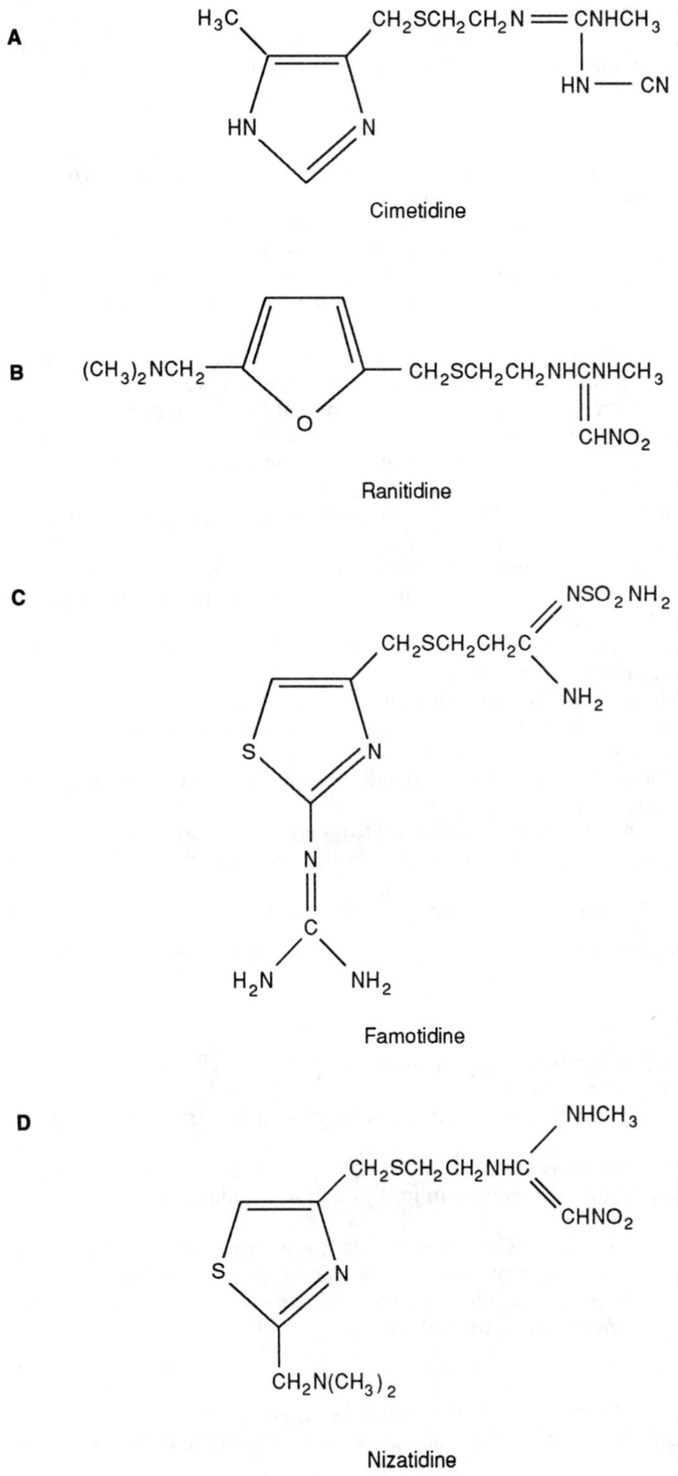

A

Cimetidine

B

Ranitidine

C

Famotidine

D

Nizatidine

Figure 8-5. Structures of H_2-receptor antagonists.

(a) The principal effect of cimetidine is to inhibit histamine-stimulated gastric acid secretion.

(b) It also inhibits gastric acid secretion induced by gastrin and acetylcholine.

(3) **Therapeutic uses.** The major therapeutic use of cimetidine is in the treatment of patients with duodenal and gastric ulcers and gastric hypersecretory states such as the Zollinger-Ellison syndrome.

(4) **Adverse effects**

(a) Generally, cimetidine is well tolerated.

(b) High doses in elderly patients, especially those with some degree of renal dysfunction, have resulted in CNS disturbances (e.g., confusion).

(c) Rarely, a weak antiandrogenic effect has been observed with very high doses, resulting in gynecomastia in men and galactorrhea in women.

(d) Cimetidine reduces liver blood flow and, thus, can markedly decrease the hepatic clearance of drugs whose metabolism is dependent on liver blood flow (e.g., propranolol).

(e) Because cimetidine reversibly inhibits the cytochrome P-450 hepatic enzyme system, a number of drug interactions have been observed. Warfarin, phenytoin, theophylline, propranolol, diazepam and phenobarbital can accumulate.

b. **Ranitidine** has a substituted furan ring.

(1) Ranitidine is 4–12 times more potent than cimetidine, and it is approved for the treatment of patients with gastroesophageal reflux disease.

(2) Ranitidine does not significantly affect the cytochrome P-450 hepatic enzyme system, but it does reduce liver blood flow.

(3) Adverse CNS effects and drug interactions have been reported.

(4) The risk of untoward antiandrogenic effects from ranitidine use appears to be minimal.

c. **Famotidine** is a thiazole derivative.

(1) Although it is most potent on a weight basis, its efficacy in patients with peptic ulcer disease is similar to that of other agents.

(2) Famotidine has a longer half-life than cimetidine or ranitidine (3 hours versus 2 hours).

(3) Pharmacodynamics and adverse reactions are similar to those of ranitidine.

d. **Nizatidine,** like famotidine, is a thiazole derivative.

(1) It has the highest bioavailability and shortest half-life (1.6 hours) of the currently available H_2-receptor antagonists.

(2) Nizatidine, like all of the currently available H_2-receptor antagonists, is principally excreted in the urine. Renal elimination involves both glomerular filtration and tubular secretion.

(3) Pharmacodynamics and adverse reactions are similar to those of ranitidine.

B. **Serotonin antagonists** are of two general classes; ergot alkaloid derivatives and phenothiazine derivatives.

1. **Methysergide**

a. **Chemistry**

(1) Methysergide is a semisynthetic ergot alkaloid congener, which lacks any intrinsic vasoconstrictor or oxytocic activity.

(2) It is a competitive antagonist of serotonin, inhibiting its vasoconstrictor and pressor effects.

b. **Therapeutic uses.** Methysergide is useful for the prophylactic treatment of migraine and other vascular headaches, but the mechanism for this action is unknown.

c. **Adverse effects**

(1) The major adverse effects seen with methysergide are gastrointestinal irritation and CNS effects, such as insomnia, restlessness, nervousness, and unsteadiness.

(2) Fibrotic changes in retroperitoneal, pleuropulmonary, and cardiac tissues are rare side effects seen after prolonged, uninterrupted use.

2. **Cyproheptadine**

a. **Chemistry**

(1) Cyproheptadine is a phenothiazine that also blocks H_1 receptors.

(2) It also has weak anticholinergic activity and possesses mild central depressant properties.

(3) It is a competitive antagonist of serotonin, blocking its vascular effects.

b. **Therapeutic uses.** Cyproheptadine is used mainly to treat pruritic dermatoses.

c. **Adverse effects** are usually mild; dry mouth and drowsiness are the most common.

C. Antagonists of the renin–angiotensin system. There are two major classes of substances that can inhibit the renin–angiotensin system: angiotensin II antagonists and inhibitors of the enzyme peptidyl dipeptidase.

    1. Angiotensin II antagonists

        a. The prototypic agent is **saralasin,** a competitive inhibitor of angiotensin II receptors.

        b. In normal individuals, the angiotensin II–receptor antagonists have partial agonist activity, resulting in both mild pressor response and increased secretion of aldosterone.

        c. In patients with malignant hypertension who are sodium (Na^+)-depleted, saralasin and congeners produce profound hypotension and decreased secretion of aldosterone.

    2. Inhibitors of peptidyl dipeptidase

        a. Captopril (the prototype), **enalapril, lisinopril,** and others of this class block the enzymatic conversion of angiotensin I to angiotensin II. Because the responsible enzyme, a peptidyl dipeptidase, is termed **angiotensin-converting enzyme (ACE),** drugs of this class are known as **ACE inhibitors.**

            (1) These agents are not angiotensin II antagonists, nor do they possess agonist activity.

            (2) They reduce systemic blood pressure in patients with increased angiotensin I levels but not in normal individuals who are in Na^+ balance.

            (3) When administered orally, these agents reduce blood pressure in hypertensive patients with high, normal, or low plasma renin levels.

            (4) Many hypertensive patients with normal renin levels respond to captopril, which suggests that other factors affecting the renin–angiotensin system (e.g., Na^+ depletion) may have a role in hypertension.

        b. These agents also increase the actions of bradykinin, since it is inactivated by peptidyl dipeptidase.

        c. They are able to depress the secretion of aldosterone by lowering angiotensin II production.

D. Eicosanoid antagonists. The sites of action of the major classes of eicosanoid antagonists are shown in Figure 8-3.

    1. Glucocorticoids inhibit the release of arachidonic acid in a number of tissues and, thus, block the production of all eicosanoids in these tissues.

        a. The effect is due to the inhibition of phospholipase A_2 by glycoproteins collectively known as **lipocortins,** produced by the steroids. One such substance is the polypeptide **macrocortin**.

        b. The consequent reduction of leukotriene synthesis may explain the efficacy of glucocorticoids in allergic disorders, such as asthma, and in inflammatory diseases.

    2. NSAIDs, discussed in Chapter 9, inhibit cyclooxygenase and, thus, inhibit the synthesis of both prostaglandins and thromboxanes.

        a. The anti-inflammatory, analgesic, and antipyretic effects of NSAIDs are attributable to the inhibition of prostaglandins, especially PGE_2.

        b. The NSAIDs vary in their cyclooxygenase-inhibiting effects because of varying effects in different tissues. For example, aspirin strongly inhibits TXA_2 but is a weaker inhibitor of prostaglandin synthesis than many newer NSAIDs.

        c. It is possible that NSAIDs promote leukotriene synthesis, by diverting arachidonic acid metabolism away from the cyclooxygenase pathway and into the lipoxygenase pathways. This might explain the allergic reactions occasionally seen with aspirin or other NSAIDs.

    3. Inhibitors of more specific sites in the arachidonic acid pathways are discussed in IV C 3 and IV D 3.

VI. AGENTS THAT REDUCE GASTRIC ACIDITY

    A. Sucralfate is a complex substance formed from a sulfated disaccharide and polyaluminum hydroxide. It polymerizes when the pH falls below 4.

        1. The condensed polymer forms a gel, which adheres to the base of a duodenal ulcer crater.

        2. When sucralfate is administered before meals, it is effective for the treatment of patients with duodenal ulcer disease.

        3. Adverse reactions are minimal because it is not systemically absorbed.

B. H$^+$,K$^+$-ATPase inhibitors. Omeprazole is the prototype of the benzimidazole sulfoxide prodrugs that diffuse across the gastric parietal cell cytoplasm, where they are protonated. It binds to parietal cell H$^+$,K$^+$-ATPase, inhibiting secretion of hydrogen ions into the gastric lumen.

1. Omepraxole is unstable in acid and is formulated in gelatin capsules. It is metabolized in the liver and excreted in the bile and urine.

2. By irreversibly inhibiting parietal cell H$^+$,K$^+$-ATPase and preventing the secretion of hydrogen ions into the gastric lumen, the drug appears to be more effective than ranitidine for treatment of patients with gastroesophageal reflux. It is also effective in the treatment of Zollinger-Ellison syndrome.

3. Omeprazole inhibits the oxidative metabolism of phenytoin, diazepam, and other drugs.

4. Although the incidence of adverse effects is low, toxicologic studies using high doses of omeprazole have demonstrated gastric carcinoid tumors in rats. Intense acid suppression leads to increased gastrin secretion, which has a trophic effect on gastric mucosa.

STUDY QUESTIONS

Directions: Each of the numbered items or incomplete statements in this section is followed by answers or by completions of the statement. Select the **one** lettered answer or completion that is **best** in each case.

1. Which of the following effects might be observed in a patient who is accidentally given an overdose of histamine while being tested for achlorhydria?

(A) Severe localized blanching of the skin
(B) Decreased capillary permeability
(C) Bronchoconstriction
(D) Relaxation of gastrointestinal smooth muscle
(E) Gastric acid suppression

2. Physiologic and pathologic roles for histamine include all of the following EXCEPT

(A) it inhibits gastric acid secretion
(B) it participates in hypersensitivity reactions
(C) it is involved in the inactivation of sensory impulses for itching
(D) it participates in the regulation of microcirculation
(E) it may be responsible for delayed vasodilation seen in inflammatory responses

3. Terfenadine is a selective H_1-receptor antagonist. Its greatest advantage over other H_1-receptor antagonists is that it

(A) is more effective in relieving seasonal rhinitis
(B) is better absorbed when given orally
(C) is less sedating
(D) has a more rapid onset of action
(E) has a much longer duration of action

4. A young child who ingests a fatal dose of dimenhydrinate will most likely die from

(A) renal dysfunction
(B) general CNS stimulation with convulsions
(C) bronchospasm and suffocation
(D) anaphylactic shock
(E) severe cardiac arrhythmia

5. Which prostaglandin agent is approved for prevention of gastric ulceration caused by NSAIDs?

(A) Dinoprostone
(B) Carboprost
(C) Misoprostol
(D) Alprostadil
(E) Doxaprost

6. True statements concerning the classic antihistamines (H_1-receptor antagonists) include all of the following EXCEPT

(A) they block histamine receptors on bronchial and intestinal smooth muscle
(B) they are substituted ethylamines
(C) they may induce hepatic microsomal enzymes
(D) overdosage in children may cause death following generalized convulsions
(E) they effectively treat bronchial asthma

7. H_2-receptor blockers have all of the following effects EXCEPT

(A) they inhibit gastric acid secretion
(B) they decrease the liver blood flow
(C) they can cause gynecomastia
(D) they are highly toxic
(E) they are used to treat patients with duodenal and peptic ulcers

8. Specific leukotriene receptor antagonists that could selectively inhibit LTC_4, LTD_4, and LTE_4 would produce all of the following pharmacologic effects EXCEPT

(A) vasodilation
(B) bronchodilation
(C) decreased permeability of postcapillary venules
(D) increased mucus secretion

1-C	4-B	7-D
2-A	5-C	8-D
3-C	6-E	

Directions: Each item below contains four suggested answers of which **one or more** is correct. Choose the answer

  A if **1, 2, and 3** are correct
  B if **1 and 3** are correct
  C if **2 and 4** are correct
  D if **4** is correct
  E if **1, 2, 3, and 4** are correct

9. True statements concerning the autacoids include which of the following?

(1) Histamine and serotonin are decarboxylated amino acids
(2) Antagonists of serotonin have not been found
(3) Angiotensin II is formed from angiotensin I by an enzyme in vascular tissue
(4) Prostaglandins are found only in reproductive organs

10. Correctly matched autacoids and their clinical uses include which of the following?

(1) Angiotensin II—diagnosis of gout
(2) Histamine—diagnosis of pernicious anemia
(3) Serotonin—peripheral vascular disease
(4) $PGF_{2\alpha}$—therapeutic abortion

11. Which of the following classes of prostaglandins can produce both platelet aggregation and potent vasoconstriction?

(1) PGF
(2) PGG
(3) PGI
(4) PGH

12. PGI_2 has which of the following properties?

(1) It is a vasodilator
(2) It is a bronchodilator
(3) It inhibits platelet aggregation
(4) It promotes TXA_2 production

13. True statements about the antihypertensive agents enalapril and captopril include which of the following?

(1) Both enalapril and captopril inhibit peptidyl dipeptidase
(2) Both agents are angiotensin II antagonists
(3) Both agents reduce blood pressure in hypertensive patients with normal renin levels
(4) Both agents reduce blood pressure in normotensive individuals

14. True statements about the effects of H_1-receptor blockers include which of the following?

(1) They increase the heart rate
(2) Their effects usually last 4–6 hours
(3) They decrease gastric secretion
(4) They cause sedation

Directions: Each group of items in this section consists of lettered options followed by a set of numbered items. For each item, select the **one** lettered option that is most closely associated with it. Each lettered option may be selected once, more than once, or not at all.

Questions 15–18

Match each of the following autacoid antagonists to the enzyme that it inhibits.

(A) Cyclooxygenase
(B) Peptidyl dipeptidase
(C) Phospholipase
(D) Thromboxane synthetase
(E) Cystathionine synthetase

15. Captopril

16. Hydralazine

17. Ibuprofen

18. Prednisolone

Questions 19–21

Match each agent with the statement that is most closely associated with it.

(A) Sucralfate
(B) Omeprazole
(C) Cimetidine
(D) Ranitidine

19. This agent is a H_2-receptor antagonist that does not significantly affect the cytochrome P-450 hepatic enzyme system.

20. This agent acts by binding to parietal cell H^+,K^+-ATPase.

21. This agent polymerizes when the pH falls below 4.

15-B   18-C   21-A
16-D   19-D
17-A   20-B

ANSWERS AND EXPLANATIONS

1. The answer is C *[II A 4 a (1), 8]*
Bronchoconstriction would be the most prominent adverse effect. The overdose of histamine would increase capillary permeability, stimulate gastrointestinal smooth muscle, and stimulate gastric acid secretion. Vasodilation and increased skin temperature would also occur.

2. The answer is A *[II A 5 a]*
Histamine stimulates gastric acid and pepsin secretion by directly affecting parietal cell H_2 receptors. All of the other roles listed in the question are true physiologic and pathologic roles for histamine.

3. The answer is C *[V A 1 f (2)]*
Terfenadine is a nonsedating antihistamine agent. It is absorbed from the gastrointestinal tract, and its duration of action and effectiveness are comparable to those of the classic antihistamines. Its greatest advantage is that it does not penetrate the CNS, and thus, it is considerably less sedating than the classic agents.

4. The answer is B *[V A 1 g]*
Dimenhydrinate is a "classic" antihistaminic agent—a H_1-receptor antagonist. A toxic dose of dimenhydrinate would result in generalized CNS stimulation with convulsions. Renal dysfunction is not a side effect of H_1-receptor antagonists. Bronchospasm, suffocation, and cardiac arrhythmias are also not adverse effects seen with acute poisoning. Allergic manifestations may be observed with topical application of the drug, but these are not severe enough to constitute anaphylactic shock and would not be lethal.

5. The answer is C *[IV B 2]*
Misoprostol, when administered chronically, can prevent gastric ulceration produced by NSAIDs. Dinoprostone and carboprost are used for abortion. Alprostadil has been used to maintain patent ductus arteriosus. Doxaprost may be useful for preventing bronchospasm.

6. The answer is E *[V A 1 a, b, c (3), e (2), g (2)]*
The classic antihistamines are substituted ethylamines. They block histamine receptors on bronchial, intestinal, and microvascular smooth muscle. They may induce hepatic microsomal enzymes. Therapeutic doses produce CNS depression, but convulsions and death can occur with toxic doses, especially in children. H_1-receptor antagonists are useful in the symptomatic treatment of patients with allergic conditions, but they are ineffective in patients with bronchial asthma.

7. The answer is D *[V A 2 a]*
H_1-receptor blockers act by inhibiting gastric acid secretion and, therefore, are used to treat patients with duodenal and peptic ulcers. They can decrease the liver blood flow, and they have a weak antiandrogenic effect that can cause gynecomastia in men. Ranitidine appears to have less of an antiandrogenic effect than cimetidine has. These agents are well tolerated and have a low incidence of adverse effects.

8. The answer is D *[IV D 2]*
The leukotrienes LTC_4, LTD_4, and LTE_4 collectively are the slow-reacting substance of anaphylaxis and are associated with vasoconstriction, bronchoconstriction, increased permeability of postcapillary venules, and increased mucus secretion. Specific leukotriene receptor antagonists could potentially reverse these pharmacologic actions.

9. The answer is B (1, 3) *[I C 1; III A 1; IV A 3, B; V B]*
Histamine and serotonin are decarboxylated amino acids. Antagonists of serotonin include methysergide and cyproheptadine. Angiotensin II is formed from angiotensin I by ACE, found on the inner surface of blood vessels. Prostaglandins are found in almost every tissue.

10. The answer is C (2, 4) *[II A 6, B 3; III A 4; IV B 2 b]*
Histamine, betazole, and pentagastrin are capable of stimulating gastric acid secretion and are useful diagnostically to distinguish between pernicious anemia, in which parietal cells are nonfunctioning, and other forms of anemia. Serotonin and angiotensin II have no current clinical use. $PGF_{2\alpha}$ is used to achieve therapeutic abortion because of its ability to cause contraction of uterine smooth muscle.

11. The answer is C (2, 4) *[IV B 1, C 1]*
PGG and PGH are endoperoxides. They cause platelet aggregation and are potent vasoconstrictors. PGF also is a vasoconstrictor; it is also luteolytic. By contrast, PGI is an inhibitor of platelet aggregation and a vasodilator, and helps to prevent thrombus formation.

12. The answer is A (1, 2, 3) *[IV C 1, 2]*
PGI_2 (prostacyclin) inhibits TXA_2 production. TXA_2 stimulates platelet aggregation and causes vasoconstriction and bronchoconstriction, whereas PGI_2 has the opposite effects. PGI_2 has been studied for its clinical value in preventing thrombus formation because of its ability to prevent platelet aggregation and adherence. PGI_2 has also been used as a heparin substitute in extracorporeal circulation procedures. In addition to its effects on platelets, PGI_2 is also a vasodilator and bronchodilator.

13. The answer is B (1, 3) *[V C 2; Ch 5 IV I 1]*
Both enalapril and captopril are ACE inhibitors; that is, they block the enzyme peptidyl dipeptidase, preventing the conversion of angiotensin I to angiotensin II. They are not angiotensin II antagonists. ACE inhibitors serve as indirect vasodilators by reducing the level of angiotensin II, a vasoconstrictor, and also by increasing the level of bradykinin, a vasodilator, because bradykinin is degraded by peptidyl dipeptidase. ACE inhibitors reduce blood pressure in hypertensive patients with high, normal, or low plasma renin levels; the reason is not yet known. ACE inhibitors do not affect blood pressure in normal persons who are in Na^+ balance.

14. The answer is C (2, 4) *[V A 1 c, d]*
The effects of H_1-receptor blockers usually begin within 30 minutes and last from 4–6 hours. H_1 blockers have minimal cardiac effects. As a class, the H_1 blockers do not alter gastric secretion, since this is primarily mediated by H_2 receptors. H_1 blockers are capable of producing sedation.

15–18. The answers are: 15-B *[V C 2]*, **16-D** *[IV C 3 a]*, **17-A** *[V D 2]*, **18-C** *[V D 1 a]*
Captopril belongs to the class of drugs known as ACE inhibitors because they inhibit peptidyl dipeptidase, the ACE that normally converts angiotensin I to angiotensin II. The autacoid angiotensin II is a potent vasoconstrictor that raises blood pressure, and thus, ACE inhibitors are used clinically to treat hypertension.

Hydralazine inhibits thromboxane synthetase, the enzyme involved in the formation of thromboxanes from PGH. TXA_2 is, like angiotensin II, a potent vasoconstrictor, and hydralazine is used clinically as an antihypertensive vasodilator.

Ibuprofen is a NSAID. These agents act by inhibiting cyclooxygenase, and thus, they inhibit the synthesis of both prostaglandins and thromboxanes. Several prostaglandins serve as mediators of the inflammatory response. Some NSAIDs inhibit 15-lipoxygenase as well as cyclooxygenase, and aspirin, by inhibiting platelet cyclooxygenase, also interrupts the thromboxane synthetase pathway.

Prednisolone and other glucocorticoids inhibit phospholipase in a number of tissues, thereby blocking all eicosanoid formation in these tissues. Thus, glucocorticoids block the synthesis of prostaglandins, leukotrienes, and thromboxanes, which probably explains their potent anti-inflammatory effects. Moreover, since leukotrienes play a role in hypersensitivity reactions, their suppression may explain the efficacy of glucocorticoids in allergic disorders.

19–21. The answers are: 19-D *[V A 2 a (4)]*, **20-B** *[VI B]*, **21-A** *[VI A]*
Cimetidine is the prototype of the H_2-receptor blockers. Cimetidine, unlike ranitidine, significantly inhibits the cytochrome P-450 hepatic enzyme system.

Omeprazole is the prototype of the benzimidazole sulfoxide prodrugs that diffuse across the gastric parietal cell cytoplasm, where they are pronated. By binding to H^+,K^+-ATPase, it inhibits secretion of hydrogen ions into the gastric lumen.

Sulcralfate is a complex substance formed from sulfated disaccharide and polyaluminum hydroxide. It polymerizes when the pH falls below 4. The polymer adheres to the base of the duodenal ulcer crater.

9

Non-Narcotic Analgesics, Nonsteroidal Anti-Inflammatory Drugs, and Drugs Used in the Treatment of Gout

I. INTRODUCTION. This chapter discusses drugs that are anti-inflammatory, analgesic, and antipyretic; their mechanisms of action differ from anti-inflammatory steroids or narcotic analgesics. Agents that modify the progression of rheumatoid arthritis and agents used in the treatment of gout are also considered.

A. Nonsteroidal anti-inflammatory drugs (NSAIDs) may be subdivided into salicylate (e.g., aspirin) and nonsalicylate (e.g., ibuprofen) categories.

1. Aspirin and most NSAIDs exert their anti-inflammatory and analgesic action via inhibition of prostaglandin (PG) biosynthesis (Figure 9-1).

2. By inhibiting the **cyclooxygenase** enzyme, these agents inhibit the formation of PGE_2, PGI_2, and $PGF_{2\alpha}$, which are putative mediators of vasodilation, pain, and edema associated with inflammation (see Chapter 8 IV B 1 f).

3. **Thromboxane A_2 (TXA_2)** formation is also inhibited, which is clinically evidenced by prolonged bleeding times (see II A 3 h). This reduced thrombus formation becomes clinically significant in the postmyocardial infarction patient; an aspirin regimen has been demonstrated to increase long-term survival.

4. Some commonly used NSAIDs are:
   a. Aspirin and other salicylates (e.g., diflunisal)
   b. Acetaminophen
   c. Indomethacin and sulindac
   d. Mefenamic acid and meclofenamate
   e. Tolmetin
   f. Propionic acid derivatives
      (1) Ibuprofen
      (2) Naproxen
      (3) Fenoprofen
      (4) Ketoprofen
      (5) Flurbiprofen
   g. Piroxicam
   h. Diclofenac
   i. Etodolac
   j. Nabumetone
   k. Phenylbutazone

B. Disease-modifying antirheumatic drugs (DMARDs) are agents typically used in conjunction with an NSAID regimen to treat rheumatoid arthritis.

1. Gold compounds (e.g., aurothioglucose, gold sodium thiomalate, auranofin)

2. Hydroxychloroquine

3. Methotrexate

4. Penicillamine

5. Azathioprine and cyclophosphamide

6. Sulfasalazine

7. Corticosteroids (intra-articular injection)

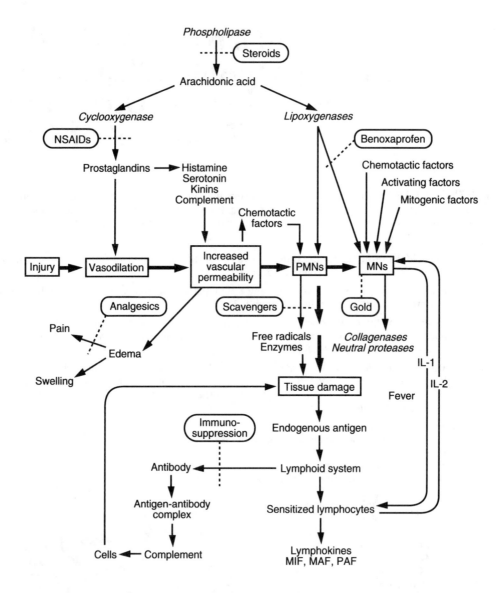

Figure 9-1. The events of the inflammatory response and mechanisms of anti-inflammatory agents. *IL-1* = interleukin-1; *IL-2* = interleukin-2; *MAF* = macrophage activating factor; *MIF* = migration inhibiting factor; *MNs* = macrophages; *NSAIDs* = nonsteroidal anti-inflammatory drugs; *PAF* = platelet activating factor; *PMNs* = polymorphonuclear leukocytes. [Adapted from Sedgwick AD, Willoughby DA: Initiation of the inflammatory response and its prevention. In *The Pharmacology of Inflammation (Handbook of Inflammation,* vol 5). Edited by Bonta IL, Bray MA, Parnham MJ. New York, Elsevier, 1985, p 40.]

C. Drugs used in the treatment of gout

1. Phenylbutazone

2. Probenecid

3. Sulfinpyrazone

4. Colchicine

5. Allopurinol

6. Certain NSAIDs

II. NONSTEROIDAL ANTI-INFLAMMATORY DRUGS (NSAIDs)

A. Aspirin (acetylsalicylic acid) and other salicylates

1. **Chemistry.** Aspirin was first isolated in 1829 by Leroux from willow bark, yielding a bitter glycoside called **salicin,** a white crystalline substance (Figure 9-2). It is stable in dry air but hydrolyzes to salicylic and acetic acids in moist air.

2. **Pharmacokinetics**
   a. Oral absorption of salicylates is fairly rapid with appreciable blood levels appearing within 30 minutes and peaking at about 2 hours.
   b. Upon oral administration of the salicylates, a portion is rapidly absorbed from the stomach. Most of an orally ingested salicylate dose, however, is absorbed from the upper portion of the small intestine.
   c. Once absorbed, the salicylates are distributed throughout the body by a pH-dependent passive diffusion process.
   d. Most of the salicylates bind avidly to serum proteins. Aspirin binds to a lesser extent.
   e. Biotransformation of salicylates occurs in the microsomal drug-metabolizing system, and the following metabolic products are seen in the urine: salicyluric acid (75%), phenolic glucuronide (10%), acyl glucuronide (5%), and free salicylic acid (10%).
   f. **Alkalinization of the urine** (pH 8) significantly increases the excretion of salicylates because of increased ionization and decreased reabsorption through the renal tubules.
   g. Rectal absorption of the salicylates is slow and unpredictable.

3. **Pharmacologic effects**
   a. **Antipyretic action**
      (1) Aspirin is rapidly effective in febrile patients, yet has little effect on normal body temperature, suggesting that prostaglandins have little influence on normal homeostatic mechanisms for body temperature.
      (2) The antipyretic action is centrally mediated; the central nervous system (CNS) action is thought to be due to inhibited PGE_2 synthesis from the hypothalamus in response to an endogenous pyrogen.
      (3) **Hyperpyrexia** can occur in salicylate toxicity, but this is partially the result of an increase in oxygen consumption and metabolic rate.
   b. **Anti-inflammatory effects**
      (1) Salicylates, and NSAIDs in general, are anti-inflammatory due to the inhibition of prostaglandin synthesis (see Figure 9-1); however, there is a wide range of potency.
      (2) The primary clinical application is in the treatment of **musculoskeletal disorders,** such as rheumatoid arthritis, osteoarthritis, and ankylosing spondylitis.
      (3) While these agents may provide symptomatic relief from pain or joint stiffness, occult joint damage may still occur to the point of necessitating an additional regimen of a DMARD.
   c. **Analgesic effects**
      (1) The analgesia is usually effective for low-to-moderate intensity pain; integumental pain is relieved better than pain from hollow visceral areas.
      (2) Relief of pain occurs through both **peripheral** and **central mechanisms**.
         (a) Peripherally, the salicylates inhibit the synthesis of prostaglandins in inflamed tissues, thus preventing the sensitization of pain receptors to both mechanical and chemical stimuli.
         (b) Centrally, the analgesic site exists in close proximity to the antipyretic region in the hypothalamus. The analgesia produced by the salicylates is not associated with mental alterations, such as hypnosis or changes in sensation other than pain.
   d. **Respiratory effects**
      (1) Salicylates stimulate respiration directly and indirectly; oxygen consumption and carbon dioxide production are increased, particularly in skeletal muscle. This effect appears to be mediated by a salicylate-induced uncoupling of oxidative phosphorylation.

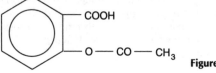

Figure 9-2. Acetylsalicylic acid.

(2) The increased carbon dioxide production stimulates respiration, but this is characterized by deep respirations rather than an increase in respiratory rate.

(3) High doses result in medullary stimulation, leading to hyperventilation and a respiratory alkalosis. Compensation rapidly occurs because the kidney is able to increase the excretion of bicarbonate, producing a **compensated respiratory alkalosis**.

(4) Toxic doses or very prolonged salicylate administration can depress the medulla, resulting in an **uncompensated respiratory acidosis**. Since renal bicarbonate excretion is elevated and since the salicylates cause the accumulation of organic acids, a **metabolic acidosis** also results.

e. **Cardiovascular effects**
(1) Therapeutic doses of salicylates have no significant cardiovascular effect.
(2) Large doses may cause peripheral vasodilation due to a direct effect on smooth muscle.
(3) Toxic doses depress circulation directly and by central vasomotor paralysis.
(4) **Noncardiogenic pulmonary edema** may also occur in older patients on long-term salicylate therapy.
(5) The **prophylactic use** of aspirin to reduce **thromboembolic events** in coronary and cerebral circulation has widened. Clinical studies have demonstrated long-term survival and reduced frequency of second myocardial infarctions.

f. **Gastrointestinal effects**
(1) Salicylates can cause epigastric distress, nausea, and vomiting due to **irritation of the gastric mucosal lining** and **stimulation of the chemoreceptor trigger zone (CTZ)** in the CNS.
(2) Salicylates, and NSAIDs in general, may cause a dose-related gastric ulceration, bleeding, exacerbation of peptic ulcer symptoms, and erosive gastritis.
(3) PGI_2, or prostacyclin, has a cytoprotective effect, particularly for gastric mucosal cells. PGI_2 has been shown to inhibit gastric acid secretion. This cytoprotection is reduced by salicylates.
(4) Salicylate-induced gastric bleeding is painless and may lead to an **iron-deficiency anemia**.

g. **Hepatic effects**
(1) Salicylates can produce at least two forms of hepatic injury.
    (a) One form is dose-dependent and usually occurs in patients with connective tissue disorders.
    (b) Usually, asymptomatic, elevated plasma transaminase levels (i.e., SGOT and SGPT) are the key indication of hepatic insult.
    (c) Salicylate-related hepatic damage is usually anicteric, mild, and reversible after discontinuation of therapy.
(2) A second form of salicylate-induced hepatic injury is more severe and associated with the encephalopathy seen in **Reye's syndrome**.
    (a) This rare, and often fatal, disorder can occur with infection from varicella (chickenpox) virus and influenza virus.
    (b) **Use of salicylates in children with chickenpox or influenza is contraindicated.**

h. **Hematologic effects**
(1) Aspirin has no effect on leukocyte count, hemoglobin, or hematocrit at therapeutic doses.
(2) There is, however, a prolongation of bleeding time with doses as small as 300 mg of aspirin.
(3) Because it can acetylate and inactivate cyclooxygenase, aspirin has important effects on the delicate balance that exists between the initiation and the inhibition of **platelet aggregation**.
    (a) Platelets are ordinarily nonadherent. However, vascular injury and exposure to subendothelial structures result in activation of the platelet cyclooxygenase enzyme system, leading to the production of TXA_2, via thromboxane synthetase. TXA_2 is capable of inducing platelet aggregation.
    (b) Concurrently opposing this physiologic process is the cyclooxygenase and prostacyclin synthetase enzyme system of the vascular endothelium. Instead of thromboxane synthetase, vascular endothelial cells contain a prostacyclin synthetase, which converts the cyclooxygenase products PGG_2 and PGH_2 to PGI_2, a potent inhibitor of platelet clumping.

       (c) It is thought that aspirin in appropriate doses can preferentially inhibit the platelet cyclooxygenase system, blocking the formation of TXA_2 and thereby suppressing platelet clumping.

       (d) By inhibiting initial platelet aggregation to subendothelial structures, aspirin also prevents the secondary release of adenosine diphosphate (ADP) from platelet granules, a process that normally occurs when platelets clump. ADP release ordinarily brings about additional waves of platelet aggregation, leading to thrombus formation. This effect persists 4–7 days after the drug has been discontinued.

    (4) In doses greater than 6 g/day, aspirin may reduce plasma prothrombin levels.

    (5) Because of its effects on the blood, aspirin should be avoided in patients with severe hepatic disease, hypoprothrombinemia, vitamin K deficiency, or hemophilia.

i. Renal effects

    (1) Salicylates can cause salt and water retention, increasing circulating plasma volume (about 20%) in patients taking large doses.

    (2) In patients with congestive heart failure, impaired renal function, or hypovolemia, salicylates can further exacerbate renal dysfunction.

    (3) The vasodilatory effects of PGI_2 on renal blood flow (and now glomerular filtration rate) may be more critical during impaired renal function.

    (4) Salicylates also affect uric acid secretion, but the effect is dose-dependent: Low doses may decrease urate excretion while large doses may induce uricosuria.

    (5) Small doses of salicylates may be enough to block the uricosuric action of probenecid and other agents that decrease tubular reabsorption of uric acid. Salicylates should not be used concomitantly with uricosuric agents in the treatment of gout (see IV F 3).

j. Metabolic effects

    (1) The salicylates uncouple oxidative phosphorylation.

    (2) Large doses of the salicylates can produce hyperglycemia, glycosuria, and deplete liver and muscle glycogen.

    (3) Aspirin, like other salicylates, can reduce lipogenesis by blocking the incorporation of acetates into fatty acids.

    (4) Toxic doses can cause significant nitrogen loss, characterized by aminoaciduria.

k. Endocrine effects

    (1) The salicylates, in very large doses, can cause stimulation of steroid secretion by the adrenal cortex. This effect is mediated through action on the hypothalamus.

    (2) Long-term salicylate therapy can decrease thyroidal uptake and clearance of iodine and can increase oxygen metabolism and the rate of disappearance of triiodothyronine (T_3) and thyroxine (T_4) from the circulation. These effects are probably due to a competitive displacement of iodinated proteins from plasma proteins by salicylates.

    (3) The salicylates may prolong the gestational period during pregnancy. This may be due to a delay in the onset of labor caused by the inhibition of prostaglandin synthesis in the uterus, since prostaglandins are believed to be involved in eliciting uterine contractions.

4. Therapeutic uses

  a. The salicylates are used in restricted situations for the symptomatic relief of fever.

    (1) They have no effect on the underlying cause of a fever, and since the hyperthermic response in an illness may be a normal protective physiologic mechanism, they should not be used routinely or trivially for this purpose.

    (2) Because of an increased incidence of Reye's syndrome in children who previously have been given aspirin for the relief of viral fevers, it is now recommended that a child with any fever be given acetaminophen instead, if medication is required.

  b. The salicylates are useful as analgesics for certain categories of pain (e.g., headache, arthritis, dysmenorrhea).

  c. The salicylates, by way of their anti-inflammatory action, provide relief of symptoms in acute rheumatic fever.

  d. The salicylates remain the standard, first-line drug in the therapy of **rheumatoid arthritis**.

    (1) Both the analgesic and the anti-inflammatory actions provide symptomatic relief in this disorder.

    (2) Relatively large doses are required, however, and these may not be well tolerated in some individuals, necessitating the use of other agents either alone or in combination with the salicylates.

e. Some clinicians recommend small daily doses of aspirin for prophylaxis of thromboembolism, stroke, or myocardial infarction, because of aspirin's antiplatelet activity.

5. Preparations and administration

a. Aspirin is available as tablets, capsules, and suppositories in a wide range of dosages. Rectal administration may be required in infants or if oral administration is impossible.

b. Nonacetylated salicylates, such as sodium salicylate, salsalate, and choline magnesium salicylate, appear to cause less gastric irritation and have less effect on platelet function. Though they may be safer than acetylated salicylates for aspirin-sensitive patients, they may not be as effective.

c. Buffered or **enteric-coated aspirin preparations** may be better tolerated, but the slightly enhanced absorption rate of buffered aspirin may not be significant.

d. Diflunisal is a salicylate that can be taken twice daily. It has four times the potency of aspirin when used in the treatment of osteoarthritis or musculoskeletal pain.

e. Mesalamine (5-aminosalicylic acid) is used for inflammatory bowel disease; it has poor oral absorption and, thus, is used for its local effect in rectal preparations.

6. Salicylate intoxication (see Chapter 14 II C 3)

a. Mild intoxication from aspirin or other salicylates is referred to as **salicylism** and usually occurs with repeated administration of large doses. Characteristic findings include:

(1) Headache, mental confusion, lassitude, and drowsiness

(2) Tinnitus and difficulty in hearing

(3) Hyperthermia, sweating, thirst, hyperventilation, vomiting, and diarrhea

b. More severe salicylate intoxication can result in more severe CNS disturbances, including hallucinations, vertigo, or convulsions. In addition, skin eruptions and, more important, marked alterations in acid–base balance are observed.

c. Fatal intoxication can be produced in children by ingestion of as little as 10 g of aspirin or as little as 5 g of **methyl salicylate,** which is widely used as a counterirritant in liniments and has the characteristic odor and taste of wintergreen.

d. Treatment of salicylate poisoning includes:

(1) Inducing emesis with syrup of ipecac or administering gastric lavage

(2) Appropriate infusion measures to correct abnormal electrolyte balance and dehydration

(3) Alkalinization of the urine

(4) Dialysis as required

B. Acetaminophen

1. Chemistry. A para-aminophenol derivative, acetaminophen (Figure 9-3) is the major active metabolite of phenacetin.

2. Pharmacokinetics

a. Acetaminophen is completely and rapidly absorbed from the gastrointestinal tract with peak plasma levels within 30–60 minutes. The plasma half-life is about 2 hours.

b. About 3% is excreted unchanged in the urine, while 80%–90% is conjugated with glucuronic or sulfuric acid in the liver and then excreted in the urine within the first day.

(1) Small amounts of hydroxylated metabolites are ordinarily excreted.

(2) At high doses, one of these metabolites undergoes spontaneous dehydration to form *N*-acetyl-*p*-benzoquinone, the metabolite thought to be responsible for hepatotoxicity (II B 6 b).

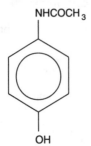

NHCOCH$_3$

OH   **Figure 9-3.** Acetaminophen.

3. **Pharmacologic effects**
   a. Acetaminophen is an effective analgesic and antipyretic agent, but it has no anti-inflammatory activity, for reasons that are not completely understood.
   b. Acetaminophen appears to be an inhibitor of prostaglandin synthesis in the brain, thus explaining its analgesic and antipyretic activity, but it is much less effective than aspirin as an inhibitor of the peripherally located prostaglandin biosynthetic enzyme system that plays such an important role in inflammation.
   c. Acetaminophen exerts little or no pharmacologic effect on the cardiovascular, respiratory, or gastrointestinal systems, on acid–base regulation, or on platelet function.

4. **Therapeutic uses**
   a. Acetaminophen provides an effective alternative when aspirin is contraindicated (e.g., in patients with peptic ulcer or hemophilia) and when the anti-inflammatory action of aspirin is not required.
   b. Acetaminophen has virtually replaced the formerly popular phenacetin because of the renal toxicity ascribed to the latter drug.

5. **Preparations and administration.** Acetaminophen is available in tablet and liquid form and is administered orally.

6. **Adverse effects**
   a. At therapeutic doses acetaminophen is well tolerated; however, untoward effects include:
      (1) Skin rash and drug fever (hyperpyrexia caused by an allergic reaction to the drug)
      (2) Rare instances of blood dyscrasias
      (3) Renal tubular necrosis and renal failure
      (4) Hypoglycemic coma
   b. An overdose of acetaminophen (about 15 g in an adult; about 4 g in a child) can result in severe hepatotoxicity, resulting in centrilobular hepatic necrosis. Doses greater than 20 g are potentially fatal.
      (1) The toxic metabolite of acetaminophen appears to be inactivated in the liver via glutathione.
      (2) It is thought that when glutathione stores are consumed, the N-acetyl-p-benzoquinone metabolite binds covalently to cellular constituents, producing hepatocellular damage.
      (3) Although clinical symptoms, such as nausea and vomiting, occur during the first 24 hours after toxic ingestion, signs of hepatic damage (e.g., enzyme abnormalities) may not occur for 2–6 days.
      (4) Treatment consists of:
         (a) Emptying the stomach and administering activated charcoal
         (b) Hemodialysis, if begun within the first 12 hours after ingestion
         (c) Administration of sulfhydryl compounds (e.g., acetylcysteine), which probably replenish hepatic stores of glutathione

C. **Indomethacin**

1. **Chemistry.** Indomethacin is a methylated indole derivative (Figure 9-4).

2. **Pharmacokinetics**
   a. Absorption from the gastrointestinal tract is rapid and virtually complete with peak plasma levels in about 2 hours. As with other drugs, absorption may be delayed when taken with meals.

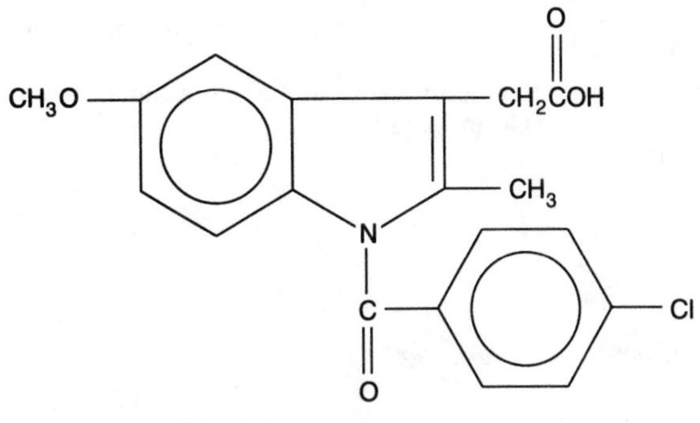

Figure 9-4. Indomethacin.

   b. Indomethacin is 90% bound to plasma proteins and also exhibits extensive tissue binding.
   c. Concentration of indomethacin in synovial fluid is equal to plasma levels within 5 hours of administration.
   d. Indomethacin is largely inactivated by O-demethylation (about 50%) and glucuronidation (about 10%); 10%–20% of unmetabolized indomethacin is eliminated in the urine. Conjugated metabolites are eliminated via feces, bile, and the urine.

3. **Pharmacologic effects**
   a. Indomethacin has prominent anti-inflammatory, antipyretic, and analgesic activity.
   b. Although indomethacin is a more potent anti-inflammatory agent than aspirin, the doses of indomethacin that are well tolerated by rheumatoid arthritis patients do not show superior results compared to the salicylates.
   c. There is evidence for both a central and peripheral action.

4. **Drug interactions**
   a. Indomethacin does not appear to alter the uricosuric effects of probenecid. It is routinely used in the treatment of gout.
   b. Indomethacin does not appear to modify the effect of oral anticoagulants, but concurrent administration could be hazardous because of increased potential for gastrointestinal bleeding.
   c. Indomethacin does antagonize the natriuretic and antihypertensive effects of furosemide, thiazide diuretics, β-adrenergic blocking agents, and angiotensin converting enzyme (ACE) inhibitors.

5. **Therapeutic uses**
   a. The major uses of indomethacin are in the treatment of rheumatoid arthritis, ankylosing spondylitis, osteoarthritis, and acute gout.
   b. It has also been used in the treatment of patent ductus arteriosus in neonates, and in the treatment of Bartter's syndrome (juxtaglomerular cell hyperplasia), characterized by hypokalemic alkalosis, hyperaldosteronism, and normal blood pressure despite high renin blood levels.
   c. Because of its toxicity and side effects, it is not routinely used for analgesia or antipyresis.

6. **Preparations and administration**
   a. Indomethacin usually is administered orally. It should be taken with meals to lessen gastric irritation.
   b. An intravenous solution is available for use in patent ductus arteriosus.

7. **Adverse effects**
   a. Overall, 35%–50% of all patients receiving indomethacin report some adverse effect; about 20% must discontinue therapy. Most adverse effects are dose-related.
   b. Gastrointestinal complaints include:
      (1) Anorexia, nausea, and abdominal pain
      (2) Ulcers, sometimes with perforations and hemorrhage
      (3) Diarrhea, sometimes associated with ulcerative lesions of the lower gastrointestinal tract
   c. CNS effects, which are the most frequently reported, including:
      (1) Severe frontal headache (25%–50%)
      (2) Dizziness and vertigo
      (3) Mental confusion
      (4) Severe depression, psychosis, hallucination, and suicide
   d. Hematologic reactions, such as neutropenia, thrombocytopenia, and, rarely, aplastic anemia. Platelet function is impaired.
   e. Hypersensitivity reactions, such as rashes, itching, urticaria, and acute asthma. Aspirin-sensitive patients may exhibit cross-reactions to indomethacin.
   f. Indomethacin is **contraindicated** in:
      (1) Pregnant or nursing women
      (2) Psychiatric disorders
      (3) Epilepsy
      (4) Parkinsonism
      (5) Renal disease
      (6) Gastrointestinal ulcerative lesions
      (7) Machine operators

D. Sulindac

1. **Chemistry.** Structurally, sulindac is an indene-derived NSAID and is closely related to indomethacin (Figure 9-5).

2. **Pharmacokinetics**
   a. About 90% of the drug is absorbed after oral administration with peak plasma levels of sulindac and its sulfide metabolite occurring at 1 hour and 2 hours, respectively.
   b. The half-life of sulindac is about 7 hours, but the sulfide metabolite half-life is about 18 hours.
   c. Sulindac and its major metabolites are all extensively bound to plasma proteins.
   d. Urinary excretion accounts for approximately 30% of a dose, while up to 25% may be excreted in the feces.
   e. Sulindac and its metabolites undergo extensive enterohepatic circulation.

3. **Pharmacologic effects**
   a. Sulindac is an anti-inflammatory, analgesic, and antipyretic drug with a relative strength of about half of indomethacin's potency.
   b. Sulindac is a **prodrug**. Its sulfide metabolite is more than 500 times more potent (than sulindac) as an inhibitor of cyclooxygenase.

4. **Therapeutic uses.** Sulindac is primarily used in the treatment of osteoarthritis, rheumatoid arthritis, ankylosing spondylitis, and acute gout.

5. **Route of administration.** Sulindac is given orally.

6. **Adverse effects**
   a. Sulindac has a lower incidence of toxicity as compared to indomethacin.
   b. Gastrointestinal effects occur in about 20% of patients, although the reactions are generally mild. Abdominal pain and nausea are the most frequent complaints.
   c. CNS effects occur in up to 10% of patients with drowsiness, dizziness, headache, and anxiety being the most commonly reported.
   d. There are reports of cross-reactivity to sulindac in aspirin-sensitive patients. Skin rash and pruritus occur at about a 5% incidence.
   e. Platelet function may be impaired, and bleeding is time prolonged.
   f. Transient elevations of hepatic enzymes in plasma are less common.
   g. Despite initial claims, sulindac does not appear to be "renal-sparing" and should be used cautiously in patients with compromised renal function.

E. Fenamates: mefenamic acid and meclofenamate

1. **Chemistry**
   a. Mefenamic acid and meclofenamate are both N-substituted phenylanthranilic acids (Figures 9-6 and 9-7, respectively).
   b. Other chemical members of this family include flufenamic, tolfenamic, and etofenamic acids.

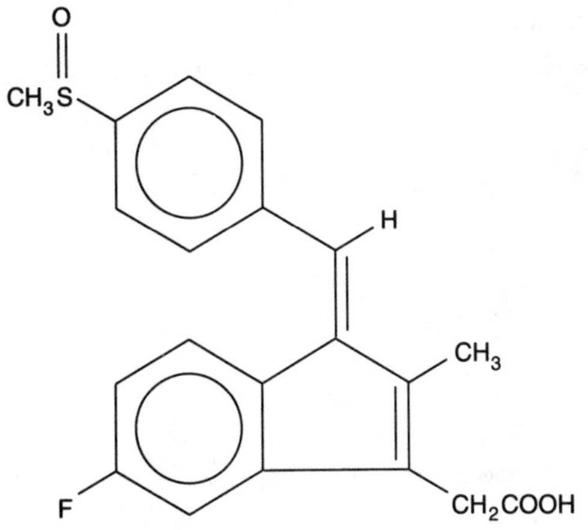

Figure 9-5. Sulindac.

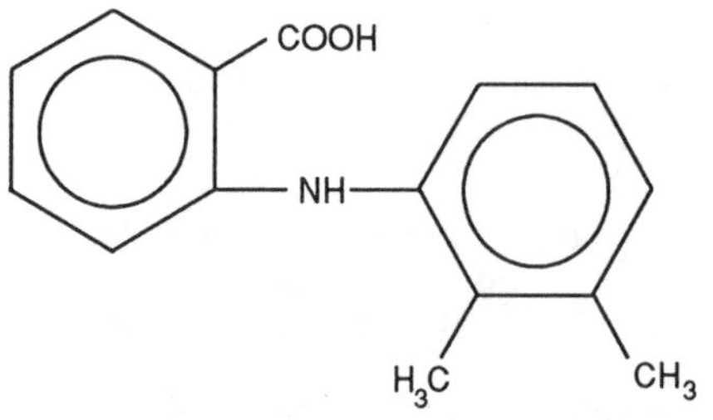

Figure 9-6. Mefenamic acid.

2. Pharmacokinetics. Peak plasma levels for meclofenamate and meclofenamic acid are about 2 hours and 2–4 hours, respectively. Plasma half-lives for these drugs are about 2–4 hours with over 50% eliminated in the urine.

3. Pharmacologic effects. The fenamates are anti-inflammatory, analgesic, and antipyretic, but unlike other NSAIDs, they appear to antagonize certain effects of prostaglandins.

4. Therapeutic uses
   a. Mefenamic acid is primarily used as an analgesic in rheumatoid arthritis, soft-tissue injury, and dysmenorrhea.
   b. Toxicity limits its utility, and it appears to have no advantage over other analgesic agents.
   c. As anti-inflammatory agents, the fenamates have been used in short-term trials for osteoarthritis and rheumatoid arthritis but, again, offer no clear advantage over other NSAIDs.

5. Adverse effects
   a. The most commonly reported effects involve the gastrointestinal system and include dyspepsia or general discomfort.
   b. Diarrhea, which may be severe and associated with steatorrhea or bowel inflammation, is also common.
   c. The fenamates are **contraindicated** in patients with a history of gastrointestinal disease.
   d. **Hemolytic anemia** is a serious side effect and may be of an autoimmune origin.
   e. There are reports of cross-reactivity to fenamates in aspirin-sensitive patients.

F. Tolmetin

   1. Pharmacokinetics. Tolmetin is rapidly and completely absorbed from the gastrointestinal tract. Peak plasma levels are achieved within 20–60 minutes after dosing, and the plasma half-life is about 5 hours. Tolmetin is extensively bound to plasma proteins and excreted virtually completely in the urine.

   2. Pharmacologic effects
   a. Tolmetin is a NSAID that is more potent than aspirin but less potent than indomethacin (Figure 9-8).
   b. It is thought to preferentially inhibit CNS cyclooxygenase.
   c. Tolmetin also produces analgesic and antipyretic effects.

   3. Therapeutic uses. The major therapeutic indication for tolmetin is the treatment of juvenile and adult rheumatoid arthritis, as well as osteoarthritis.

   4. Adverse effects are those common to most of the other NSAIDs, including:
   a. Gastrointestinal discomfort
   b. CNS symptoms

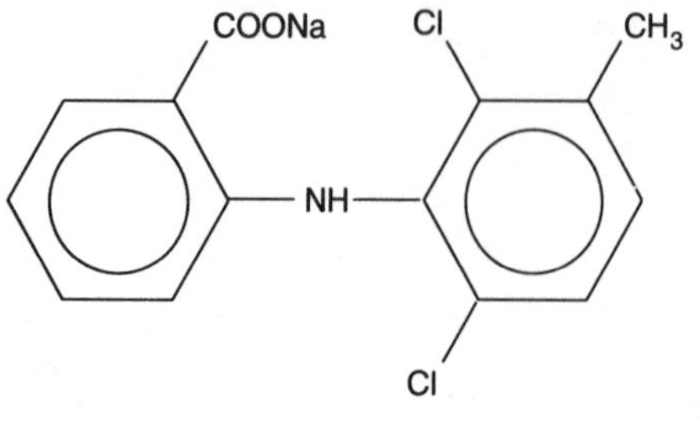

Figure 9-7. Meclofenamate.

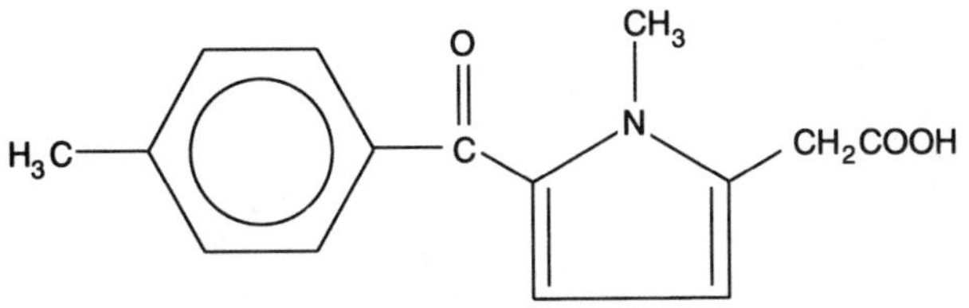

Figure 9-8. Tolmetin.

   c. Cross-reactivity in aspirin-sensitive patients
   d. Anaphylactoid reactions in some patients who are not aspirin-sensitive.

G. Propionic acid derivatives

1. General considerations

  a. This group of compounds includes:

    (1) Ibuprofen
    (2) Naproxen
    (3) Fenoprofen
    (4) Ketoprofen
    (5) Flurbiprofen

  b. These agents offer significant advantages over aspirin and indomethacin because they are better tolerated at anti-inflammatory doses.

  c. All of these compounds can induce gastrointestinal side effects or alter platelet function; some may alter leukocyte function and motility.

2. Drug interactions

  a. Potential adverse drug interactions may result from the high degree of plasma albumin binding and the impact that this may have on **oral anticoagulants**.

  b. Propionic acid derivatives do not alter the effects of **oral hypoglycemic agents** or **warfarin**.

  c. Propionic acid derivatives may reduce the diuretic and natriuretic effects of furosemide, as well as the antihypertensive effects of thiazides, β-adrenergic antagonists, and ACE inhibitors.

3. Ibuprofen

  a. **Pharmacokinetics.** Oral absorption is rapid with peak plasma levels appearing within 1–2 hours and a half-life of about 2 hours. Excretion is rapid and complete with more than 90% appearing in the urine, mostly as metabolites or conjugates.

  b. **Pharmacologic effects.** Ibuprofen is equal to aspirin in its anti-inflammatory effect, but it is a more effective analgesic than aspirin or acetaminophen (Figure 9-9).

  c. **Therapeutic uses.** As an NSAID, ibuprofen is used for the treatment of arthritis and osteoarthritis.

  d. **Adverse effects**

    (1) Ibuprofen should be used cautiously in patients with known peptic ulceration or gastric intolerance to other aspirin-like drugs.

    (2) Gastrointestinal effects occur in about 5%–15% of patients, but the incidence of these events is less than with aspirin or indomethacin.

    (3) Ibuprofen should not be used during pregnancy or nursing.

    (4) Ibuprofen is a potent inhibitor of cyclooxygenase and prolongs bleeding time.

4. Naproxen

  a. **Pharmacokinetics.** Peak concentrations occur within 2–4 hours, but naproxen's half-life is about 14 hours, allowing an advantage of twice a day dosing. Naproxen is highly bound to plasma proteins. Excretion is primarily in the urine (Figure 9-10).

  b. **Therapeutic uses.** As an NSAID, naproxen is used for the treatment of rheumatoid arthritis and osteoarthritis.

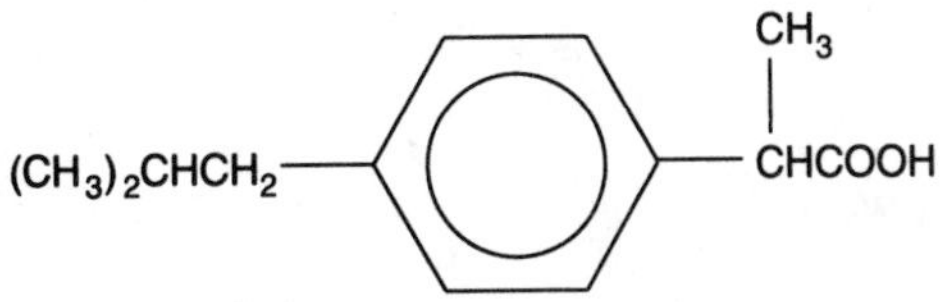

Figure 9-9. Ibuprofen.

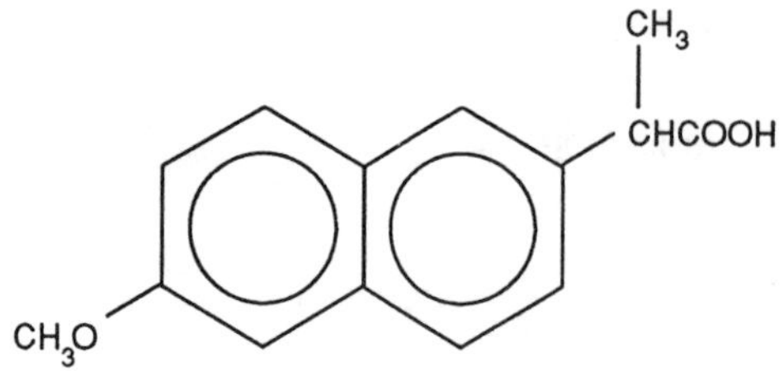

Figure 9-10. Naproxen.

c. Adverse effects
(1) While the the incidence of gastrointestinal and CNS effects approximate those of indomethacin, naproxen is better tolerated.
(2) Less commonly seen are pruritus and dermatologic problems.
(3) Isolated cases of jaundice, renal dysfunction, angioneurotic edema, thrombocytopenia, and agranulocytosis have been reported.
(4) Naproxen does cross the placenta and appears in the milk of lactating women at about 1% of the maternal plasma level.

5. Fenoprofen
a. Pharmacokinetics. Oral absorption is rapid, though not as complete (85%) as ibuprofen; peak plasma levels appear at about 2 hours with a half-life of about 3 hours. Similarly, there is a high degree of plasma protein binding and virtually complete elimination via the urine (Figure 9-11).
b. Adverse effects
(1) Gastrointestinal effects account for the majority (15%) of reports, but these are generally milder than with equal doses of aspirin, and few require discontinuation.
(2) CNS effects reported include tinnitus, vertigo, lassitude, confusion, and anorexia.

6. Ketoprofen
a. Pharmacokinetics. Ketoprofen exhibits a profile similar to ibuprofen, but slightly longer half-lives are seen in elderly patients (Figure 9-12).
b. Adverse effects
(1) Gastrointestinal effects (30%) are generally less severe than those seen with aspirin and may be reduced further by taking the drug with food, milk, or antacids.
(2) Renal function should be monitored in patients over 60 or with impaired renal function as ketoprofen can cause fluid retention and transient increases in plasma creatinine levels.
(3) Patients treated concurrently with ketoprofen and methotrexate can develop life-threatening methotrexate hepatotoxicity.

7. Flurbiprofen
a. Pharmacokinetics. Flurbiprofen has a profile similar to ibuprofen, but its plasma half-life is about 6 hours (Figure 9-13).
b. Therapeutic uses
(1) Flurbiprofen tablets are used to treat the signs and symptoms of rheumatoid arthritis and osteoarthritis.
(2) Additionally, flurbiprofen is available in an ophthalmic dosage form for the treatment of postoperative miosis. It is the only NSAID approved for ophthalmic use.
(a) Trauma of intraocular surgery releases prostaglandins, which cause progressive miosis.
(b) Flurbiprofen decreases miosis without affecting intraocular pressure.

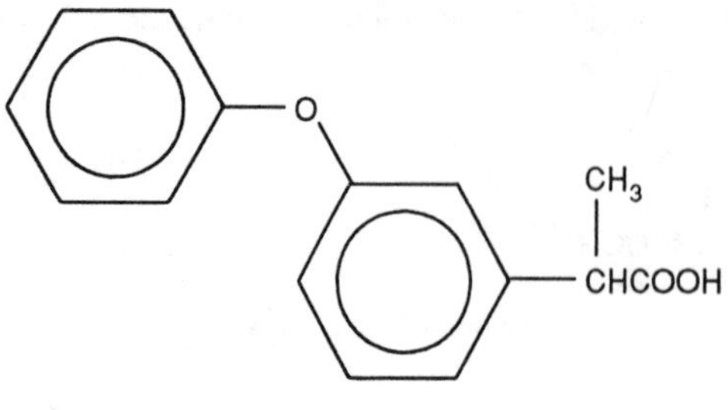

Figure 9-11. Fenoprofen.

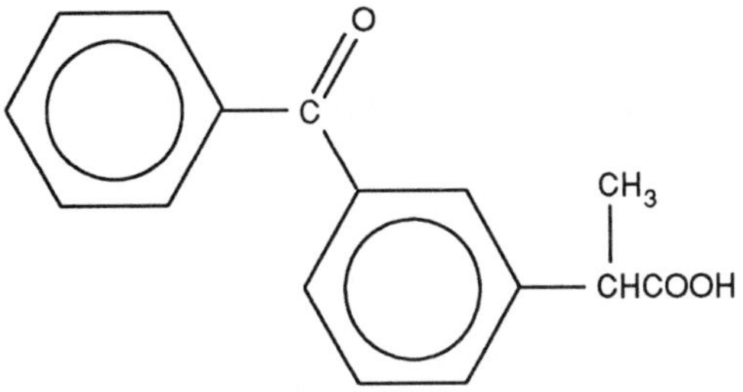

Figure 9-12. Ketoprofen.

c. Adverse effects

(1) The profile is similar to other propionic acid derivatives with regard to the incidence of gastrointestinal and CNS effects.

(2) Flurbiprofen may exacerbate herpes simplex keratitis and delay wound healing. A foreign body sensation is the most common adverse effect.

H. Piroxicam

1. **Chemistry.** Piroxicam is one of the oxicam derivatives, a class of enolic acids (Figure 9-14).

2. **Pharmacokinetics**
   a. Oral absorption is virtually complete with peak plasma levels appearing 3–5 hours later.
   b. The plasma half-life is estimated to be about 50 hours, which allows once-daily dosing.
   c. Steady-state plasma levels are achieved within 7–12 days, and maximal therapeutic responses occur within 2 weeks.

3. **Pharmacologic effects**
   a. As an anti-inflammatory agent, piroxicam is equipotent to indomethacin, aspirin, and naproxen.
   b. Piroxicam may also inhibit activation of neutrophils, suggesting an additional mode of anti-inflammatory action.
   c. As with other cyclooxygenase inhibitors, piroxicam is both analgesic and antipyretic.

4. **Therapeutic uses.** Piroxicam is approved for use in the treatment of rheumatoid arthritis and osteoarthritis, but it has also been used in ankylosing spondylitis, musculoskeletal disorders, dysmenorrhea, postoperative pain, and gout.

5. **Adverse effects**
   a. Piroxicam is better tolerated than aspirin or indomethacin; however, approximately 20% of patients taking piroxicam report an adverse effect, and about 5% discontinue therapy.
   b. Gastrointestinal side-effects are most common with an incidence of less than 1% for peptic ulcer.
   c. Piroxicam may have cross-reactivity in patients who are aspirin-sensitive.

I. Etodalac and nabumetone

1. **Etodolac** is a NSAID that causes significantly less gastrointestinal irritation. It is rapidly and well absorbed and has a plasma half-life of about 7 hours. A single dose provides postoperative analgesia for about 6–8 hours. About 5% of patients discontinue etodolac due to adverse effects.

2. **Nabumetone** is a NSAID chemically similar to naproxen with significantly less potential gastric irritation than other NSAIDs. Its lower incidence of gastric irritation may be explained by hepatic conversion to an active metabolite, similar to the hepatic activation of sulindac.

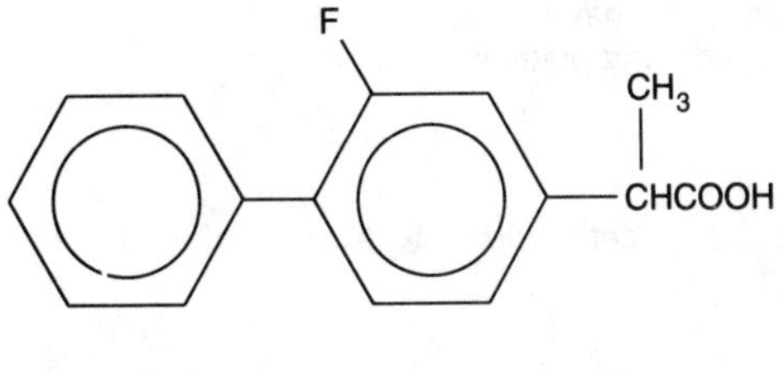

Figure 9-13. Flurbiprofen.

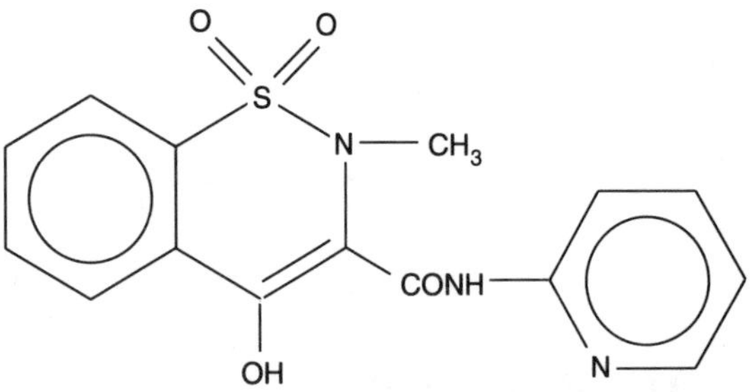

Figure 9-14. Piroxicam.

J. Phenylbutazone

1. **Chemistry.** Phenylbutazone, one of a group of drugs derived from pyrazolon, is a congener of antipyrene.

2. **Pharmacokinetics.** Phenylbutazone is rapidly and completely absorbed with peak plasma levels within 2 hours. The half-life is notably very long, 50–65 hours. Significant concentrations may persist in synovial fluid up to 3 weeks following treatment.

3. **Pharmacologic effects**
   a. Phenylbutazone is an effective anti-inflammatory agent, but toxicity prohibits its long-term use.
   b. Phenylbutazone possesses anti-inflammatory and analgesic activity that is qualitatively similar to that of aspirin. Its analgesic effect against nonrheumatic pain, however, is less than that produced by aspirin.

4. **Drug interactions**
   a. Phenylbutazone may displace:
      (1) Oral anticoagulant drugs
      (2) Oral hypoglycemic drugs
      (3) Sulfonamides
      (4) Protein-bound thyroid hormone, thus complicating interpretations of thyroid function tests
   b. Induction of hepatic enzymes, or mixed function oxidases, can disturb the metabolism of other active moieties.
   c. The effects of **insulin** may be potentiated by phenylbutazone.

5. **Therapeutic uses**
   a. Phenylbutazone is chiefly used in the short-term therapy of acute gout and in acute exacerbations of rheumatoid arthritis but only after other agents have failed.
   b. Because phenylbutazone is poorly tolerated by many patients, it is not used as an antipyretic or general analgesic agent.
   c. Brief courses of the drug may be beneficial in the treatment of osteoarthritis and ankylosing spondylitis with the same reservations as in other indications.

6. **Route of administration.** Phenylbutazone is administered orally. It should be taken with meals to lessen gastric irritation.

7. **Adverse effects**
   a. Significant salt and water retention occurs through a direct effect on renal tubules; this can cause cardiac decompensation and acute pulmonary edema.
   b. Phenylbutazone can cause agranulocytosis or aplastic anemia.
   c. As many as 10%–50% of patients experience nausea, vomiting, or skin rashes.
   d. Peptic ulceration has been reported.
   e. Because phenylbutazone binds to plasma proteins and displaces other drugs (e.g., warfarin), a number of undesirable drug interactions may occur.
   f. Phenylbutazone also has a direct effect in reducing platelet function.

K. Diclofenac

1. **Chemistry.** Diclofenac is the first of a series of phenylacetic acid derivatives developed as anti-inflammatory agents (Figure 9-15).

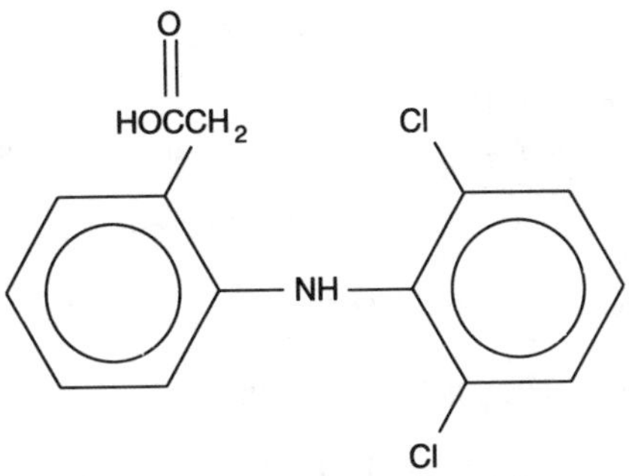

Figure 5-15. Diclofenac.

2. Pharmacokinetics

a. Oral absorption is rapid and complete with peak plasma levels within 2 hours; food slows the rate, but not extent, of absorption.

b. There is a substantial first-pass effect, reducing systemic levels by as much as 50%.

c. Diclofenac is highly protein-bound in plasma, and its half-life is 1–2 hours.

d. Diclofenac accumulates in synovial fluid, which may account for its long-lived therapeutic effect, despite its short plasma half-life.

3. Pharmacologic effects

a. Diclofenac is a potent anti-inflammatory, antipyretic, and analgesic agent; it is a more potent inhibitor of cyclooxygenase than indomethacin or naproxen.

b. Additionally, diclofenac appears to alter the release or uptake of fatty acids, reducing intracellular levels of arachidonate in leukocytes.

4. Therapeutic uses. Diclofenac is approved for use in the treatment of rheumatoid arthritis, osteoarthritis, and ankylosing spondylitis. It may also be useful for short-term treatment of acute musculoskeletal injury, tendinitis, bursitis, postoperative pain, and dysmenorrhea.

5. Adverse effects

a. Approximately 30% of diclofenac patients report an adverse event with about 2% discontinuing therapy.

b. Gastrointestinal symptoms (20%) are the most common; bleeding, ulceration, and perforation have been reported.

c. Elevated hepatic transaminase levels occur in about 15% of diclofenac patients. Hepatic transaminases should be monitored for the first 8 weeks of therapy. Hepatitis and jaundice have been reported.

d. Diclofenac is not recommended for children, nursing mothers, or women who are pregnant.

III. DISEASE-MODIFYING ANTIRHEUMATIC DRUGS (DMARDs)

A. General considerations

1. DMARDs encompass a wide range of compounds used in conjunction with NSAIDs to modify the immunologic response.

2. While NSAIDs may provide symptomatic relief for joint pain and morning stiffness, occult joint damage may still be occurring. Radiologic assessments of joint involvement and erosions are a valuable corroboration of the clinical efficacy of any drug regimen.

3. Since degenerative lesions do not regress once formed, there is an increasing tendency to institute **DMARD** therapy early in progressive cases.

B. Gold

1. Chemistry. Most gold preparations used are aurous salts in which the gold is attached to sulfur.

2. Pharmacokinetics

a. With long-term **chrysotherapy,** gold deposits build up. Gold can be detected in the urine up to a year after cessation of chrysotherapy.

b. **Aurothioglucose** and **gold sodium thiomalate** are given by intramuscular injection.

      (1) Peak plasma levels are seen within 2–6 hours, and virtually all (95%) is protein bound.

      (2) The plasma half-life is about 7 days for a 50-mg dose.

      (3) The pharmacokinetics of these compounds are complex and varied, mostly depending upon the dose and duration of treatment.

  c. Auranofin is given orally with about 25% absorption. Steady-state concentrations are achieved within 8–12 weeks of treatment.

      (1) A 6-month regimen of 6 mg/day yields about 20% gold accumulation as compared to injectable gold compounds.

      (2) With auranofin, the half-life of gold in the body is about 80 days.

3. Pharmacologic effects

  a. Gold preparations (i.e., aurothioglucose, gold sodium thiomalate, auranofin) have minimal anti-inflammatory activity.

  b. The primary mechanisms of action may be in the inhibition of mononuclear phagocyte maturation and function.

      (1) Gold is sequestered in mononuclear phagocytes within the inflamed synovium.

      (2) Gold thiomalate reduces migration and phagocytic activity of macrophages in inflammatory exudates, as well as lysozomal enzyme activity.

      (3) Gold may suppress cellular immunity.

4. Therapeutic uses

  a. Gold compounds are most effective in early, progressive rheumatoid arthritis that is unresponsive to other regimens.

  b. Gold therapy is of little use in advanced arthritis or in mild disease.

  c. It has been estimated that chrysotherapy will have the following effects:

      (1) It induces a protracted remission in 15% of patients.

      (2) It improves symptoms in 60%–70% of the patients.

      (3) It must be discontinued in 15%–20% of the patients.

      (4) It fails to elicit a response in 10%–15% of patients.

  d. Chrysotherapy is sometimes beneficial in juvenile rheumatoid arthritis, palindromic rheumatism, psoriatic arthritis, and other connective tissue disorders.

5. Preparations and route of administration

  a. Aurothioglucose

      (1) Aurothioglucose is water-soluble (50% gold), but it is given by intramuscular injection as a sterile suspension in fixed oil; each dose contains 50 mg/ml.

      (2) Dosing is usually a 10-mg test dose in the first week, followed by 25 mg in the second and third weeks. Thereafter, 50-mg doses may be given weekly until the cumulative dose equals 1 g.

  b. Gold sodium thiomalate

      (1) Water-soluble gold sodium thiomalate (50% gold) is also given by intramuscular injection.

      (2) Dosing is almost identical to aurothioglucose, but after the third week, 25–50 mg is given. Some physicians use the same dosage regimen as for aurothioglucose (50 mg).

      (3) Remission dosing. For both injectables, if a remission occurs, the dose (25–50 mg) may be given every 2 weeks for up to 20 weeks. This is followed by a dose every 3 weeks for an additional 18 weeks; after this, a monthly schedule may be followed indefinitely.

      (4) In the absence of clinical response, gradually increasing weekly doses may be used, but these **should not exceed 100 mg/week**.

  c. Auranofin

      (1) Auranofin (29% gold) is taken orally (3-mg tablets); for active rheumatoid arthritis, the daily dose is 6 mg. Some patients may require 9 mg three times daily.

      (2) Initial clinical responses may not be detected until 10–12 weeks of therapy. Patients should be on 6 mg/day for at least 6 months prior to increasing doses to 9 mg/day.

      (3) Therapy should be discontinued if, after 3 additional months, response is still inadequate.

      (4) Auranofin may be somewhat less effective than injectable gold for rheumatoid arthritis, but it is less toxic and better tolerated.

6. Adverse effects occur in 25%–50% of patients on chrysotherapy.

  a. Cutaneous reactions, ranging from vasodilation and "nitroid" reactions to exfoliative dermatitis and lesions of the mucous membrane, are often observed with gold thiomalate but rarely with aurothioglucose.

    b. Eosinophilia is quite common.

    c. Proteinuria occurs frequently, although this nephrosis is reversible.

    d. Blood dyscrasias, including potentially serious thrombocytopenia, leukopenia, agranulocytosis, and aplastic anemia, have occurred.

    e. Auranofin causes diarrhea in nearly one-half the patients taking it, but it is less likely to cause renal or mucocutaneous toxicity than injectable gold.

    f. Other untoward effects of gold therapy include encephalitis, hepatitis, and peripheral neuritis.

C. Other DMARDs used for rheumatoid arthritis. Although this diversified group of drugs is collectively associated with the disease-modifying aspects of gold, these drugs are unlikely to induce remissions or retard synovial erosions as effectively as gold. These drugs include: immunosuppressive agents, glucocorticoids, penicillamine, hydroxychloroquine, and sulfasalazine.

  1. Immunosuppressive agents

    a. Azathioprine and **cyclophosphamide** are immunosuppressive drugs that have been used to treat refractory rheumatoid arthritis.

      (1) Azathioprine rarely causes severe toxicity with the dosage used for rheumatoid arthritis.

      (2) Cyclophosphamide's adverse effects are so severe that most clinicians reserve it for life-threatening rheumatoid vasculitis.

    b. Methotrexate (oral) produces an antirheumatic effect within 6 weeks of treatment.

      (1) At recommended doses, severe toxicity is rare; however, the drug is teratogenic.

      (2) Aspirin and other NSAIDs increase its toxicity by slowing its rate of excretion.

      (3) Methotrexate is contraindicated in patients with renal insufficiency or hemodynamic instability.

    c. Cyclosporine is a fungus-derived cyclic peptide.

      (1) Therapeutic uses

        (a) Cyclosporine is a highly selective **inhibitor of helper T cells**. It inhibits the production of interleukin-2 (IL-2) by helper T cells and reduces the production and release of other lymphokines in response to an antigenic stimulus.

        (b) Cyclosporine also **binds to** lymphoid proteins called **cyclophilins** and **to isomerase enzymes,** which aid in the folding of certain proteins.

        (c) Cyclosporine is used in combination with prednisone to **sustain cardiac, renal, and hepatic transplants**. One-year survival is about 75%.

      (2) Pharmacokinetics. Oral bioavailability of cyclosporine ranges from 20%–50% and its half-life is about 6 hours. It is metabolized in the liver and most is then excreted in the bile.

      (3) Adverse effects. The major adverse effect is nephrotoxicity, a dose-related phenomenon which occurs in 25%–75% of patients treated with the drug. Both the glomerular filtration rate (GFR) and renal plasma flow (RPF) are reduced, but these effects are usually reversible. Neurologic toxicity, hypertension, and increased incidence of infections can also be seen.

  2. Glucocorticoids

    a. Patients with severe rheumatoid arthritis may benefit from 5–10 mg/day of oral **prednisone,** while patients with vasculitis may require higher doses. The adverse effects of long-term systemic corticosteroids usually preclude their use for all but the most severe forms of rheumatoid arthritis.

    b. An acutely inflamed rheumatoid joint may be helped by an intra-articular injection.

  3. Penicillamine

    a. Penicillamine in high doses can be effective in patients with refractory rheumatoid arthritis and may delay progression of erosions. It is highly toxic and teratogenic.

    b. Therapy is initiated with single daily doses of 125–250 mg, gradually increased at 1–3-month intervals to a maximum of 1–1.5 g/day. Many patients respond to 500–750 mg/day.

  4. Hydroxychloroquine

    a. Therapy is initiated with 400–600 mg/day taken with food or milk. After a clinical response (usually within 1–3 months), the daily dose is reduced to 200–400 mg/day.

    b. This antimalarial drug can produce adverse effects on the skin, CNS, and bone marrow and irreversible retinal damage as a result of ocular deposition. Ophthalmic examinations prior to therapy and every 3 months afterwards are recommended.

5. Sulfasalazine appears to be as effective as penicillamine but is less toxic. Gastrointestinal disturbances and rash are common. Sulfasalazine may prevent progression of joint damage.

IV. DRUGS USED IN THE TREATMENT OF GOUT

A. General considerations. Because the drugs used in gout act by various mechanisms, a brief review of some aspects of this condition is in order.

1. Gout is the most readily treated of all the rheumatic disorders.

2. Hyperuricemia is not always accompanied or followed by gout, but when gout occurs, it is preceded by hyperuricemia.

3. Causes of hyperuricemia include the following:

   a. Excessive uric acid synthesis associated with myeloproliferative disorders and malignancies, especially after antineoplastic or radiation therapy (conditions that lead to high rates of cell formation and destruction will lead to increased serum levels of purines, derived from cellular nucleic acids, and will, thus, result in hyperuricemia)

   b. A primary defect in the rate of purine synthesis

   c. Decreased renal excretion of uric acid caused by certain drugs (e.g., thiazides) or due to genetic deficiency

   d. Sex-linked uricaciduria (e.g., in Lesch-Nyhan syndrome) due to a lack of the enzyme hypoxanthine–guanine phosphoribosyltransferase

4. Acute gouty arthritic episodes can be precipitated by excessive alcohol consumption, by kidney disease, and possibly by high-purine diets or external stresses. If the gout is a secondary phenomenon unrelated to a genetic defect, the underlying cause of the hyperuricemia must be determined.

5. Twenty-five percent of the body's uric acid is degraded in the gastrointestinal tract by bacterial enzymes. Seventy-five percent is renally excreted. Ninety-eight percent of the filtered uric acid is reabsorbed in the proximal tubule and then secreted in the distal portion of the proximal tubule.

6. Mechanism of gouty inflammation

   a. When the plasma is supersaturated with urate, needle-shaped crystals of monosodium urate precipitate in joint tissue.

   b. An acute inflammatory reaction occurs, resulting in the ingestion of monosodium urate crystals by polymorphonuclear leukocytes.

   c. Lysosomal enzymes are released by the granulocytes, producing a decrease in the local pH in the joint tissue.

   d. With a decreased pH, further urate precipitation occurs in joints and cartilage.

B. Probenecid

1. Mechanism of action and pharmacologic effects

   a. At therapeutic doses, probenecid lowers serum levels of uric acid by inhibiting the proximal tubular reabsorption of uric acid.

     (1) In low doses, probenecid blocks the tubular secretion of uric acid, while at therapeutic doses probenecid is uricosuric.

     (2) When approximately 1 g of probenecid is administered daily, urinary excretion of uric acid increases by 50%, resulting in a corresponding fall in serum urate.

     (3) The metabolic products of probenecid are also uricosuric.

   b. As a general inhibitor of the tubular secretion of organic acids, probenecid will also increase serum levels of other organic acids, such as penicillin.

   c. Probenecid has no analgesic activity.

2. Pharmacokinetics. Probenecid is rapidly absorbed from the gastrointestinal tract.

3. Therapeutic uses

   a. By virtue of its uricosuric effects, probenecid is useful for the treatment of chronic gout.

   b. By virtue of its effects on organic acid excretion, probenecid is also used to prolong the effects of penicillin [see Chapter 12 II B 2 e (1) (b) (ii)].

4. Administration. Probenecid is administered orally.

   a. The action of probenecid is blocked by the administration of aspirin.

b. Because of its biphasic action [see IV B 1 a (1)], therapy with probenecid should not be initiated during an acute attack of gout.

5. Adverse effects. Probenecid is well tolerated, the most common adverse effects being gastrointestinal disturbances and hypersensitivity reactions, such as skin rash and drug fever.

C. Sulfinpyrazone

1. Chemistry. Sulfinpyrazone is a sulfoxide derivative of phenylbutazone.

2. Mechanism of action and pharmacologic effects
  a. Sulfinpyrazone inhibits the proximal tubular reabsorption of uric acid. A hydroxy metabolite is also a potent uricosuric substance.
  b. Sulfinpyrazone also inhibits prostaglandin synthesis and interferes with a number of platelet functions, including adherence to subendothelial cells.

3. Pharmacokinetics. After oral administration, sulfinpyrazone is well absorbed from the gastrointestinal tract and most is excreted unchanged in the urine.

4. Therapeutic uses
  a. Sulfinpyrazone is used for the treatment of chronic gout.
  b. Because of its effects on platelets, it is being examined as an antithrombotic agent.

5. Administration. Sulfinpyrazone is given orally. Administration with meals is recommended. As with probenecid, sulfinpyrazone therapy should not be initiated during an acute gouty attack.

6. Adverse effects are similar to those seen with probenecid.

D. Colchicine. This alkaloid derivative is effective in the treatment of acute attacks of gout and is also effective if given prophylactically to prevent such attacks.

1. Mechanism of action
  a. Colchicine inhibits the migration of polymorphonuclear leukocytes to the inflammatory area. It is proposed that colchicine produces ultrastructural alterations in leukocytes by attaching to the microtubular protein (tubulin) that is involved in cell motility and, thus, prevents the migration of granulocytes and inhibits phagocytic activity.
  b. Colchicine also blocks cell division by binding to mitotic spindles (mitotic blockade).

2. Pharmacokinetics
  a. Colchicine is rapidly absorbed from the gastrointestinal tract.
  b. Large amounts of the drug and its metabolites re-enter the intestinal tract in the bile and intestinal secretions.
  c. This high local concentration of drug, together with the rapid turnover of intestinal epithelial cells, which makes the cells particularly susceptible to mitotic blockade by colchicine, leads to altered function of the intestinal mucosa and produces one of the drug's major untoward effects, diarrhea.

3. Administration. In an acute attack of gout, colchicine is usually administered orally in intermittent doses until pain disappears or gastrointestinal symptoms occur.
  a. The patient usually experiences a marked improvement in joint symptoms within 12 hours.
  b. A total of no more than 10 mg should be administered in one such course of therapy.
  c. Colchicine is excreted unchanged by the liver and kidney; therefore, the dosage may have to be reduced if renal or liver disease is present.

4. Adverse effects
  a. Nausea, vomiting, and abdominal pain with diarrhea are warning signs that more serious toxicity could result and may indicate a need to discontinue colchicine therapy.
  b. The most serious untoward effects that occur with chronic administration are agranulocytosis, aplastic anemia, myopathy, and alopecia.
  c. A fatal dose of colchicine can be as little as 8 mg in 24 hours.

E. Allopurinol

1. Chemistry. Allopurinol is an isomer of hypoxanthine, a purine.

2. Mechanism of action
  a. Allopurinol, together with its primary metabolite alloxanthine, prevents the terminal steps

in uric acid synthesis by inhibiting the enzyme xanthine oxidase, which converts xanthine or hypoxanthine to uric acid. Hyperuricemia is, thus, reversed by the blockade of uric acid production.

b. Allopurinol acts as a competitive inhibitor, while alloxanthine acts noncompetitively.

c. The inhibition of xanthine oxidase causes serum levels of the catabolic intermediates xanthine and hypoxanthine to increase. Renal clearance of these substances, however, is rapid and their increased plasma concentrations do not exceed their solubility. Thus, crystallization within joint tissue does not occur as it would with comparable levels of uric acid.

3. **Administration.** Allopurinol is administered orally. Starting with a low dose may lessen the probability of precipitating recurrent acute gouty attacks.

4. **Adverse effects**

a. Allopurinol is well tolerated. The most common untoward effects are hypersensitivity reactions, including cutaneous reactions.

b. **Acute attacks of gout** occur more frequently during initial therapy with allopurinol.

(1) This may be due in part to the active dissolution of microcrystalline deposits of sodium urate (tophi) within subcutaneous tissue, resulting in transient periods of hyperuricemia and crystal deposition in joint tissue.

(2) To reduce this complication, simultaneous prophylactic therapy with colchicine is indicated.

F. Nonsteroidal anti-inflammatory agents used in the treatment of gout

1. **Indomethacin** may provide symptomatic relief in acute attacks. The dosage of indomethacin must be reduced for patients who are also taking probenecid, since the latter increases the plasma levels of indomethacin (see II C).

2. **Phenylbutazone** is an alternative drug to indomethacin in the treatment of acute gouty arthritis (see II J).

3. Aspirin and other salicylates, although they may provide symptomatic relief, actually antagonize the action of the uricosurics probenecid and sulfinpyrazone. Therefore, the salicylates are contraindicated when probenecid or sulfinpyrazone is being administered.

STUDY QUESTIONS

Directions: Each of the numbered items or incomplete statements in this section is followed by answers or by completions of the statement. Select the **one** lettered answer or completion that is **best** in each case.

1. All of the following are undesirable effects of the salicylates EXCEPT

(A) exfoliation of gastric mucosal cells
(B) inhibition of peripheral PGE_2 and $PGF_{2\alpha}$ synthesis
(C) stimulation of the chemoreceptor trigger zone
(D) salicylism
(E) decreased gastric mucus secretion

2. A hemophiliac patient has rheumatoid arthritis. Which drug might be prescribed to relieve the pain?

(A) Acetaminophen
(B) Acetylsalicylic acid
(C) Phenylbutazone
(D) Ibuprofen
(E) Naproxen

3. The prophylactic use of aspirin could find therapeutic benefit in which of the following applications?

(A) Noncardiogenic pulmonary edema
(B) Thromboembolic events
(C) Metabolic acidosis
(D) Gastric cytoprotective effect
(E) Hypertension

4. True statements concerning characteristics of anti-inflammatory drugs include all of the following EXCEPT

(A) aspirin is uricosuric in high doses
(B) sulindac has a long half-life
(C) indomethacin causes frontal headaches
(D) ibuprofen has more potent anti-inflammatory effects than aspirin
(E) brief courses of phenylbutazone may have value in the treatment of ankylosis spondylitis

5. Which of the following drugs used in the treatment of gout has as its primary effect the reduction of uric acid synthesis?

(A) Allopurinol
(B) Sulfinpyrazone
(C) Colchicine
(D) Aspirin
(E) Indomethacin

6. A patient is diagnosed as having inflammatory bowel disease. Which preparation listed below could be effective therapy?

(A) Choline magnesium salicylate
(B) Diflunisal
(C) 5-Aminosalicylic acid
(D) Salsalate
(E) Sodium salicylate

7. A patient with rheumatoid arthritis who had a previous myocardial infarction and now has congestive heart failure wants more effective therapy for his arthritis. Which of the following agents is contraindicated?

(A) Aspirin
(B) Indomethacin
(C) Sulindac
(D) Phenylbutazone
(E) Ibuprofen

8. Ibuprofen can now be bought over-the-counter for use as an analgesic. All of the following statements concerning this drug are true EXCEPT that

(A) it is a more effective analgesic than aspirin
(B) it is a more effective anti-inflammatory agent than aspirin
(C) it is used for the treatment of rheumatoid arthritis
(D) it is used for the treatment of osteoarthritis
(E) it can cause gastrointestinal complaints

1-B   4-D   7-D
2-A   5-A   8-B
3-B   6-C

9. Characteristics of piroxicam include all of the following EXCEPT

(A) it is similar to aspirin in analgesic efficacy
(B) it has a long half-life
(C) it is given once a day
(D) it is not as well tolerated as aspirin
(E) it can cause gastrointestinal toxicity

10. The major therapeutic use for gold is in the treatment of

(A) advanced rheumatoid arthritis
(B) acute gout
(C) chronic ankylosing spondylitis
(D) early progressive rheumatoid arthritis
(E) chronic gout

11. Characteristics of probenecid include all of the following EXCEPT

(A) it promotes the renal tubular secretion of penicillin
(B) it is useful in the treatment of gout
(C) at appropriate doses, it promotes the excretion of uric acid
(D) it has a mechanism of action similar to that of sulfinpyrazone
(E) the metabolic products of probenecid are uricosuric

Directions: Each item below contains four suggested answers of which **one or more** is correct. Choose the answer

A if **1, 2, and 3** are correct
B if **1 and 3** are correct
C if **2 and 4** are correct
D if **4** is correct
E if **1, 2, 3, and 4** are correct

12. Characteristics of acetaminophen include which of the following?

(1) It does not inhibit prostaglandin synthesis
(2) It can be used to treat headaches in a patient with hemophilia
(3) An overdose depletes glucuronide stores
(4) It is capable of reducing pain in a patient with arthritis

13. Colchicine exhibits which of the following properties?

(1) It is a uricosuric agent
(2) It inhibits the migration of granulocytes
(3) It can cause constipation
(4) It can produce agranulocytosis

Directions: The group of items in this section consists of lettered options followed by a set of numbered items. For each item, select the **one** lettered option that is most closely associated with it. Each lettered option may be selected once, more than once, or not at all.

Questions 14–18

For each of the characteristics listed below, choose the drug that is most likely to show that characteristic.

(A) Aspirin
(B) Acetaminophen
(C) Phenylbutazone
(D) Probenecid
(E) Ibuprofen

14. Produces significant fluid retention

15. Possesses no analgesic activity

16. Is a uricosuric whose action is antagonized by salicylates

17. Possesses no anti-inflammatory activity but is a central prostaglandin inhibitor

18. Increases depth of respiration

9-D	12-C	15-D	18-A
10-D	13-C	16-D	
11-A	14-C	17-B	

ANSWERS AND EXPLANATIONS

1. The answer is B *[I A 2; II A 3 f, 6 a]*
Salicylates (e.g., aspirin) inhibit prostaglandin synthesis and, thus, have excellent anti-inflammatory properties. For example, the enzyme cyclooxygenase is irreversibly inactivated by aspirin, and this blocks the synthesis of PGE_2 and $PGF_{2\alpha}$. Both of these prostaglandins are thought to be involved in inflammation-associated vasodilation, pain, and edema. The salicylates can cause epigastric distress and stimulate the chemoreceptor trigger zone in the CNS. Dose-related gastric ulceration and hemorrhage can occur, caused in part by exfoliation of gastric mucosal cells. Because the formation of PGI_2 (prostacyclin), which is known to inhibit gastric acid secretion, is suppressed, protective gastric mucus secretion is suppressed and gastric secretion increases. Salicylism is a mild salicylate intoxication and usually occurs with repeated ingestion of moderately large doses of salicylates.

2. The answer is A *[II A 3 h (5), B 3 c, G 3 d (4), J 7 f]*
All of the agents listed in the question except acetaminophen are capable of reducing platelet aggregation and, thus, prolonging bleeding times. Acetaminophen might be useful, therefore, in relieving the pain of arthritis in the hemophiliac patient, who is already at risk for deficient hemostasis.

3. The answer is B *[II A 3 e (5)]*
The prophylactic use of aspirin to reduce thromboembolic events has widened. Long-term salicylate therapy in older patients can cause noncardiogenic pulmonary edema. Toxic doses of aspirin depress the medulla and ultimately cause the accumulation of organic acids, resulting in a metabolic acidosis. Salicylates depress prostacyclin, which inhibits gastric acid secretion, thereby reducing cytoprotection. It has no use in the treatment of hypertension.

4. The answer is D *[II A 3 i, C 7 c, D 2 b, G 3 b, J 5 c]*
High doses of aspirin are uricosuric, and sulindac has a long half-life. CNS complaints, including frontal headache, frequently occur with indomethacin. Ibuprofen is not a more potent anti-inflammatory agent than aspirin; it is equipotent. Phenylbutazone is quite toxic, and its use is reserved for the short-term treatment of gout and ankylosis spondylitis.

5. The answer is A *[II A 3 i; IV C 2, D 1, E 2, F 1]*
The only agent listed in the question that interferes with the synthesis of uric acid is allopurinol. It does this by inhibiting xanthine oxidase, which converts xanthine and hypoxanthine to uric acid. Sulfinpyrazone is a uricosuric agent, while colchicine acts by preventing the migration of granulocytes. Indomethacin is a nonsteroidal anti-inflammatory agent; it is useful for symptomatic relief in acute attacks of gout. Aspirin is also anti-inflammatory and analgesic; in high dosages it can be uricosuric.

6. The answer is C *[II A 5 e]*
The only preparation listed in the question that is used for the treatment of inflammatory bowel disease is 5-aminosalicylic acid. It is poorly absorbed orally and, therefore, is used for its local effect in rectal preparations.

7. The answer is D *[II J 7 a]*
Although all NSAIDs have salt-retaining properties, phenylbutazone has the greatest liability and should be avoided. This drug exerts a direct effect on renal tubules, which can cause cardiac decompensation and acute pulmonary edema. Thus, it should not be used in a patient already experiencing decreased cardiac function.

8. The answer is B *[II G 3 a–d]*
Ibuprofen is equivalent to aspirin in its anti-inflammatory effect, although it is a more effective analgesic than aspirin. As a NSAID, ibuprofen would be used for the treatment of rheumatoid arthritis and osteoarthritis. Ibuprofen can cause gastrointestinal and CNS untoward effects, but it appears to be better tolerated than aspirin gastrointestinally. It is also safer than aspirin when taken in overdose amounts.

9. The answer is D *[II H]*
Piroxicam is a nonsteroidal anti-inflammatory agent that is similar in efficacy to aspirin, indomethacin, and naproxen. Because it has a long half-life, it can be given once a day. Although it is generally better tolerated than aspirin or indomethacin, piroxicam can cause severe gastrointestinal toxicity.

10. The answer is D *[III B 4]*
The major therapeutic use of gold is in the treatment of early, progressive rheumatoid arthritis, particularly when it is unresponsive to salicylates and other types of nonsteroidal anti-inflammatory therapy. Gold therapy is of little use in advanced rheumatoid arthritis. Gold is not used in the treatment of acute or chronic gout or ankylosing spondylitis. Therapeutic drugs for gout include probenecid, sulfinpyrazone, colchicine, allopurinol, indomethacin, and phenylbutazone. Drugs used for the treatment of ankylosing spondylitis include sulindac, phenylbutazone, and indomethacin.

11. The answer is A *[IV B, C 2 a]*
Probenecid prolongs penicillin blood levels by inhibiting its secretion. Probenecid is a uricosuric agent that is useful in the treatment of gout because it blocks the reabsorption of uric acid in the kidney. Sulfinpyrazone has a similar mechanism of action, namely, inhibiting the renal tubular reabsorption of uric acid. The metabolic products of probenecid are uricosuric.

12. The answer is C (2, 4) *[II B 3, 4, 6]*
Acetaminophen does inhibit prostaglandin synthesis centrally. It is capable of reducing the pain, but not the inflammation, associated with arthritis. Due to its lack of effect on hemostasis, it can be used for the treatment of headache in a patient with hemophilia. An overdose depletes glutathione stores, not glucuronide. This depletion may play an important role in the severe hepatotoxicity that can occur with an overdose of acetaminophen.

13. The answer is C (2, 4) *[IV D 1 a, 4 a, b]*
Colchicine is not a uricosuric agent. It appears to attach to microtubular proteins, thus preventing the migration of granulocytes. Diarrhea, not constipation, is a characteristic untoward effect and is an indicator for discontinuation of the drug. Chronic administration can lead to agranulocytosis.

14–18. The answers are: 14-C *[II J 7 a]*, **15-D** *[IV B 1 c]*, **16-D** *[IV B 1 a, 4 a]*, **17-B** *[II B 3 a]*, **18-A** *[II A 3 d (2)]*
Phenylbutazone, by a direct effect on renal tubules, causes salt and water retention. Probenecid is the only agent listed that has no analgesic activity. Probenecid at therapeutic doses is uricosuric; it acts by inhibiting proximal tubular reabsorption of uric acid. Its action is antagonized by the salicylates. Acetaminophen is a central prostaglandin inhibitor, but it exerts no anti-inflammatory activity. Aspirin in full therapeutic doses causes an increase in alveolar ventilation characterized by an increase in the depth of respiration. Higher doses lead to hyperventilation and respiratory alkalosis. Toxic doses result in respiratory and metabolic acidosis.

10
Hormones, Antagonists, and Other Agents Affecting Endocrine Function

I. ENDOCRINE FUNCTION

A. Hypothalamic–pituitary relationship

1. Releasing hormones. Pituitary (**adenohypophyseal**) function is mediated by neurohumoral substances, or releasing hormones, from the hypothalamus, which are transported via a rich capillary network in the region of the median eminence. These releasing hormones affect both the synthesis and release of pituitary hormones. Five hypothalamic releasing hormones have been well characterized.

  a. Gonadotropin-releasing hormone (GnRH)
  b. Growth hormone-releasing hormone (GHRH)
  c. Melanocyte-stimulating hormone (MSH)
  d. Thyrotropin-releasing hormone (TRH)
  e. Corticotropin-releasing hormone (CRH)

2. Vasopressin and oxytocin, bound to a large carrier protein, neurophysin, are also produced by the hypothalamus. The active hormone is released from the posterior pituitary.

3. Some hypothalamic hormones are inhibitory, such as somatostatin and dopamine, which suppress prolactin release.

B. Pituitary hormones

1. Pituitary hormones are comprised of three major groups:

  a. Somatomammotropins
    (1) Growth hormone
    (2) Prolactin
    (3) Placental lactogen
  b. Glycoproteins
    (1) Luteinizing hormone (LH)
    (2) Follicle-stimulating hormone (FSH)
    (3) Human chorionic gonadotropin (hCG)
    (4) Thyroid-stimulating hormone (TSH)
  c. Corticotropin and related peptides
    (1) Adrenocorticotropic hormone (corticotropin, ACTH)
    (2) α-Melanocyte-stimulating hormone (α-MSH)
    (3) β-Melanocyte-stimulating hormone (β-MSH)
    (4) β-Lipoprotein (β-LPH)
    (5) γ-Lipoprotein (γ-LPH)

2. Mechanism of action

  a. Many hormones affect signal transduction through one of three major mechanisms.
    (1) Cyclic adenosine monophosphate (cyclic AMP), or the **second messenger,** is increased via adenyl cyclase; cyclic AMP activates protein kinases, which phosphorylates cellular constituents. Calcium (Ca^{2+}) levels are also affected. It appears that guanine nucleotide proteins (G proteins) may activate membrane-bound phospholipase C and account for the increased membrane fluidity, Ca^{2+} flux, and "flip-flop" of lipids in the membrane bilayer.
    (2) Insulin and certain growth factors may act as membrane-bound receptors, which are also protein kinases.

(3) Steroid hormones bind to a membrane-bound receptor and become internalized via endocytosis. These hormone-receptor complexes access cytosolic or nuclear receptor proteins to act on DNA.

b. Feedback inhibition of hormone synthesis and release can be manipulated for therapeutic goals or used diagnostically to determine the level of endocrine dysfunction.

II. ENDOCRINE DYSFUNCTION

A. Pituitary anterior lobe disorders

1. Hypopituitarism in the adult (Sheehan's syndrome)

2. Pituitary dwarfism (in children)

3. Selective pituitary hormone deficiencies

4. **Hypersecretion of pituitary hormones**
   a. Acromegaly and gigantism (growth hormones)
   b. Cushing's syndrome (ACTH)
   c. Galactorrhea (prolactin)

B. Pituitary posterior lobe disorders. Diabetes insipidus (vasopressin, or antidiuretic hormone, ADH)

C. Thyroid dysfunction

1. **Hypothyroidism**
   a. Cretinism and juvenile in children
   b. Myxedema in adults

2. **Hyperthyroidism**
   a. Thyrotoxicosis, Graves' disease, Plummer's disease
   b. Thyroid storm or crisis

3. **Goiter**

4. **Thyroiditis**
   a. Hashimoto's disease (autoimmune)
   b. Subacute granulomatous thyroiditis
   c. Riedel's (fibrous) thyroiditis

5. **Thyroid neoplasms**

D. Adrenal dysfunction

1. **Hyposecretion**
   a. Addison's disease (primary insufficiency)
   b. Secondary adrenal insufficiency

2. **Hypersecretion**
   a. Cushing's syndrome
   b. Congenital adrenal hyperplasia
   c. Adrenal virilism (adrenogenital syndrome)
   d. Hyperaldosteronism

3. **Pheochromocytoma**

4. **Nonfunctional adrenal masses**

E. Parathyroid dysfunction

1. Hypoparathyroidism (postoperative tetany)

2. Hyperparathyroidism

3. Calcitonin

F. Gonadal dysfunction

1. Male hypogonadism

2. Testicular feminization syndrome

3. Precocious puberty

G. Carbohydrate metabolism disorders

1. Diabetes mellitus

2. Hypoglycemia

3. Genetic disorders
  a. Galactosemia
  b. Fructose intolerance
  c. Glycogen storage disorders

III. HORMONES AND AGENTS AFFECTING ENDOCRINE FUNCTION

A. Growth hormone is a somatomammotropin, as are prolactin and placental lactogen. They are structurally similar and probably evolved from a common ancestral gene.

1. Activity, regulation, and mechanism of action
  a. Growth hormone synthesis and release is controlled by both GHRH and somatostatin.
  b. Growth hormone is secreted by pituitary somatotrophic cells, which comprise up to 50% of all pituicytes; growth hormone is the most abundant and may comprise 10%–15% of the gland's dry weight.
  c. Growth hormone secretion is pulsatile with about 0.5 mg/day released in 6–8 distinct but irregular bursts.
  d. Secretion may be elicited by hypoglycemia, exercise, stress, emotional excitement, a protein-rich meal, and after the onset of deep sleep.
  e. Physiologic actions
    (1) Statural growth, as well as balanced systemic growth
    (2) Retention of protoplasmic nitrogen, increased amino acid transport, and decreased plasma urea levels
    (3) A diabetogenic effect on carbohydrate and lipid metabolism, which shifts the source of fuel from carbohydrates to lipids
  f. The mechanism of action for growth hormone is unknown but does not appear to involve changes in cyclic nucleotide levels, intracellular Ca^{2+} or other familiar mechanisms of signal transduction.
    (1) Growth hormone may act by stimulating synthesis or release of **somatomedins,** which are identical to polypeptides known as **insulin-like growth factors (IGF) 1 and 2.**
    (2) IGF-1 appears to mediate growth hormone activity, enhancing sulfate incorporation into proteoglycans, increasing protein synthesis, RNA, and DNA.
    (3) Low levels of IGF-1 are associated with **dwarfism.**
    (4) Like insulin, the IGF-1 receptor has protein kinase activity, which mediates the hormonal signal transduction.

2. Growth hormone deficiency may be a result of:
  a. Adult hypopituitarism (Sheehan's syndrome) where, in conjuction with low cortisol levels, may lead to hypoglycemia.
  b. Juvenile hypopituitarism due to either craniopharyngioma or an idiopathic etiology, resulting in **pituitary dwarfism.**
    (1) Recombinant DNA (rDNA)–derived growth hormone is used to treat pituitary dwarfism.
    (2) Growth hormone is contraindicated in subjects with:
      (a) Closed epiphyses
      (b) Active tumors or neoplasia
      (c) Active or unhealed intracranial lesions
    (3) There are two synthetic versions of growth hormone. Somatropin (191 amino acids) is the same as endogenous growth hormone; Somatrem (192 amino acids) has an extra methionine on the *N*-terminus.
    (4) Adverse reactions
      (a) Development of antibodies to growth hormone, the clinical significance of which is uncertain
      (b) Occasional headache, myalgia, mild hyperglycemia, and glucosuria
      (c) Leukemia in a small percentage of treated children
      (d) Hypothyroidism
      (e) Glucose intolerance due to insulin resistance
      (f) Reduction of growth-promoting effects as a result of interference from glucocorticoid therapy
      (g) Development of a limp due to slipped capital femoral epiphysis

3. Hypersecretion of growth hormone can result in **acromegaly** and **gigantism**.
   a. The use of **bromocriptine,** a dopaminergic agonist, in acromegaly is paradoxical since dopamine stimulates growth hormone secretion in normal individuals.
   b. Analogs of somatostatin, such as **octreotide,** offer therapeutic promise with minimal side effects.
   c. Over 90% of the cases of acromegaly are caused by growth hormone–secreting adenomas, or somatotropinomas.

B. Prolactin

1. Activity, regulation, and mechanism of action
   a. Prolactin is synthesized and stored in pituitary lactotrophs, but secretion is primarily under negative control by the hypothalamus.
   b. **Dopamine** is putatively considered the **prolactin release-inhibiting hormone (PRIH)**.
   c. Prolactin release mirrors that of growth hormone with regards to stimuli, such as sleep, exercise, circadian rhythms, and estrogen levels.
   d. Dopamine may not be the only PRIH as opioid peptides and TRH affect prolactin secretion.
   e. The primary physiologic action of prolactin is lactation. Prolactin, in a complex interaction with hormones of the adrenal cortex, thyroid, and ovaries, prepares the breast for secretion postpartum. Insulin, growth hormone, and oxytocin are also involved.
   f. During pregnancy, high estrogen and progestin levels inhibit prolactin activity, but after birth, these hormone levels drop, leaving prolactin's actions unopposed.
   g. Breast-feeding elevates prolactin levels, which mediates an antigonadotropic effect, causing a lack of ovulation. This natural contraception diminishes over several months as the prolactin release to the sucking response wanes.
   h. Prolactin induces rapid increases in RNA synthesis for milk production proteins and lactose synthesis.

2. Prolactin-secreting disorders
   a. Hyperprolactinemia may be due to:
      (1) Dopaminergic antagonist drug therapy
      (2) Infiltrative disorders of the hypothalamus or pituitary
      (3) Hypothyroidism
      (4) Use of oral contraceptives
      (5) Prolactin-secreting tumors
   b. Treatment of the resulting galactorrhea, amenorrhea, and infertility
      (1) Levodopa (l-dopa), a precursor to dopamine synthesis, has been used with initial and variable success, but some patients become refractory.
      (2) Bromocriptine, an ergot derivative and dopaminergic agonist, is often used in treating pituitary adenomas.
         (a) Galactorrhea and amenorrhea usually abate within weeks, and pregnancy is possible.
         (b) Bromocriptine should be discontinued during pregnancy.
         (c) Tumor regression has been noted, but the mechanism is unknown.
         (d) Cessation of bromocriptine therapy generally allows a recurrence of symptoms (and tumors).
         (e) Bromocriptine restores ovulatory menses in about 80% of women with hyperprolactinemia.
   c. Prolactin may be contributory in the development of mammary tumors.
      (1) In animal models, drugs that enhance prolactin secretion (e.g., reserpine, haloperidol, phenothiazines) facilitate tumor growth.
      (2) In patients with breast tumors, prolactin levels are normal; however, there may be a permissive role.

C. Human placental lactogen

1. Activity
   a. Placental lactogen has both growth-promoting and lactogenic activity.
   b. Its amino acid sequence is 83% identical to growth hormone and 30% identical to prolactin.

2. Function
   a. The function is not clearly defined but placental lactogen is synthesized by the syncytiotrophoblasts of the placenta for release into maternal circulation.

     b. Placental lactogen stimulates growth and development of the mammary gland.

     c. Placental lactogen is also luteotropic and may stimulate steroid production by the corpus luteum.

D. Gonadotropic hormones, FSH, LH, hCG, and inhibin, are also collectively known as glycoprotein hormones.

  1. Activity, regulation, and mechanism of action

     a. FSH and LH are produced and secreted by the gonadotropic cells of the pituitary. As with other hormones under hypothalamic control, their release is modulated by plasma steroid concentrations, or the combined effect of their action (feedback inhibition).

     b. At puberty, gonadotropin secretion doubles, reflecting increases in frequency and amplitude of GnRH pulses.

     c. In men, FSH and LH plasma levels are fairly stable; in women, plasma levels vary with the stage of the menstrual cycle.

     d. Hormonal control of ovulation and the menstrual cycle is complex due to several levels of interaction and feedback inhibition.

       (1) The **preovulatory,** or **follicular, phase** is characterized by rising LH and FSH levels, which mediate ovulation and follicular growth, respectively. Ovarian estrogen production increases.

       (2) **Ovulation** is associated with LH and FSH spikes, often three- to sixfold higher than during menstruation. Estrogen production peaks also.

       (3) The **postovulatory,** or **luteal, phase** is characterized by proliferation of vaginal and uterine mucosae. Menstruation is then determined by the cessation of progesterone production.

       (4) As the **corpus luteum** involutes, estrogen and progesterone levels decline, causing endometrial and uterine degeneration, and menstruation begins.

       (5) The degeneration of the corpus luteum may be mediated by a luteolytic substance, prostaglandin $F_{2\alpha}$ ($PGF_{2\alpha}$), or it may be programmed to degenerate at a fixed interval without external signals.

     e. hCG is secreted by the syncytiotrophoblasts of the fetal placenta as early as 1 week after ovulation.

       (1) hCG maintains luteal function and suppresses LH release.

       (2) hCG can be detected in the urine; levels peak at about 6 weeks after conception and stabilize at a lower level during pregnancy.

  2. Oral contraceptives

     a. Types of formulations

       (1) **Combination preparations** are the most common oral contraceptives used and contain both an **estrogen** and a **progestin.**

         (a) The estrogen used is either **ethinyl estradiol** or **mestranol.**

         (b) The progestin used is **norethindrone acetate, or norgestrel, or ethynodiol diacetate.**

         (c) The primary mechanism of action appears to be suppression of the midcycle surge of LH and FSH, thereby suppressing ovulation and ovarian follicle growth.

       (2) **Sequential preparations** (estrogen for 14–16 days followed by 5–6 days of combined estrogen and progestin) were removed from the market due to reports of increased incidence of endometrial tumors.

         (a) A **biphasic** or **triphasic** preparation, which replaces these, has a fixed estrogen level, but varies the progestin level to reflect changes in the menstrual cycle.

         (b) This approach may minimize "breakthrough" or irregular bleeding.

       (3) **Single-entity preparations**

         (a) The "minipill" contains progestin alone and may act by thickening the consistency of cervical mucus, which is a barrier to sperm. It has a high failure rate and may cause irregular bleeding.

         (b) The "morning after" pill, or postcoital preparation, contains diethylstilbestrol (DES). DES must be started within 72 hours and continued (25 mg twice daily) for 5 days in spite of nausea and vomiting. If DES is not effective, abortion may be considered due to the increased risk of vaginal carcinoma in children exposed in utero to estrogen and DES.

     b. Adverse effects

       (1) Estrogen increases the risk of thrombotic events, presumably by increasing levels of clotting factors and platelet aggregation.

(a) Thrombophlebitis and thromboembolism are significantly increased and appear to be estrogen dose-dependent.

(b) The incidence of cerebral and coronary thrombosis is increased and reflects age, smoking, hypertension, or other comorbid disease, and duration of estrogen therapy.

(c) Mortality may increase 15–18 times in women over 45 years old who smoke.

(d) The use of preparations with low estrogen (35 ng or less) and progestin decreases the risk of thrombotic events.

(2) Moderate-to-severe hypertension occurs in about 5% of all women on oral contraceptives but is generally reversible. Estrogen and progestin facilitate salt and water retention due to increased plasma renin and consequent angiotensin activity.

(3) The development of certain types of **cancer** has been studied with oral contraceptives, but actual culpability is clouded by the long latency period and multiple risk factors.

    (a) Estrogens are tumorigenic, causing tumors of the breast, uterus, testis, bone, and other tissues.

    (b) There is an increased incidence of vaginal and cervical cancer in women who were exposed in utero to DES.

    (c) **Postmenopausal women** taking only estrogen may have a 5–15-fold **increased risk** of developing endometrial cancer. Epidemiologic studies show a **lower incidence** when estrogen levels are reduced or accompanied by progestin.

    (d) Interestingly, **premenopausal women** taking combination oral contraceptives may have a **reduced risk** of endometrial and ovarian cancer.

    (e) Studies examining breast cancer rates among birth control users are conflicting and complicated by multiple risk assessment. Presently, there is no confirmed evidence of increased risk, but oral contraceptives are **contraindicated** in patients with known or suspected neoplasms. Close monitoring of patients with fibrocystic disease, history of breast cancer, or breast nodules is advised.

(4) Nausea, vomiting, breast tenderness, weight gain, dizziness, and headaches are all associated with oral contraceptive use.

(5) Depression, irritability, ocular disturbances, and an increased incidence of gallbladder disease have been noted.

(6) Oral contraceptives may cause birth defects if taken during the first trimester of pregnancy.

3. Levonorgestrel implants (Norplant)

a. Activity and mechanism of action

(1) Contraception is achieved by subdermal implantation of six flexible silastic tubes containing a progestin, levonorgestrel. Effective contraception may last up to 5 years.

(2) The amount of hormone initially released is about 85 ng/day but drops to about 50 ng/day at 9 months. At 18 months, the level is about 35 ng/day, which eventually bottoms out to about 30 ng/day.

(3) **The mechanism of action** is due to inhibition of ovulation and thickening of cervical mucus. Effective contraception may be achieved within 1 day when implanted during the first 7 days of menstruation.

(4) Altered lipoprotein levels have been noted.

    (a) Total cholesterol levels decreased in all studies and significantly so in several trials.

    (b) High-density lipoprotein (HDL) levels have been noted to go both up or down but with no definite trend.

    (c) Low-density lipoprotein (LDL) and triglyceride levels decreased.

    (d) Increases have been noted in the ratio of total cholesterol to HDL-cholesterol, but they were not statistically significant.

b. Adverse effects

(1) **Bleeding irregularities** are common but diminish over time; hemoglobin levels generally increase, probably due to diminished loss of menstrual blood.

(2) **Delayed follicular atresia** has been noted but rarely caused complications.

(3) Ectopic pregnancies have occurred with levonorgestrel implant use, but the rate (1.3/1000 woman-years) was less than that seen in noncontraceptive users (2.7–3.0/1000 woman-years). **Increased weight** may increase the possibility of ectopic pregnancy. Patients with lower abdominal/pelvic pain should be evaluated to rule out ectopic pregnancy.

(4) Levonorgestrel has been identified in **breast milk**. Children followed up to 3 years show no significant effects on growth or health. Levonorgestrel implants or other steroids, are not the contraceptives of first choice for lactating mothers.

(5) Thromboembolic disorders may require removal of the steroid implants. Removal should also be considered in cases of prolonged immobilization or illness.

(6) Cardiovascular side effects are increased in women who smoke.

(7) Elevated blood pressure may occur.

(8) There is an increased risk of thrombosis, stroke, or heart attack.

(9) Carcinoma risk assessment may show reduced ovarian and endometrial cancer ratios but increased risk of breast cancer.

(10) Hepatic tumors have been reported.

(11) Ocular lesions have been reported.

c. Contraindications include:

   (1) Active **thrombophlebitis** or **thromboembolic disease**

   (2) Undiagnosed abnormal **genital bleeding**

   (3) Known or suspected **pregnancy**

   (4) Hepatic disease; benign or malignant **liver tumors**

   (5) Known or suspected **breast cancer**

4. Noncontraceptive uses (estrogens and progestins)

  a. Prevention of heart attacks

   (1) Estrogens have a beneficial effect in postmenopausal women in reducing myocardial infarction morbidity and mortality.

   (2) Estrogens have a deleterious effect, increasing risk in men and possibly in premenopausal women.

   (3) Estrogens decrease LDL and increase HDL levels; progestins have the opposite effect. Atherosclerosis is correlated with elevated LDL and lower HDL levels.

  b. Postmenopausal osteoporosis

   (1) Osteoporosis is due to loss of both hydroxyapatite (calcium phosphate complexes) and protein matrix (colloid), resulting in compromised skeletal integrity.

   (2) Several months of estrogen therapy may be necessary to effect a positive Ca^{2+} balance. Doses of 15–25 ng/day are required to maintain or increase bone density.

   (3) The positive effects may be rapidly lost when estrogen therapy is discontinued.

   (4) The risk-to-benefit ratio is highest for women who have undergone hysterectomy or oophorectomy because endometrial carcinoma (from estrogens) is no longer an issue.

  c. Estrogen replacement therapy

   (1) Estrogen during and after **menopause** is used to relieve vasomotor symptoms, hot flashes, and atrophic vaginitis.

   (2) Dysmenorrhea can also be treated with a nonsteroidal anti-inflammatory drug (NSAID).

   (3) Failure of **ovarian development** (dysgenesis) may result in dwarfism due to hypopituitarism. Estrogen therapy at puberty in combination with an androgen for growth spurt can satisfactorily emulate endogenous release.

  d. Antineoplastic uses of certain hormones have evolved, allowing manipulation of cancer development.

   (1) Progestins are used in endometrial, breast, and prostate carcinomas and in hypernephromas.

   (2) Antiandrogens and DES are used in prostatic cancer.

   (3) Antiestrogens, such as tamoxifen, and androgens are used in the treatment of breast cancer.

    (a) Tamoxifen, after oral dosing, reaches peak blood levels within 4–7 hours; it has a biphasic half-life of 7–14 hours and 4–7 days. Steady-state levels are achieved within 4 weeks.

    (b) Tamoxifen is primarily indicated for:

     (i) Initial endocrine control of breast cancer

     (ii) Palliative treatment of advanced breast cancer in postmenopausal women. Premenopausal women do not respond as well as women who have been postmenopausal for years.

    (c) Tamoxifen has a relatively safe toxicity profile but **adverse effects** include:

     (i) Hot flashes, nausea, and vomiting

     (ii) Menstrual irregularities, vaginal bleeding, and discharge

     (iii) Pruritus vulvae and dermatitis

(iv) Pain or inflammation at the tumor site, which is associated with a good response

(d) GnRH agonists have also been used in conjunction with antiandrogens for treatment of prostate cancer.

(i) Leuprolide, a peptide analog, inhibits LH and FSH release by chronically stimulating, desensitizing and down-regulating pituitary GnRH receptors.

(ii) Leuprolide produces responses equal to DES with less toxicity.

(iii) A leuprolide-induced transient flare-up of the disease can be prevented by concurrent use of flutamide, an antiandrogen.

(iv) Leuprolide is given as an injectable depot or by single administration.

5. **Fertility drugs**

a. **Clomiphene** is a nonsteroidal partial antagonist, which induces ovulation presumably by blocking hypothalamic estrogen receptors.

(1) The disrupted feedback inhibition results in enhanced gonadotropin secretion.

(2) In premenopausal women, ovulation may be accompanied by formation of ovarian cysts and ovarian hypertrophy.

(3) In men, gametogenesis and steroidogenesis are also increased.

(4) Clomiphene has little or no effect in postmenopausal women.

(5) After clomiphene treatment, 80% of the patients ovulate, 30%–40% become pregnant, and about 10% of these pregnancies are multiple births.

b. **Gonadotropins**

(1) Human menopausal gonadotropin (**Pergonal**) contains equal amounts of FSH and LH, whereas urofollitropin (**Metrodin**) contains only FSH. They stimulate ovarian follicle development but require a sequential dose of hCG to induce ovulation. They are administered parenterally.

(2) This treatment is reserved for:

(a) Women with low basal gonadotropin levels and low endogenous estrogen

(b) Women who do not respond to clomiphene or cannot tolerate it

(c) Men (with hCG) to augment spermatogenesis

(3) These agents are **contraindicated** in:

(a) Women with primary ovarian failure

(b) Uncontrolled thyroid or adrenal dysfunction

(c) Intracranial lesions, such as a pituitary tumor

(d) Pregnancy

(e) Abnormal bleeding

(f) Ovarian cysts or enlargement not due to polycystic ovary syndrome

(4) An important **adverse effect** to note is the development of **ovarian hyperstimulation syndrome (OHSS)**.

(a) OHSS is clinically distinct from ovarian enlargement and is characterized by a dramatic increase in vascular permeability.

(b) Acute fluid retention in the peritoneal cavity, thorax, and pericardium may yield pelvic pain, nausea, vomiting, and weight gain.

(c) OHSS occurs in about 1%–6% of all patients treated and most often starts after therapy is discontinued.

(5) Multiple births have been reported in 17%–20% of all treated pregnancies.

6. **Progestins (noncontraceptive uses) and antiprogestins**

a. **Progestins** may be indicated for:

(1) Dysfunctional uterine bleeding

(2) Dysmenorrhea

(3) Premenstrual syndrome

(4) Endometriosis

(5) Suppression of postpartum lactation

(6) Carcinoma

(7) Hypoventilation

b. **Antiprogestins,** such as mifepristone (RU-486), are under clinical investigation for use as a contraceptive and abortifacient.

(1) Mifepristone is a competitive antagonist at both progesterone and glucocorticoid receptors. Its actions include:

(a) Inhibition of ovulation during the follicular phase by blocking hypothalamic-pituitary progesterone receptors, which suppresses midcycle gonadotropin release

(b) During the luteal phase, inhibition of progesterone action on the uterus, which induces prostaglandin release from the endometrium

(c) Termination of pregnancy by facilitating luteolysis, menstruation, uterine motility, softening of the cervix, and detachment of the embryo

(2) Mifepristone is also being studied for use in:

(a) Induction of labor after intrauterine death

(b) Cervical ripening in anticipation of a second-trimester abortion

(c) The treatment of progesterone-sensitive tumors, as an adjunct

7. Androgens and antiandrogens

a. Testosterone is synthesized in the testis, ovary, and adrenal cortex.

(1) In target tissues, like the seminiferous tubules or Sertoli cells, testosterone is reduced to dihydrotestosterone.

(2) The actions of the androgenic hormones manifest in early embryonic growth (sex differentiation), early neonatal life (anabolic growth), puberty, and adult sexual life.

(3) The gonadotropin, LH, appears to mediate its effect through cyclic AMP on the Leydig cells to convert cholesterol to androgens.

(4) The major effect of FSH is on the Sertoli cells of the seminiferous tubules and, thus, spermatogenesis. FSH also affects LH-mediated actions on the Leydig cells.

(5) Growth hormone and estrogen may have synergistic and antagonistic actions, respectively, on LH-mediated effects.

b. Feedback inhibition of gonadotropin release may encompass not only plasma cerebral spinal fluid (CSF) levels of hormones but also estrogens formed locally in the brain and **inhibin,** a peptide produced in the Sertoli cells and ovary.

c. Therapeutic uses include:

(1) Replacement therapy to induce puberty and maintain sex characteristics in adults with testicular failure, accidental castration, or hypogonadism

(2) In some types of refractory anemia to stimulate erythropoietin secretion

(3) For desired anabolic effects (weight gain) in undernourished patients or in the terminally ill (This application is a controversial and dangerous form of abuse among professional athletes.)

(4) Replacement therapy in women with hypopituitarism; androgens are given in conjunction with other hormones (i.e., thyroid, growth, adrenal corticosteroid, estrogen hormones)

(5) Breast cancer therapy due to an antiestrogenic effect

(6) Short stature, not due to pituitary insufficiency (growth hormone) (Androgen treatment in children less than 9 years old may have negative consequences.)

(7) Hereditary angioneurotic edema, a condition where complement activation is unopposed, leading to increased vascular permeability and angioedema (The benefit of androgens is likely manifested on liver function rather than an androgenic action per se.)

d. Preparations are available for oral, injectable, or transdermal (scrotal skin) administration.

(1) The greatest androgenic potency is with agents that are 17-β esters of testosterone and given by injection.

(a) Substitution at the 17-β position affects lipid solubility and duration of action.

(b) In order of decreasing duration, the 17-β esters are testosterone ethanate > cypionate > propionate > acetate.

(2) The 17-α alkylated derivatives are orally active and less androgenic. Some are 17-α methyltestosterone, Fluoxymesterone, oxandrolone, and norethindrone.

e. Adverse effects are divided into three major areas.

(1) Virilizing effects

(a) Acne, facial hair, and deepening of the voice in women

(b) Menstrual irregularities

(c) Male-pattern baldness, altered musculature, and hypertrophy of the clitoris

(d) Premature closing of epiphyseal plates and altered bone development in children

(e) Masculinization of the female embryo after in utero exposure

(f) Inhibition of gonadotropin release (in normal men) and reduction spermatogenesis for months after discontinuation

(2) Feminizing effects

(a) Gynecomastia in men but the mechanism is poorly understood

(b) Exacerbation of feminizing effects in children and men with poor liver function

(3) Toxic effects
(a) Edema
(b) Jaundice and cholestatic hepatitis, especially with all of the 17-α alkyl substituted androgens
(c) Peliosis hepatitis (rare)
(d) Hepatic carcinoma
(e) Effects on laboratory and diagnostic tests

f. Antiandrogens
(1) Androgen receptor antagonists, like cyproterone and flutamide, are potentially useful in treating prostate cancer, acne, male-pattern baldness, virilizing syndromes, precocious puberty, and inhibiting the sex drive in men who are sex offenders.
(2) Finazteride, a 5α-reductase inhibitor, acts by blocking the metabolic activation of testosterone to dihydrotestosterone. This agent is being studied in benign prostatic hypertrophy.

g. Male contraceptives
(1) Gossypol, a phenolic derivative of the cotton plant, is a potent azoospermic agent and also impairs sperm motility, both of which are reversible effects. Adverse effects include those seen in cottonseed poisoning:
(a) Hypokalemia and weakness
(b) Diarrhea, edema, dyspnea, and neuritis
(c) Paralysis at high doses
(2) Gonadal steroids, like **estrogen** and **progesterone,** are azoospermic but depress libido and potency; gynecomastia can occur.
(3) An experimental regimen with variable results is a combination of an **androgen** and a **progestin**. Azoospermia develops over months and takes as long to recover following discontinuation.
(4) Potent agonists and antagonists of GnRH, given with testosterone, produce variable azoospermia.

E. Thyroid hormones

1. Synthesis
a. Thyroglobulin, a large protein of 600,000 molecular weight, is synthesized in the thyroid gland.
b. The tyrosines on the molecule are iodinated and coupled by a peroxidase. The iodinated thyroglobulin is secreted into the lumen of the gland.
c. The hypothalamus releases TRH, which stimulates the pituitary gland to release thyrotropin. In the thyroid gland, thyrotropin stimulates the uptake of thyroglobulin from the lumen back into the cell where it is broken down to yield the thyroid hormones.
d. There are two active forms of thyroid hormone (Figure 10-1): **thyroxine (T_4)** and **triiodothyronine (T_3),** which is the more potent form.

2. Physiology
a. Thyroid hormones regulate growth and development.
b. They exert a calorigenic effect by increasing the basal metabolic rate.
c. Thyroid hormones accelerate carbohydrate utilization and enhance lipolytic reactions, one consequence of which is a decrease in plasma cholesterol.
d. They inhibit pituitary secretion of thyrotropin by negative feedback.
e. They are cardiovascular stimulants.

3. Therapeutic uses
a. Thyroid hormone therapy is used for the treatment of hypothyroidism (myxedema), including myxedema coma.
b. If thyroid hormone therapy is begun early after birth in hypothyroid infants, the consequences of cretinism are prevented.
c. Thyroid hormone is used in patients with simple goiter and in patients with nodular goiter who are deficient in the secretion of thyroid hormone. In the case of nodular goiter, carcinoma should be ruled out.

4. Preparations and administration
a. Thyroid tablets are made from extracts of the thyroid gland.
b. Thyroglobulin is a purified extract of pig thyroid.
c. Levothyroxine sodium is the sodium salt of L-thyroxine.

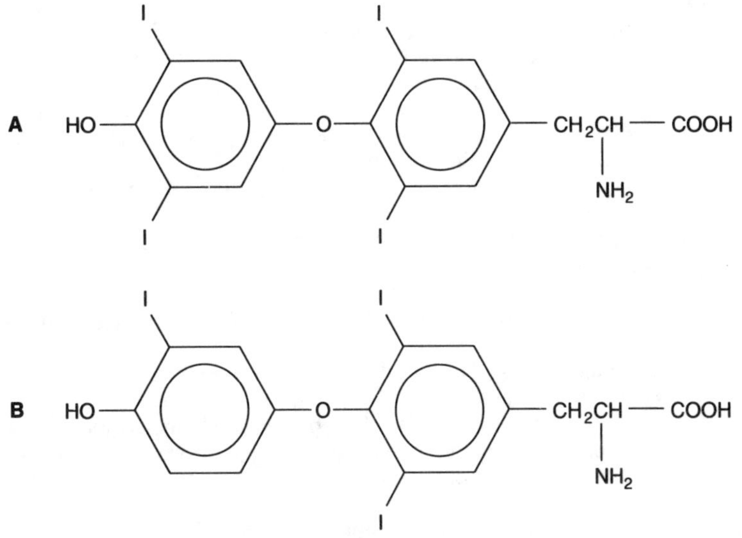

Figure 10-1. Structures of thyroxine (*A*) and triiodothyronine (*B*).

   d. Liothyronine sodium is the sodium salt of L-triiodothyronine.
   e. Equivalent clinical responses are obtained from the daily administration of about 60 mg of thyroid, 60 mg of thyroglobulin, 100 μg of levothyroxine, or 25 μg of liothyronine.

5. Adverse effects
   a. Cardiac effects are the most important and call for care in initiating therapy.
   b. Palpitations caused by thyroid hormones can be treated with β-adrenergic blocking agents.
   c. Levothyroxine can cause thyrotoxicosis. During long-term administration, serum T_4 levels may rise without a change in dose.

6. Thyroid hormone inhibitors
   a. Types and their mechanisms of action
      (1) Antithyroid agents. Propylthiouracil and methimazole both inhibit the organification of iodine by inhibition of peroxidase. Propylthiouracil also inhibits the peripheral conversion of T_4 to T_3.
      (2) Ionic inhibitors competitively inhibit iodine uptake. They are seldom used today.
      (3) Iodide in high concentrations can suppress the thyroid by mechanisms that are not clear.
      (4) Radioactive iodine concentrates in the thyroid gland and, in sufficient amounts, can damage the gland through the cytotoxic effects of ionizing radiation.
   b. Antithyroid agents
      (1) Pharmacokinetics
         (a) The prototype agent, **propylthiouracil,** is rapidly absorbed and has a short half-life (2 hours). It has a shorter duration of action than methimazole. Both drugs concentrate in the thyroid and are excreted renally.
         (b) Antithyroid agents cross the placenta and are found in breast milk, methimazole to a greater extent than propylthiouracil.
      (2) Therapeutic uses. Antithyroid agents are most frequently used to treat children, young adults, and pregnant women with hyperthyroidism due to Graves' disease. They may be used:
         (a) Alone
         (b) With radioiodine, while awaiting the beneficial effects of radiation to appear
         (c) Prior to the surgical treatment of hyperthyroidism
      (3) Adverse effects
         (a) The most serious adverse effect, though rare, is agranulocytosis.
         (b) The most common adverse effect is transient leukopenia.
         (c) Other common complaints are maculopapular rash and fever.
         (d) Joint pain and hair depigmentation can occur.

c. Iodide
(1) Therapeutic uses in hyperthyroidism
(a) Iodide is used preoperatively to control hyperthyroidism in Graves' disease because it reduces the size of the gland and makes the gland firmer.

(b) It is best to control the hyperthyroidism first with an antithyroid agent, such as propylthiouracil. Iodide is then begun 10 days prior to the operative procedure.

(2) Preparations and administration
(a) Lugol's solution contains 5% iodine, which is reduced to iodide in the intestine, and 10% postassium iodide.

(b) Potassium iodide is available for oral use in both solution and solid forms.

(3) Adverse effects
(a) Preparations containing iodine or iodide can produce an acute hypersensitivity reaction, resulting in angioedema, cutaneous hemorrhages, and symptoms of serum sickness.

(b) Chronic iodide administration can result in **iodism.**

   (i) This is characterized by a brassy taste, increased salivation, and soreness of the teeth and gums. Swelling of the eyelids and symptoms resembling an upper respiratory tract infection can be observed.

   (ii) Inflammation of the pharynx and larynx can occur, as well as severe frontal headache.

   (iii) Several types of skin lesions have been observed.

   (iv) All of the above symptoms usually resolve within a few days after the discontinuance of iodide.

d. Radioactive iodine
(1) Pharmacokinetics
(a) The most commonly used isotope is iodine-131 (^{131}I), which has a half-life of 8 days and emits both β particles and γ rays.

(b) Radioiodine is rapidly incorporated into the colloid of the thyroid follicles.

(2) Therapeutic uses
(a) Radioactive iodine is highly effective in the treatment of hyperthyroidism, especially in older patients with heart disease.

(b) It is also a useful diagnostic tool to delineate thyroid disorders.

(3) Preparations and route of administration. Sodium iodide labeled with either ^{131}I or iodine-125 (^{125}I) is available as a solution and as capsules and can be administered orally or intravenously.

(4) Adverse effects
(a) The treatment of hyperthyroidism with radioactive iodine is associated with a relatively high incidence of delayed hypothyroidism.

(b) Usually, there is a delayed onset in the control of hyperthyroidism.

(c) There is no conclusive evidence that radioiodine causes cancer in adults, but most physicians are hesitant to use it in patients less than 30 years old, not only because of this possible risk but also because of potential unknown effects on future offspring.

(d) Radioiodine is contraindicated in pregnancy and in nursing mothers.

F. Parathyroid hormones

1. General considerations
a. Physiologic role of parathyroid hormone
(1) Parathyroid hormone (PTH, parathormone) is a single peptide chain of 84 amino acids, which regulates the concentration of Ca^{2+} and phosphate levels in the extracellular fluid. Plasma Ca^{2+} is the most important regulator of PTH secretion.

(2) PTH acts on various peripheral tissues to mobilize Ca^{2+} into the extracellular fluid and restore the concentration to normal when it has been lowered.

(3) PTH increases the active absorption of Ca^{2+} from the small intestine. This is a vitamin D–dependent process.

(4) PTH increases the rate of bone resorption of Ca^{2+} and phosphate.

(5) At physiologic doses PTH increases the renal tubular reabsorption of Ca^{2+} and the excretion of phosphate.

(6) The effects on both bone and kidney are probably mediated via cyclic AMP.

(7) PTH has a plasma half-life of about 2–5 minutes and is rapidly removed by the liver and kidney.

b. Diseases of the parathyroid gland
    (1) Hypoparathyroidism
        (a) Hypoparathyroidism is one of many causes of hypocalcemia.
        (b) Symptoms include paresthesias of the extremities, tetany, laryngospasm, and eventually generalized convulsions. Spasms of smooth muscle can also occur. Electrocardiographic changes can include marked tachycardia.
        (c) Dietary supplementation of vitamin D and Ca^{2+} is the principal form of treatment.
    (2) Hyperparathyroidism
        (a) The primary form is due to parathyroid hyperplasia or adenoma or to tumors at other sites.
        (b) The secondary form is a result of conditions producing a negative Ca^{2+} balance, such as malabsorption or renal disease.
        (c) Symptoms and signs include hypercalciuria (which can result in renal calculi), muscle weakness, constipation, nausea, and vomiting.
        (d) Treatment is usually by surgical resection, although long-term therapy with neutral phosphate, a low-calcium diet, and plenty of fluids may be given to those patients who are poor surgical candidates.

2. Calcitonin
  a. General considerations
    (1) Parafollicular C cells of the thyroid are the site of production and secretion of calcitonin. Parafollicular C cells are also found in the parathyroid and thymus.
    (2) The synthesis and secretion of calcitonin are regulated by the plasma Ca^{2+} concentration. Cyclic AMP, epinephrine, glucagon, gastrin, and cholecystokinin all play a role by stimulating calcitonin release following the ingestion of Ca^{2+} salts.
    (3) By altering osteoclastic and osteocytic activity, calcitonin can directly inhibit bone resorption.
    (4) Calcitonin, in part by a cyclic AMP–mediated reaction, increases kidney excretion of Ca^{2+}, phosphate, and sodium (Na^+).
  b. Therapeutic uses
    (1) The major uses of calcitonin are to decrease hypercalcemia and hyperphosphatemia in patients with:
        (a) Hyperparathyroidism
        (b) Idiopathic hypercalcemia of pregnancy
        (c) Vitamin D intoxication
        (d) Osteolytic bone metastases
    (2) Calcitonin may decrease the rate of bone loss in patients with postmenopausal osteoporosis.
    (3) Though calcitonin is effective for the treatment of Paget's disease of bone, patients may become resistant to therapy in several months.
  c. Preparations and route of administration
    (1) Calcitonin used clinically is salmon calcitonin.
    (2) It is administered subcutaneously or intramuscularly.
  d. Adverse effects include occasional edema and nausea and the stimulation of antibody formation.

3. Sodium etidronate
  a. Mechanism of action. It is thought to slow the formation and dissolution of hydroxyapatite crystals.
  b. Pharmacologic effects. Its advantages over calcitonin include oral efficacy and lack of antigenicity.
  c. Therapeutic uses. Sodium etidronate is used in the treatment of Paget's disease of bone.
  d. Route of administration. Etidronate disodium is given orally. Daily doses, given for not more than 6 months, may produce a long-lasting remission.

G. Corticotropin and adrenal corticosteroids

1. General considerations
  a. The adrenal cortex serves as a homeostatic organ, regulating reactions to stress.
  b. Corticosteroid pathway. The release of adrenal corticosteroids is controlled by a pathway (Figure 10-2) that includes the central nervous system (CNS). Corticosteroid secretion shows a diurnal rhythm; peak secretion occurs between 4 A.M. and 8 A.M.

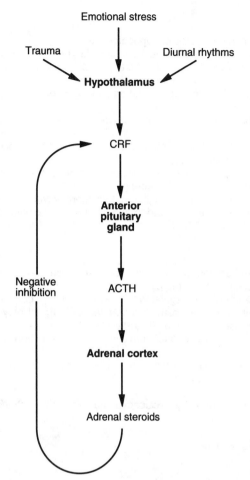

Figure 10-2. The pathway of adrenocorticotropic hormone (*ACTH*) and adrenal steroid secretion. *CRF* = corticotropin-releasing factor.

(1) A number of stimuli, including trauma, chemicals, diurnal rhythms, and emotion, can cause the hypothalamus to release **corticotropin-releasing factor (CRF)**.

(2) CRF traverses the hypophyseal portal system and stimulates the anterior pituitary gland.

(3) The anterior pituitary gland, in turn, is stimulated to release ACTH.

(4) ACTH circulates in the bloodstream and stimulates the production of **glucocorticoids** from the adrenal cortex. The major endogenous glucocorticoid is cortisol (hydrocortisone) with 10–25 mg secreted daily. About 0.5–2 mg of corticosterone and 30–150 μg of aldosterone are secreted daily. In stressful situations, these values can increase tenfold.

(5) **Aldosterone** secretion is stimulated by serum angiotensin and serum potassium (K^+) levels.

(6) A **negative feedback pathway** maintains homeostasis. When the levels of endogenous corticosteroids increase, the **pituitary–adrenal axis** is suppressed, and the production of ACTH is reduced, as is that of CRF.

   c. **Endogenous corticosteroids** released by the adrenal cortex

     (1) **Glucocorticoids** chiefly affect carbohydrate and protein metabolism. Endogenous glucocorticoids include:

       (a) Cortisol (hydrocortisone)

       (b) Cortisone

       (c) Corticosterone

     (2) **Mineralocorticoids** chiefly affect electrolyte and water metabolism. Endogenous mineralocorticoids include:

       (a) Aldosterone

       (b) Desoxycorticosterone

2. **Adrenocorticotropic hormone (ACTH)**
   a. **Chemistry**
      (1) Human ACTH is a polypeptide hormone consisting of 39 amino acids.
      (2) Synthetic derivatives have fewer amino acids but still possess the action of endogenous ACTH.
   b. **Mechanism of action**
      (1) ACTH is thought to stimulate specific protein receptor sites on the adrenal cortical cell membrane.
      (2) This membrane receptor is believed to be linked with a system for generating cyclic AMP. When the receptor is occupied by ACTH, the cyclic AMP system is activated and the synthesis of corticosteroids is initiated. ACTH is thought to increase the amount of cholesterol entering the mitochondria.
      (3) The binding of ACTH to the receptor stimulates the rate-limiting step in the corticosteroid synthetic pathway (which originates with cholesterol).
      (4) Although ACTH is required for the synthesis of mineralocorticoids, it stimulates the synthesis of glucocorticoids more than that of mineralocorticoids.
   c. **Therapeutic uses.** The development of synthetic steroids limited the use of ACTH principally to serving as a **diagnostic tool** for distinguishing the two types of adrenal insufficiency.
      (1) In **primary adrenal insufficiency (Addison's disease),** the administration of ACTH produces no effect because of the underlying adrenal cortex dysfunction.
      (2) In **secondary adrenal insufficiency,** the dysfunction occurs in the anterior pituitary. If ACTH is administered, the adrenal cortex will respond by synthesizing and releasing the adrenocorticosteroids.
   d. **Route of administration.** Since ACTH is a polypeptide hormone, it must be administered parenterally, and most often is given intramuscularly. It is rapidly hydrolyzed in the tissues with a half-life of 15 minutes.
   e. **Adverse effects** from ACTH are rare, but hypersensitivity reactions have occurred on occasion. Toxicity is dose-related and results from corticosteroid excess.

3. **Adrenal corticosteroids**
   a. **Structure-activity relationships.** The general structure of a corticosteroid is shown in Figure 10-3. Certain structural features are especially relevant to activity:
      (1) Position 11: Oxygen or halogen is essential for corticoid function to exist.
      (2) Position 17: The presence of OH or C = O increases corticoid activity.
      (3) A double bond at 1,2 increases glucocorticoid activity.
      (4) Position 6 or 9: Halogenation increases activity.
      (5) Position 6 or 16: The presence of an alkyl group increases glucocorticoid activity.
   b. **Mechanism of action**
      (1) The steroid receptor is nuclear, not cytoplasmic as previously thought.
      (2) Once the steroid traverses the cell membrane and binds to the receptor, the steroid–receptor complex in the cell nucleus then binds to chromatin.
      (3) The drug-receptor-chromatin complex stimulates the formation of messenger RNA (mRNA).
      (4) The mRNA stimulates the synthesis of enzymes that control rate-limiting reactions in the synthetic pathway of the steroids.
   c. **Pharmacokinetics**
      (1) Adrenal corticosteroids are readily absorbed from the gastrointestinal tract.

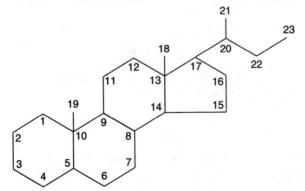

Figure 10-3. General structure of the adrenal corticosteroids.

(2) Some 90% of a dose becomes bound to plasma proteins.

(3) Steroids are metabolized in the liver and are often bioactivated by reduction reactions. The final or phase II metabolic reaction results in the conjugation of the steroid with sulfate or glucuronide, and the conjugate then is excreted by the kidney.

d. Glucocorticoid effects

(1) Physiologic doses of cortisol are released into the circulation. Transport occurs via transcortin, which is a high-affinity, low-capacity carrier. Physiologic doses can result in:

(a) Increased liver glycogen stores

(b) Increased gluconeogenesis

(c) Increased lipolysis

(d) CNS effects, at times including euphoria

(e) Maintenance of cardiovascular function by potentiation of norepinephrine

(f) Maintenance of skeletal muscle function (in Addison's disease, there is wasting of skeletal muscle)

(g) Increased hemoglobin synthesis, resulting in an elevation of the red blood cell count

(2) Pharmacologic doses of cortisol bind to albumin, a low-affinity, high-capacity carrier. Pharmacologic doses can result in:

(a) Anti-inflammatory and antiallergic effects, in which steroids:

(i) Suppress leukocyte migration

(ii) Stabilize lysosomal membranes

(iii) Reduce the activity of fibroblasts, which are involved in collagen and tissue repair in inflamed areas

(iv) Reverse the capillary permeability that is associated with histamine release

(v) Suppress the immune response by inhibiting antibody synthesis

(b) Inhibition of growth and cell division

(3) The anti-inflammatory and antiallergic effects result from glucocorticoid inhibition of prostaglandin and leukotriene synthesis (see Chapter 8 V D 1; Figure 8-3).

e. Mineralocorticoid effects. Unlike the case with glucocorticoids, physiologic and pharmacologic doses of mineralocorticoids produce similar effects; it is the intensity of the effects that differs.

(1) Mineralocorticoids cause retention of Na^+, phosphate, Ca^+, and bicarbonate (HCO_3^-) and reduction of serum K^+.

(2) Control of serum Na^+ depends primarily upon the juxtaglomerular apparatus, where a low Na^+ level in the blood causes the release of renin from the kidney. Renin cleaves angiotensinogen to form angiotensin (see Chapter 8 III A); angiotensin II triggers aldosterone release.

(3) Aldosterone acts on Na^+ and K^+ transport in the distal tubule of the kidney to enhance Na^+ reabsorption.

f. Route of administration. Corticosteroid dosing varies greatly, depending on the patient's condition.

(1) It is best if oral steroids are taken around 8 A.M. to mimic the natural secretion of the adrenal cortex.

(2) A major concern is to avoid suppression of the pituitary–adrenal axis.

(a) If the axis is suppressed, the adrenal cortex will not respond to stress by releasing steroids; the consequences can be fatal.

(b) Once the axis is suppressed, it may take more than a year for normal function to return.

(c) Less than 25 mg of prednisone per day (or equivalent; see Table 10-1) taken at 8 A.M. for fewer than 5–10 days usually will not suppress the pituitary–adrenal axis.

(d) To minimize the effects of pituitary–adrenal axis suppression, when steroid treatment ceases, doses should be tapered off rather than stopped abruptly.

(3) When steroids are used in children, alternate-day therapy is recommended. With this regimen, normal growth patterns can be maintained and suppression of the pituitary–adrenal axis by negative feedback is less likely.

g. Preparations

(1) Systemic

(a) Mineralocorticoids

(i) Aldosterone is an endogenous mineralocorticoid but is not available as a medicinal agent.

(ii) Desoxycorticosterone and **fludrocortisone** are the agents used as replacements for aldosterone in Addison's disease.

Table 10-1. Glucocorticoids: Anti-Inflammatory Potency, Relative Oral Potency, and Potential for Sodium Retention

Glucocorticoid	Anti-Inflammatory Potency	Equivalent Oral Potency (mg)	Sodium Retention
Short-acting (12 hr or less)			
Hydrocortisone	1.0	20	2+
Cortisone	0.8	25	2+
Intermediate-acting (12–24 hr)			
Prednisolone	5.0	5	1+
Prednisone	4.0	5	1+
Methylprednisolone	5.0	4	0
Triamcinolone	5.0	4	0
Long-acting (over 24 hr)			
Betamethasone	40.0	0.6	0
Dexamethasone	30.0	0.75	0

(b) **Glucocorticoids**
   (i) **With some mineralocorticoid activity. Hydrocortisone** and **cortisone** are examples. Though they possess primarily glucocorticoid activity, they do cause some Na^+ retention. This becomes significant only in patients who are not able to tolerate the additional Na^+ load.
   (ii) **Without mineralocorticoid activity.** These are semisynthetic analogs of the natural substances and are very important, since an anti-inflammatory dose can be given without the adverse effect of Na^+ retention. Examples include **prednisone, prednisolone, methylprednisolone, triamcinolone, betamethasone,** and **beclomethasone.** Beclomethasone was the first corticosteroid available in inhalation form; it is used to treat acute bronchial asthma.
(c) Table 10-1 lists the commonly used corticosteroids, divided on the basis of their duration of action, with their anti-inflammatory potency, equivalent milligram potency, and Na^+ retention potential.

(2) **Topical** (Table 10-2)
   (a) For mild pruritus or inflammation, or for maintenance treatment of some dermatoses, 1% topical hydrocortisone is adequate.
   (b) For active acute dermatoses or resistant chronic dermatitis, a higher potency steroid may be more effective.
   (c) **Clobetasol propionate** is a high potency topical steroid, which appears to be effective for the treatment of psoriasis and other dermatoses. Clobetasol can cause adrenal suppression and, therefore, should be reserved for severe, refractory dermatoses.

h. **Therapeutic uses**
   (1) **Replacement therapy for adrenal insufficiency**
      (a) For acute adrenal insufficiency, cortisol (hydrocortisone) Na^+ succinate is given first by intravenous injection; it is then given in intravenous fluids.
      (b) For chronic adrenal insufficiency, cortisone acetate is taken on arising and in the late afternoon, and the mineralocorticoid fludrocortisone acetate is taken daily.
   (2) **Management of rheumatoid arthritis**
      (a) Before systemic steroids are used, therapy with nonsteroidal agents is tried (see Chapter 9 II). The patient also should be exhibiting progressive disability.
      (b) Steroids can also be administered by intra-articular injection for the temporary relief of especially painful joints.
   (3) **Other uses.** Corticosteroids are also widely used in the treatment of:
      (a) Rheumatic carditis
      (b) Renal diseases, including the nephrotic syndrome
      (c) Most collagen vascular diseases
      (d) Severe allergic reactions
      (e) Ocular disorders involving inflammation
      (f) Various skin diseases, usually by topical administration

Table 10-2. Potency of Topical Steroids

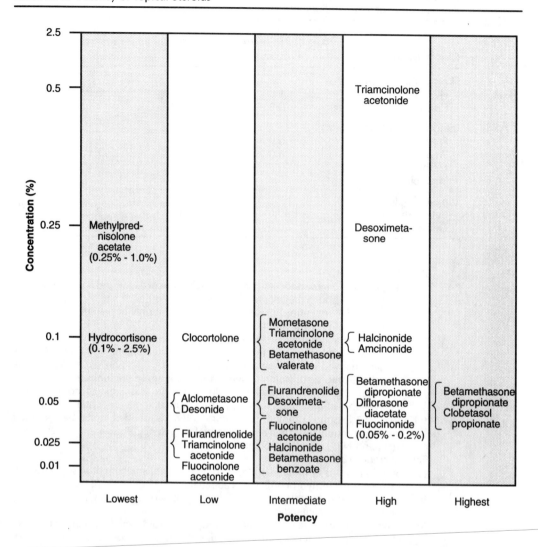

< >

Concentration (%)	Lowest	Low	Intermediate	High	Highest
0.5			Triamcinolone acetonide		
0.25	Methylpred-nisolone acetate (0.25% - 1.0%)			Desoximeta-sone	
0.1	Hydrocortisone (0.1% - 2.5%)	Clocortolone	{ Mometasone Triamcinolone acetonide Betamethasone valerate	{ Halcinonide Amcinonide	
0.05		{ Alclometasone Desonide	{ Flurandrenolide Desoximeta-sone	{ Betamethasone dipropionate Diflorasone diacetate Fluocinonide (0.05% - 0.2%)	{ Betamethasone dipropionate Clobetasol propionate
0.025 / 0.01		{ Flurandrenolide Triamcinolone acetonide Fluocinolone acetonide	Fluocinolone acetonide Halcinonide Betamethasone benzoate		

Potency

(g) Chronic ulcerative colitis
(h) Cerebral edema
(4) The use of corticosteroids in cancer patients is discussed in Chapter 11 V D.
i. **Adverse effects**
(1) Prolonged therapy with corticosteroids can result in the following:
(a) Suppression of pituitary–adrenal function
(b) Increased susceptibility to infection
(c) Peptic ulceration, which may be the result of altered mucosal defense mechanisms
(d) Myopathy characterized by proximal arm and leg weakness
(e) Psychological disturbances, including suicidal tendencies or "steroid psychosis"
(f) Posterior subcapsular cataracts, especially in children
(g) Osteoporosis, which can lead to vertebral fractures
(i) Glucocorticoids directly inhibit osteoblast formation as well as intestinal Ca^{2+} absorption.
(ii) They also increase secretion of parathyroid hormone.
(h) Hyperglycemia
(2) Glucocorticoids can arrest growth in small children receiving small doses. Both DNA synthesis and cell division are inhibited.

4. Adrenal steroid inhibitors

a. **Metyrapone** reduces cortisol production by inhibiting the 11-β-hydroxylation reaction.

(1) It is used in diagnosing primary and secondary adrenal insufficiency. When cortisol production is blocked, negative feedback should increase ACTH and the production of precursors of cortisol if the pituitary and adrenal glands are functional.

(2) Metyrapone has also been used to treat hypercortisolism that results from adrenal neoplasms.

b. **Ketoconazole** (see Chapter 12 III E) inhibits adrenal steroidogenesis and is being studied as an investigational drug for use in hyperadrenal states.

IV. DIABETES MELLITUS AND INSULIN THERAPY

A. General considerations

1. In 1921, Banting and Best extracted insulin from the pancreas and demonstrated its therapeutic effects in diabetic dogs and human subjects.

2. It is important to remember that diabetes mellitus involves not only a deficiency of insulin but also an excess of certain other hormones, such as growth hormone, glucocorticoids, and glucagon. Thus, not only the pancreas is involved in glucose homeostasis, but also the anterior pituitary gland and the adrenal cortex.

3. Etiology of diabetes mellitus

a. It is currently believed that the juvenile-onset (insulin-dependent) form has an autoimmune etiology.

b. Viruses may also play a role in the etiology of diabetes. Coxsackie B, mumps, and rubella viruses all have been shown to produce morphologic changes in the islet-cell structure.

c. The genetic role in the etiology of diabetes is controversial. Possibly a genetic trait makes an individual's pancreas more susceptible to one of the above viruses.

4. Syndromes of diabetes mellitus

a. **Type I (juvenile-onset, insulin-dependent, IDDM) diabetes**

(1) In this type of diabetes, there is no circulating insulin in the plasma and, thus, insulin replacement is required.

(2) There is complete failure of pancreatic β-cell function.

(3) The patient is prone to both hyperglycemia and ketoacidosis.

b. **Type II (maturity-onset, non–insulin-dependent, NIDDM) diabetes**

(1) This type may be due to a defect in the receptor on the pancreatic β-cell membrane.

(2) In the earliest forms of the disease, there is a delay in the initial secretion of insulin after stimulation by glucose.

(3) Also, less insulin than normal is secreted at any given glucose concentration.

(4) The patient is not prone to ketoacidosis.

c. In both types of diabetes mellitus, plasma immunoreactive glucagon concentrations are increased, especially during ketoacidosis. The normal suppression of glucagon by hyperglycemia is also impaired.

d. The pathognomonic finding of capillary basement membrane thickening occurs early in the course of diabetes mellitus. It is this change that is probably responsible for the major **complications of diabetes,** including:

(1) Microangiopathy

(2) Nephropathy

(3) Neuropathy

(4) Retinopathy

(5) Atherosclerosis

(a) This disorder occurs more often in diabetics than in nondiabetics.

(b) Tibial and peroneal artery sclerosis are almost the *sine qua non* of diabetes.

B. Chemistry of insulin

1. Insulin consists of two amino acid chains joined together by disulfide linkages; it has a molecular weight of about 6000.

2. Pancreatic β cells form insulin from a single-chain precursor, proinsulin, which possesses little biologic activity.

3. Insulin can exist as a monomer, a dimer, or a hexamer consisting of three dimers.
   a. Two molecules of zinc are coordinated in the hexamer form, and it is this form that is stored in the granules of the β cell.
   b. The biologically active form is thought to be the monomer.

4. There are species variations in the amino acid sequence of insulin.

C. Mechanism of action

1. The initial action of insulin is at the cell surface, where the hormone interacts with a highly specific receptor.

2. Exactly how insulin facilitates the transport of glucose and amino acids is not known.

D. Pharmacokinetics

1. Regulation of insulin secretion (Figure 10-4)
   a. Insulin is synthesized in the β cells of the islets of Langerhans as a single polypeptide precursor, preproinsulin, which is subsequently converted to proinsulin.
   b. Proinsulin, is synthesized in the rough endoplasmic reticulum and packaged, through the Golgi apparatus, into secretory granules. Along the way, an enzymatic process converts proinsulin to insulin and C peptide.
   c. Stored granules containing many insulin molecules are released by exocytosis.
   d. Oral glucose has a greater ability to stimulate insulin secretion than intravenously administered glucose. Fatty acids, amino acids, and ketone bodies all increase insulin secretion.

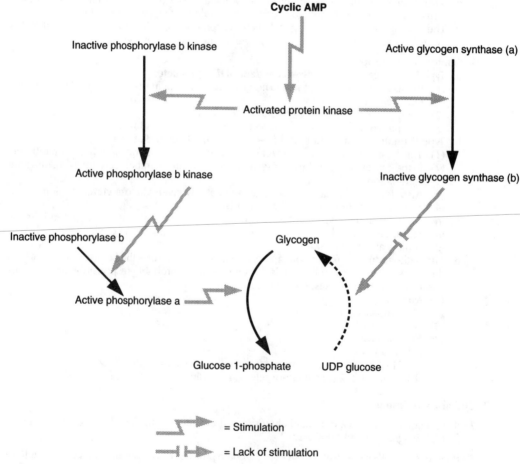

Figure 10-4. Regulation of insulin secretion. (Adapted from the work of Huijing and Larner and of Soderling et al.)

    e. Gastrointestinal hormones, such as secretin, pancreozymin, and gastrin, can stimulate insulin secretion.

    f. Autonomic control of insulin secretion

      (1) β-Adrenergic agonists increase insulin secretion by increasing intracellular cyclic AMP.

      (2) Cyclic AMP plus Ca^{2+} may activate a microtubular–microfilament system that promotes the release of the insulin granule.

    g. Glucose-induced insulin release appears to occur in two phases:

      (1) An initial-burst phase, which peaks in minutes and then rapidly declines

      (2) A slow phase, which takes an hour to reach a peak

  2. Most secreted insulin circulates in the blood and lymphatic system as the free hormone.

  3. Though small quantities of insulin can be detected in the urine, the kidney normally filters and reabsorbs the hormone.

  4. Both the liver and the kidney are of primary importance in the degradation of insulin by a proteolytic enzyme. Each is capable of destroying 40% of the insulin produced per day.

E. Metabolic effects of insulin deficiency

  1. When insulin is deficient, there is a reduction in the rate of transport of glucose across the membranes of certain cells, including muscle and adipose cells.

  2. Insulin does not significantly influence the rate of glucose transport across liver cells, erythrocytes, or leukocytes, and the rate of entry of glucose into the brain is only affected in ketoacidosis.

  3. There is a reduction in the activity of the enzyme systems necessary for catalyzing glucose to glycogen.

  4. Hyperlipemia, ketonemia, and acidosis can all occur with insulin deficiency. The lack of insulin allows hormone-sensitive lipase to mobilize fatty acids, which leads to elevated circulating levels of ketones, acetoacetate, and β-hydroxybutyrate.

  5. Insulin deficiency combined with glucagon excess results in the conversion of large amounts of protein to glucose, resulting in an increased excretion of urea and ammonia (azoturia).

F. Route of administration

  1. The usual route of administration for all insulin preparations is subcutaneous. The limitation of the route is the variability on insulin absorption from the depot injection site.

  2. Insulin is administered intravenously during emergency circumstances. If administration is via this route, the crystalline form is used. Recently, peritoneal infusion and intranasal administration with adjuvants have resulted in successful hormone replacement.

  3. Intensified treatment regimens, including multiple daily injections and continuous subcutaneous infusion have been employed to mimic the physiologic replacement of insulin.

  4. Since insulin is a protein, it cannot be given orally because it would be digested.

G. Preparations. Various types of insulin are made that differ in their onset and duration of action. The potency of insulin is expressed in USP units.

  1. Crystalline zinc insulin (regular insulin)

    a. Regular insulin is a short-acting, soluble insulin, which is prepared in a phosphate buffer with zinc at a pH of 3.5.

    b. Its peak action occurs in 2–4 hours and its duration is 5–7 hours.

    c. It can be administered subcutaneously or intravenously and is a good agent for exerting rapid control for diabetic ketoacidosis.

    d. The frequency of injections (4–5/day) is not very convenient.

  2. Protamine zinc insulin

    a. Adding the basic protein protamine to crystalline zinc insulin causes the formation of large crystals. This produces a compound that is less soluble.

    b. When injected, this formulation serves as a tissue depot, producing slow absorption into the bloodstream.

    c. The action of protamine zinc insulin peaks in 16–18 hours and lasts up to 36 hours.

    d. Fine control of hyperglycemia is difficult with such a long-acting preparation.

  3. Isophane insulin (NPH, neutral protamine Hagedorn)

    a. This intermediate-acting insulin is similar to protamine zinc insulin, but it contains only a small amount of protamine (0.5 mg/100 units of insulin).

    b. Therefore, NPH insulin has an earlier onset and earlier peak effects than protamine zinc insulin, but the duration of action is similar for both preparations.

    c. The effects of NPH insulin peak in 8–12 hours and have a duration of 24–48 hours.

    d. These effects are clinically equivalent to combining 2–3 units of crystalline zinc insulin with 1 unit of protamine zinc insulin.

  4. Lente insulins

    a. These insulins do not contain protamine; their insolubility results from the addition of excess zinc in an acetate rather than a phosphate buffer.

    b. The onset of action for the lente insulins varies greatly and depends upon the physical state, the ambient zinc concentration, and the pH.

    (1) A microamorphous crystalline form, known as **prompt insulin zinc suspension (semilente insulin),** peaks in 4–8 hours and has a duration of action of 12–16 hours.

    (2) A large crystalline form with a high zinc content, known as **extended insulin zinc suspension (ultralente insulin),** has an onset and duration of action similar to those of protamine zinc insulin.

    (3) Combining 7 parts of ultralente with 3 parts of semilente produces **insulin zinc suspension (lente insulin),** which is quite similar to NPH insulin in its onset and duration of action.

  5. Human insulins

    a. Human insulins are produced by semisynthetic and recombinant DNA techniques.

    b. Recently, the human proinsulin gene was synthesized, and human proinsulin is now produced on a large scale as the precursor to human insulin.

    c. Human insulin's biologic activity and intravenous pharmacokinetics are quite similar to porcine insulin.

    d. Human insulins are useful for individuals with an allergy to insulin from animal sources.

    e. It is absorbed more quickly than porcine insulin after subcutaneous injection, thereby improving glycemic control after meals.

H. Factors altering insulin requirements

  1. Other drugs. Salicylates inhibit the enzymes necessary for gluconeogenesis and also accelerate their utilization. Anticoagulants tend to stimulate insulin secretion, thereby decreasing insulin requirements.

  2. Hormones. Glucagon, epinephrine, and growth hormone all increase insulin requirements.

  3. Exercise. This decreases insulin requirements by making muscle more permeable to glucose and releasing muscle-bound insulin.

  4. Stress. Both physiologic (i.e., fever, infection, pregnancy) and psychological stress increase insulin requirements, possibly secondary to epinephrine release.

  5. Eating patterns. Alterations in the diet or a change in eating time may increase or decrease insulin requirements.

  6. Obesity. This increases insulin requirements, perhaps as the result of an increase in the number of insulin-binding sites on the greater surface area of the adipose tissue.

I. Adverse effects

  1. Hypoglycemia

    a. The worst sequela is **insulin shock,** characterized by abnormalities of the CNS, including hypoglycemic convulsions.

    b. Early symptoms of hypoglycemia, such as sweating, tachycardia, and hunger, are thought to be brought about by the compensatory secretion of epinephrine.

    c. Hypoglycemia is best treated by administering glucose intravenously, or by giving fruit juice or other soluble carbohydrates. Glucagon may be administered parenterally as an alternative to glucose.

2. **Local reactions.** Irritation at the site of insulin injection can lead to lipohypertrophy or lipo-atrophy. Sites of injection should be rotated. Subcutaneous infusion can result in infection and local allergic reactions to components of the infusion system.

3. **Antigenic response**
   a. With the development of new, more highly purified animal insulins and the advent of human insulin, the production of insulin antibodies and the hypersensitivity reactions are less of a problem. Insulin antibodies may attenuate responses to regular insulin injected subcutaneously and delay recovery from hypoglycemia.
   b. The order of antigenic potency, in descending order, is beef > pork > highly purified ("single-peak") pork > human insulin. Antigenicity increases as the duration of action of the insulin is increased. Thus, protamine zinc insulin is the most antigenic because of its long duration of action and also because it contains a large amount of the basic protein protamine.

4. **Growth-promoting properties** of insulin may be a factor in the macrovascular complications of diabetes.

5. **Weight gain** is an undesirable effect of intensive insulin therapy.

V. ORAL HYPOGLYCEMIC AGENTS (SULFONYLUREAS)

A. Mechanism of action

1. Sulfonylureas stimulate insulin secretion from pancreatic β cells without entering the cell. This occurs in the absence of glucose.

2. Sulfonylureas may also sensitize the pancreatic β cells to glucose and inhibit the efflux of K^+ from pancreatic β cells.

3. Sulfonylureas induce increased activity of peripheral insulin intracellular receptors.

4. Sulfonylureas may act to reduce glucagon secretion.

5. High-affinity sulfonylurea receptors have been demonstrated on pancreatic β cells. The order of potency of sulfonylurea in binding to β cells approximates its potency in stimulating the release of insulin and inhibiting the effects of K^+.

B. Preparations and pharmacokinetics. All sulfonylurea agents are readily absorbed from the small intestine and are avidly bound by plasma proteins. Their onset of action varies from 30 minutes to 3 hours. The duration of action also varies from agent to agent. The general structure of a sulfonylurea is illustrated in Figure 10-5.

1. **Tolbutamide**
   a. The onset of action occurs in 30 minutes, while the duration of action is 6–12 hours.
   b. Tolbutamide is the shortest-acting and least potent sulfonylurea and is readily metabolized in the liver to inactive products. Excretion occurs via the kidney.

2. **Acetohexamide**
   a. Onset of action is rapid; effects peak in 3 hours and last for 12–18 hours.
   b. The major metabolite, hydroxyhexamide, is thought to possess most of the activity of this agent. It is excreted renally.

3. **Tolazamide**
   a. Tolazamide is slowly absorbed. Effects do not peak for 6 hours, and the drug has a duration of action of 24 hours.
   b. Its metabolic products are weaker hypoglycemics than the parent compound.
   c. Metabolic products are excreted by the kidney.

4. **Glyburide** and **glipizide** are second-generation sulfonylureas. They are the most potent sulfonylurea agents available. Both are metabolized by the liver to products with little activity. Both drugs have a duration of action of 24 hours.

5. **Chlorpropamide**
   a. Though rapidly absorbed, this agent has a duration of action of 24–60 hours because of its binding to plasma proteins.
   b. It is metabolized in the liver and is excreted slowly by the kidney as unchanged drug and as metabolites.

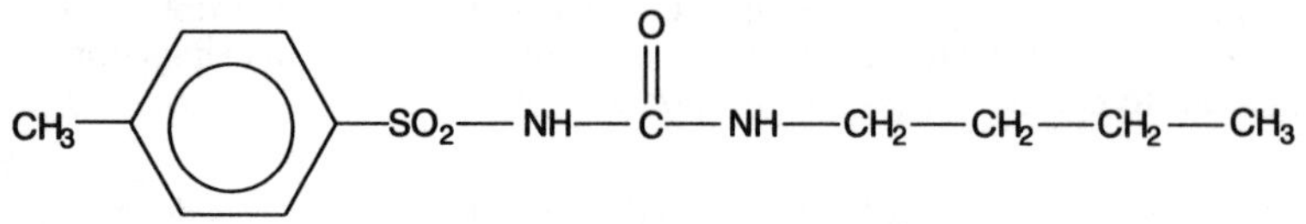

Tolbutamide

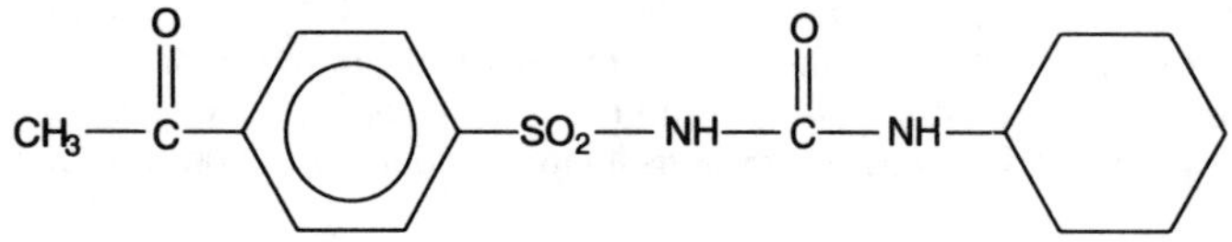

Acetohexamide

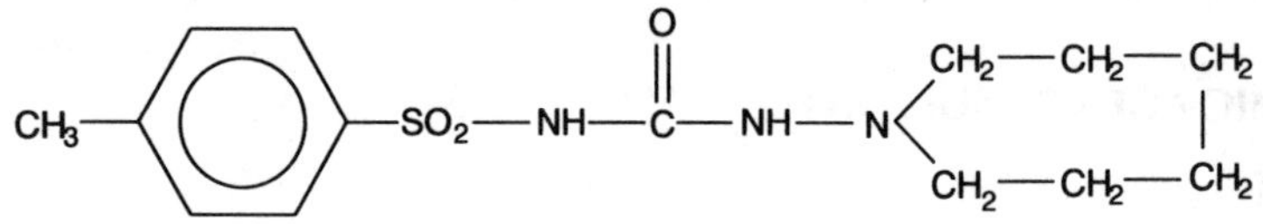

Tolazamide

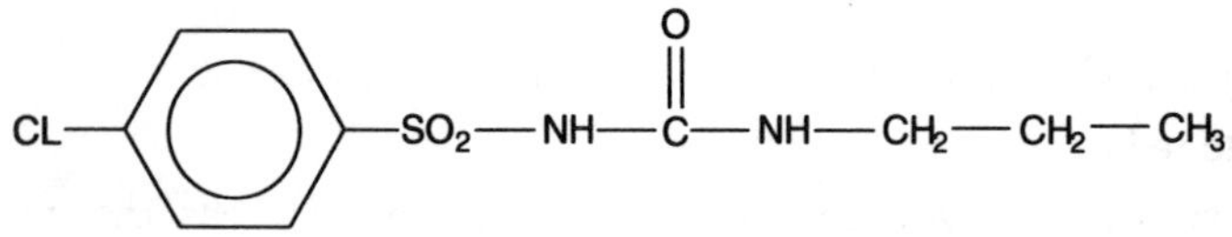

Chlorpropamide

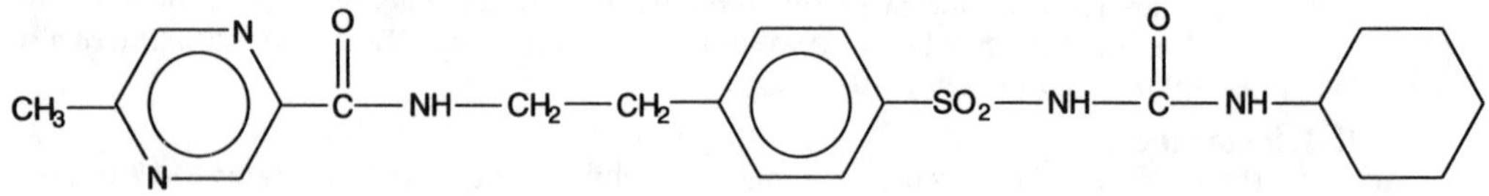

Glipizide

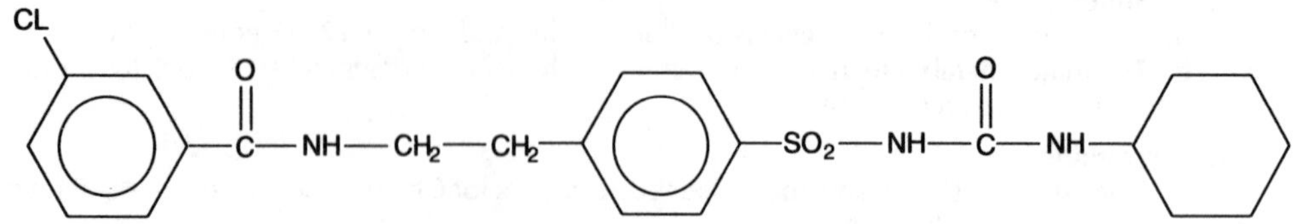

Glyburide

Figure 10-5. Structure of sulfonylurea agents.

C. Therapeutic uses

1. The sulfonylureas are used in the treatment of patients who have NIDDM and who cannot be treated with diet alone or who are unwilling to take insulin if dietary control fails.

2. The findings of the University Group Diabetes Program (UGDP), though controversial, support the above statement, and many physicians have had success using the sulfonylurea agents. The UGDP study did suggest that use of these agents was associated with a higher cardiovascular mortality rate than that occurring with dietary control alone or with insulin therapy.

3. No study to date has demonstrated that sulfonylurea agents prevent the long-term complications of diabetes.

4. Combining a sulfonylurea with a suboptimal insulin regimen in patients with NIDDM may provide better glycemia control than the suboptimal insulin regimen alone or reduced insulin requirements.

D. Adverse effects

1. These are seen in 3%–5% of patients treated with a sulfonylurea agent.

2. Hypoglycemia can occur in elderly patients with hepatic or renal insufficiency because the agent will have a longer than expected duration of action. Its frequency is related to potency and duration of action of the drug. The highest incidence occurs with glyburide and chlorpropamide.

3. Cutaneous reactions include rashes and photosensitivity.

4. Gastrointestinal reactions include nausea and vomiting.

5. Hematologic reactions—leukopenia, agranulocytosis, thrombocytopenia, pancytopenia, and hemolytic anemia—have occurred.

6. Transient cholestatic jaundice occurs rarely.

7. Inappropriate secretion of antidiuretic hormone has been observed, especially with chlorpropamide, which can cause hyponatremia.

8. A disulfiram-like reaction has been reported with chlorpropamide.

9. Other drugs may influence the hypoglycemic actions of sulfonylureas through pharmacodynamic and pharmacokinetic interactions. Since sulfonylureas are highly bound to plasma proteins, any drug that displaces them could enhance their hypoglycemic activity.

STUDY QUESTIONS

Directions: Each of the numbered items or incomplete statements in this section is followed by answers or by completions of the statement. Select the **one** lettered answer or completion that is **best** in each case.

1. An adrenocortical drug that is anti-inflammatory in pharmacologic doses is

(A) desoxycorticosterone
(B) aldosterone
(C) cortisol
(D) vasopressin
(E) oxytocin

2. All of the following statements about growth hormone are true EXCEPT

(A) it may stimulate the synthesis or release of somatomedins
(B) low levels of IGF-1 are associated with dwarfism
(C) Sheehan's syndrome may result in growth hormone deficiency
(D) hyposecretion can result in acromegaly
(E) it is contraindicated in subjects with closed epiphyses

3. Which of the following agents is incorrectly matched with the descriptive phrase that follows?

(A) Dopaminergic antagonist drug therapy—may result in hyperprolactinemia
(B) Bromocriptine—restores ovulatory menses in women with hyperprolactinemia
(C) hCG—peaks 2 weeks after conception
(D) Sequential oral contraceptive preparations—associated with an increased incidence of endometrial tumors
(E) "Minipill"—contains progestin alone

4. All of the following statements about oral contraceptives are true EXCEPT

(A) the "combination pill" contains both estrogen and progestin
(B) ethinyl estradiol and mestranol are commonly used in oral contraceptives
(C) the "minipill" contains progestin alone
(D) the "triphasic pill" is a variant of the combination pill
(E) the triphasic pill contains estrogen, progestin, and luteinizing hormone

5. Thrombophlebitis and thromboembolism have been associated with the use of oral contraceptives that have an excess of

(A) progestin
(B) estrogen
(C) testosterone
(D) aldosterone
(E) prostaglandins

6. Which adverse effect is incorrectly matched with the statement about oral contraceptives?

(A) Thrombotic events—high estrogen, low progestin decreases the risk
(B) Hypertension—occurs in 5% of all women on oral contraceptives
(C) Tumorigenic—estrogen dose-dependent
(D) Combination oral contraceptives—reduce risk of endometrial and ovarian cancer in premenopausal women
(E) Smoking—increases cardiovascular side effects in women who take oral contraceptives

7. Correct statements about ACTH include all of the following EXCEPT

(A) endogenous ACTH is also called corticotropin
(B) ACTH stimulates the synthesis of corticosteroids
(C) release of ACTH can be inhibited by cortisol
(D) ACTH is most useful clinically as a diagnostic tool in adrenal insufficiency
(E) the oral route is the preferred route of administration

8. Endogenous corticosteroids released by the adrenal cortex include all of the following EXCEPT

(A) cortisol
(B) cortisone
(C) beclomethasone
(D) aldosterone
(E) corticosterone

1-C	4-E	7-E
2-D	5-B	8-C
3-C	6-A	

9. Which of the following statements about adrenal steroids is true?

(A) "Glucocorticoid activity" implies an effect on electrolyte homeostasis
(B) ACTH and cortisol both have the basic steroid nucleus
(C) Pharmacologic doses of glucocorticoids cause few toxic effects
(D) Steroid receptors mediate the metabolic effects of steroids
(E) Aldosterone secretion is inhibited by serum angiotensin

10. Which of the following synthetic steroids shows predominantly mineralocorticoid action?

(A) Hydrocortisone
(B) Spironolactone
(C) Dexamethasone
(D) Fludrocortisone
(E) Cortisone

11. Effects of physiologic doses of cortisol (glucocorticoids) include all of the following EXCEPT

(A) an increase of liver glycogen stores
(B) maintenance of normal cardiovascular function
(C) changes in mood and behavior
(D) increased lipogenesis from protein
(E) increased hemoglobin synthesis

12. Prolonged therapy with corticosteroids can lead to all of the following adverse effects EXCEPT

(A) suppression of the pituitary–adrenal axis
(B) increased susceptibility to infection
(C) peptic ulceration
(D) muscle hypertrophy
(E) psychological disturbances

13. Correct statements about crystalline zinc (regular) insulin include all of the following EXCEPT

(A) it can serve as replacement therapy for juvenile-onset diabetes
(B) it can be administered intravenously
(C) it is a short-acting insulin
(D) it can be administered orally
(E) it is a good agent for the rapid control of diabetic ketoacidosis

14. The primary reason for a physician to prescribe human insulin is that

(A) it has a faster onset of action than other insulins
(B) it has a shorter duration of action than other insulins
(C) it can be given to patients who have an allergy to animal insulins
(D) it is more effective in preventing the complications of diabetes than animal insulins
(E) it is cheaper than other insulins because it is produced by recombinant technology

---

9-D	12-D
10-D	13-D
11-D	14-C

Directions: Each item below contains four suggested answers of which **one or more** is correct. Choose the answer

    A if **1, 2, and 3** are correct
    B if **1 and 3** are correct
    C if **2 and 4** are correct
    D if **4** is correct
    E if **1, 2, 3, and 4** are correct

15. A patient who is undergoing menopause complains that the "hot flashes" are extremely disturbing. Which of the following drugs could relieve her symptoms?

(1) Ethinyl estradiol
(2) Ethynodiol
(3) Mestranol
(4) Fluoxymesterone

16. A poorly controlled diabetic patient is complaining of hunger, sweating, and palpitations. Examination reveals a moist, pale skin and hypothermia. Which of the following can be deduced from this patient's symptoms?

(1) The patient's symptoms are due to hyperglycemia
(2) The insulin dose is probably too high
(3) The patient is probably "spilling" sugar in her urine
(4) The symptoms are premonitory of insulin shock

Directions: The group of questions below consists of lettered choices followed by several numbered items. For each numbered item select the **one** lettered choice which it is **most** closely associated. Each lettered choice may be use once, more than once, or not at all.

Questions 17–19

For each indication listed below, select the drug that is most appropriate.

(A) Levothyroxine
(B) Propylthiouracil
(C) Iodide
(D) Parathyroid hormone
(E) Calcitonin

17. Useful in the treatment of hyperparathyroidism

18. Useful in conjunction with radioiodine therapy

19. Useful in the treatment of myxedema

15-B   18-B
16-C   19-A
17-E

ANSWERS AND EXPLANATIONS

1. The answer is C *[I A 2; III G 1 c (2), 3 d (2) (a), g (1) (a); Table 10-1]*
Both desoxycorticosterone and aldosterone are mineralocorticoids and, thus, have no anti-inflammatory effects. Vasopressin and oxytocin are produced by the hypothalamus and have no anti-inflammatory properties. ACTH and cortisol possess anti-inflammatory properties, ACTH because it stimulates glucocorticoid synthesis and cortisol because it is a glucocorticoid.

2. The answer is D *[III A 1 f, 2 a, b, 3]*
Acromegaly and gigantism result from hypersecretion, not hyposecretion, of growth hormone. Over 90% of cases are caused by growth hormone–secreting adenomas. All of the other statements in the question are true.

3. The answer is C *[III B 2 a, b (2), D 1 e (2), 2 a (2), (3)]*
Hyperprolactinemia may result from dopaminergic antagonist drug therapy, infiltrating disorders of the hypothalamus or pituitary, hypothyroidism, use of oral contraceptives, and prolactin-secreting tumors. Bromocriptine, an ergot alkaloid derivative and dopaminergic agonist, is often used to treat pituitary adenomas. Estrogen for 14–16 days followed by 5–6 days of combined estrogen: progestin (sequential) were removed from the market due to reports of an increased incidence of endometrial tumors. The "minipill" contains progestin alone, which acts by thickening the consistency of cervical mucus, creating a barrier to sperm. hCG can be detected in the urine. Levels peak 6 weeks after conception and stabilize at a lower level during pregnancy.

4. The answer is E *[III D 2 a (2) (a)]*
The "triphasic pill" does not contain leutinizing hormone. It provides estrogen in constant dosage and a progestin in varying dosage to reflect the changing progesterone levels of the normal menstrual cycle. All of the other statements in the question are true.

5. The answer is B *[III D 2 b]*
Estrogen excess can be associated with nausea, monilial infections, cholasma and increased areolar pigmentation, edema, leg cramps, thrombophlebitis, and, in predisposed individuals (i.e., smokers, hypertensives), an increased incidence of cerebral and coronary thrombosis.

6. The answer is A *[III D 2 b (1)–(3)]*
Preparations with low estrogen (35 mg or less) and progestin decrease the risk of thrombotic events. Estrogen can increase the risk of thrombotic events by increasing levels of clotting factors and platelet aggregation. All of the other statements listed in the question are true.

7. The answer is E *[III G 1 b (1)–(6), 2 c, d]*
ACTH cannot be administered orally. Since it is a polypeptide hormone, it must be administered parenterally, most often intramuscularly. All of the other statements in the question are true.

8. The answer is C *[III G 1 c]*
Cortisol, cortisone, aldosterone, and corticosterone are endogenous corticosteroids released by the adrenal cortex. Beclomethasone was the first steroid available in a form suitable for inhalation and is used to treat acute bronchial asthma.

9. The answer is D *[III G 1 b (5), c (2), 2 a (1), 3 b, i]*
Mineralocorticoids, not glucocorticoids, affect electrolyte homeostasis. ACTH does not have a basic steroid nucleus; it is a polypeptide with 39 amino acids. Pharmacologic doses of glucocorticoids often result in a number of adverse effects. Steroid receptors do indeed mediate the metabolic effects of steroids. Aldosterone secretion is stimulated by serum angiotensin.

10. The answer is D *[III G 3 g (1) (a) (ii); Ch 6 IX B]*
Hydrocortisone and cortisone are short-acting glucocorticoids with some mineralocorticoid activity. Spironolactone is an aldosterone antagonist. Dexamethasone has no Na^+-retaining potency. Fludrocortisone shows predominantly mineralocorticoid action.

11. The answer is D *[III G 3 d (1)]*
Glucocorticoids produce a dose-dependent increase in liver glycogen with consequent hyperglycemia. Glucocorticoids participate in blood pressure homeostasis by maintaining normal blood volume and peripheral vascular reactivity. They can affect thought processes and CNS metabolism. Glucocorticoids can

increase hemoglobin synthesis, resulting in an elevation of the red blood cell count. Glucocorticoids facilitate the conversion of protein to carbohydrate and facilitate the effect of adipokinetic peptides, causing lipolysis and triglycerides in adipose tissue.

12. The answer is D *[III G 3 i]*
Corticosteroids, especially when used for long periods, can result in a variety of unwanted effects. Some of these include suppression of the pituitary–adrenal axis, increased susceptibility to infection, peptic ulceration, osteoporosis, and psychological disturbances including suicidal tendencies. Muscle hypertrophy is not an adverse effect of prolonged corticosteroid therapy. Rather, a myopathy can occur that is characterized by proximal arm and leg weakness.

13. The answer is D *[IV F, G 1]*
Crystalline zinc (regular) insulin is a short-acting insulin that can serve as a replacement therapy in juvenile-onset diabetes. However, its early onset of action and the fact that it can be given intravenously are particularly advantageous when rapid control is important, as in diabetic ketoacidosis. Crystalline zinc insulin, like any insulin preparation, can only be administered parenterally because it is a protein and would be digested in the gastrointestinal tract. It is the only form of insulin that can be given intravenously as well as by the usual subcutaneous route.

14. The answer is C *[IV G 5 d]*
Clinically available human insulins are produced by semisynthetic and recombinant DNA techniques. They are more expensive than the traditional insulin preparations. Some forms of human insulin may have a faster onset of action and shorter duration than conventional preparations, but this may or may not be advantageous. The major advantage of human insulin is that it can be administered to patients who are allergic to insulin made from animal sources. Human insulins are no more effective in preventing the complications of diabetes than any other insulin preparation.

15. The answer is B (1, 3) *[III D 2 a (1) (a), (b), 4 c (1)]*
Estrogens are used during and after menopause to relieve vasomotor symptoms such as hot flashes. Ethinyl estradiol and mestranol are estrogens. Ethynodiol is a progestin, and fluoxymesterone is an androgen.

16. The answer is C (2, 4) *[IV I 1]*
The patient described in the question has symptoms of hypoglycemia, not hyperglycemia, and is rapidly approaching insulin shock. The insulin dose is probably too high. Because of the low glucose level, the patient would not be "spilling" sugar into the urine. Early symptoms of hypoglycemia can be treated with soluble oral carbohydrates (e.g., fruit juice). Insulin shock calls for emergency treatment with intravenous glucose or parenteral glucagon.

17–19. The answers are: 17-E *[III F 2 b]*, **18-B** *[III E 6 b (2)]*, **19-A** *[III E 3]*
Calcitonin is chiefly used therapeutically to decrease hypercalcemia and hyperphosphatemia in patients with hyperparathyroidism and other disorders associated with hypercalcemia.

Propylthiouracil may be used with radioiodine to control the effects of hyperthyroidism until the benefits of radiation take effect. Unlike iodide, which would block thyroidal uptake of the radioiodine, propylthiouracil interferes with the synthesis of thyroid hormone.

Levothyroxine is used for the treatment of hypothyroidism, including myxedema coma and neonatal hypothyroidism.

11
Cancer Chemotherapy

I. INTRODUCTION

A. General considerations. Cancer, or neoplastic disease, is characterized by uncontrolled cell division, invasion, and metastasis. Most of the current clinical antineoplastic agents act on the proliferating population of cells; none acts primarily to influence tumor cell invasion or metastases.

1. There may be as many as 100 different types of cancer, each with its own response rate to a given drug. The sensitivity of a given cancer to a given drug depends upon its location, its degree of differentiation, its size, and, presumably, other biochemical factors that are poorly understood.

2. Most tumors are **clonal,** arising from a single altered cell. Tumor progression frequently results from a series of acquired genetic changes within the neoplastic clone, giving rise to subpopulations of tumor cells with increasingly aggressive characteristics. This evolution may occur, in part, because the genetic apparatus of tumor cells is abnormally unstable. A new class of "tumor-suppressor" genes is presumed to inhibit the growth of tumors; thus, the loss of function in a cell, by a combination of inherited and somatic deletions or other mechanisms, allows abnormal proliferation.

B. Combination therapy

1. Combinations of anticancer agents with different mechanisms of action are often used in an attempt to destroy all of the malignant cells. Acronyms for these combinations are frequently employed; for example, **MOPP** stands for mechlorethamine, vincristine (Oncovin), procarbazine, and prednisone.

2. Antineoplastic agents kill a *constant fraction* of the tumor cells rather than a *fixed number* of cells. In an attempt to eliminate all of the malignant cells, cancer chemotherapeutic agents are often administered as an **adjunct** to surgery or irradiation.

C. Cell cycle and anticancer therapy

1. **Growth of a tumor** is a function of the:
   a. Fraction of the total cell population that is proliferating
   b. Time required for an individual cell to divide (cell cycle time)
   c. Rate of cell loss

2. **Cell cycle**
   a. Both normal and malignant cells that are proliferating pass through four discrete phases (Figure 11-1):
   (1) Mitosis, or M phase
   (2) Gap 1, or G_1 phase
   (3) DNA synthesis, or S phase
   (4) Gap 2, or G_2 phase
   b. G_0 is a resting phase in which the cells are not proliferating.
   c. Interphase is any period between episodes of mitosis.

3. **Antitumor therapies**
   a. Some antitumor therapies, such as irradiation, carmustine, or mechlorethamine, are cytotoxic to proliferating and nonproliferating cells. These **proliferation-independent agents** kill both normal and malignant cells.

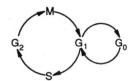

Figure 11-1. The cell cycle. M = mitosis; G_1 = gap 1 phase; S = DNA synthesis phase; G_2 = gap 2 phase; G_0 = resting phase.

    b. Most antitumor agents are preferentially toxic to proliferating cells.

        (1) There are two general classes:

            (a) Phase-specific agents act at specific phases of the cell cycle. For example, hydroxyurea and cytarabine kill only cells in the S phase.

            (b) Phase-nonspecific agents kill proliferating cells preferentially but do not act on cells at a specific phase in the cell cycle. Examples of these drugs are 5-fluorouracil and cyclophosphamide.

        (2) Some agents exert their major cytotoxic action in one phase of the cell cycle but also have a more limited activity in other phases.

        (3) Some agents are **self-limiting** because they are not only phase-specific but also block the cell in another phase of the cell cycle. For example, methotrexate kills cells in the S phase, but also inhibits RNA synthesis in the G_1 and G_2 phases, thereby limiting its own cytotoxicity.

D. Toxicity

    1. Antineoplastic agents generally have a slight selectivity for tumor cells as opposed to normal tissues. Therefore, many of the clinically used antineoplastic agents cause severe toxicity to the patient's normal tissues.

    2. Because rapidly proliferating cells are likely to be the ones most severely affected, the common side effects are:

        a. Myelosuppression

        b. Gastrointestinal bleeding and ulcers; nausea and vomiting

        c. Alopecia

        d. Nephrotoxicity

        e. Teratogenesis; abortion

        f. Immunosuppression

    3. Anticancer agents can also be carcinogenic.

E. Dosage calculations. The doses of antineoplastic agents are usually calculated on the basis of the patient's body surface area (in square meters) rather than body weight.

F. Classification. The major classes of antineoplastic agents are grouped primarily by chemical structure, source, or mechanism of action. The five major groups are:

    1. Alkylating agents

    2. Antimetabolites

    3. Natural products

    4. Hormones and antagonists

    5. Miscellaneous agents

II. ALKYLATING AGENTS

A. General considerations

    1. All of the drugs in this category have or can form an alkyl group that becomes covalently bound to cellular constituents.

    2. All alkylating agents are phase-nonspecific. In addition to killing rapidly proliferating cells, these drugs also kill nonproliferating cells as a result of alkylation of RNA, DNA, and essential proteins. Thus, some nitrogen mustards are proliferation-independent.

3. **Alkylation of DNA** is responsible for the cytotoxic antitumor activity of most alkylating agents.
   a. The 7-nitrogen and 6-oxygen of guanine are the most favored sites in DNA for alkylation.
   b. Once one of these sites has been alkylated, several events may follow:
      (1) **Cross-linking. Bifunctional alkylating agents** (those which have two chloroethyl moieties) may form a second covalent bond with an adjacent DNA substituent, a protein, or RNA, resulting in inhibition of DNA replication.
      (2) **Mispairing of bases.** Alkylated guanine forms base pairs with thymine rather than cytosine. This leads to miscoding of the gene and the possible production of defective proteins.
      (3) **Depurination of DNA.** Alkylation of the 7-nitrogen in guanine causes cleavage of the imidazole ring, which leads to a weakened sugar–phosphate backbone of DNA and strand breakage.

4. Enzymes involved in DNA repair may limit the responsiveness of some tumors to the alkylating agents.

5. The major classes of alkylating agents are:
   a. Nitrogen mustards
   b. Nitrosoureas
   c. Alkyl sulfonates
   d. Triazenes

B. Nitrogen mustards

1. **Chemistry.** The basic structure of the nitrogen mustards is shown in Figure 11-2.

2. **Mechanism of action**
   a. One chloroethyl moiety undergoes cyclization with the release of a chloride ion.
   b. The resulting highly reactive carbonium ion can attack nucleophilic groups on protein, DNA, RNA, and other cellular constituents.
   c. As with all alkylating agents, the nitrogen mustards are phase-nonspecific.
   d. **Tumor cell resistance** to nitrogen mustards can occur due to an increased cellular capacity for DNA repair with resulting cross-resistance to other alkylating agents.

3. **Mechlorethamine** is the prototype of the nitrogen mustards.
   a. **Chemistry.** In the mechlorethamine structure, R $= CH_3$ (see Figure 11-2).
   b. **Pharmacokinetics**
      (1) Mechlorethamine was the first clinically used nitrogen mustard.
      (2) It is highly reactive with a chemical and biologic half-life in plasma of 10 minutes.
      (3) It is proliferation-independent.
   c. **Therapeutic uses**
      (1) It is used to treat Hodgkin's disease and non-Hodgkin's lymphomas.
      (2) In the treatment of Hodgkin's disease, mechlorethamine is combined with vincristine, procarbazine, and prednisone to form the MOPP regimen.
      (3) It has also been used topically for the treatment of mycosis fungoides.
   d. **Route of administration**
      (1) Because it causes severe tissue damage when given by other routes, mechlorethamine **must be given intravenously** in a rapidly flowing infusion of saline.
      (2) Care must be taken to avoid extravasation during administration.
   e. **Adverse effects**
      (1) Myelosuppression
      (2) Nausea and vomiting
      (3) Alopecia
      (4) Menstrual irregularities

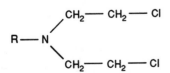

Figure 11-2. Basic structure of the nitrogen mustards.

4. Cyclophosphamide is an essential part of many effective drug combinations.
  a. Chemistry. The R structure of cyclophosphamide is shown in Figure 11-3.
  b. Pharmacokinetics
   (1) Cyclophosphamide is well absorbed orally. It must be activated in the liver by the mixed-function oxidase system.
   (2) The metabolites **phosphoramide mustard** and **acrolein** are believed to be the final cytotoxic species.
   (3) Alkylating activity levels in the blood remain high for 2–10 hours.
   (4) Cyclophosphamide and its metabolites are eliminated primarily by the kidneys, and thus, renal failure greatly increases their retention.
  c. Therapeutic uses
   (1) Cyclophosphamide is used alone and in combination with other agents in the treatment of a variety of neoplastic disorders, including:
      (a) Hodgkin's disease
      (b) Burkitt's lymphoma
      (c) Ovarian and breast carcinomas
      (d) Oat cell lung cancer
      (e) Neuroblastoma
   (2) Cyclophosphamide has also been used as an immunosuppressing agent for organ transplants.
  d. Route of administration
   (1) Cyclophosphamide is administered orally or intravenously.
   (2) The total leukocyte count is monitored, and the dose is adjusted accordingly.
  e. Adverse effects
   (1) Unlike other nitrogen mustards, cyclophosphamide rarely induces thrombocytopenia.
   (2) Alopecia occurs frequently but is modest.
   (3) Up to 10% of treated patients develop a sterile hemorrhagic cystitis, which is probably due to chemical irritation of the bladder mucosa by the metabolite acrolein. A liberal fluid intake dilutes the urinary concentration of acrolein and decreases this side effect.
   (4) Prolonged cyclophosphamide treatment can occasionally produce interstitial pulmonary fibrosis.
   (5) Prolonged use has also resulted in fatal cardiomyopathy, especially when cyclophosphamide was used with other cardiotoxic drugs.

5. Melphalan (ʟ-sarcolysin)
  a. Chemistry. The R structure of melphalan is shown in Figure 11-4.
  b. Pharmacokinetics and therapeutic uses
   (1) Melphalan is well absorbed from the gastrointestinal tract.
   (2) Its major use is in the treatment of multiple myeloma, but it is also used with breast and ovarian cancer.
  c. Route of administration. Melphalan is administered orally. Close hematologic monitoring is essential.
  d. Adverse effects
   (1) Like other alkylating agents, melphalan causes prominent myelosuppression.
   (2) Nausea, vomiting, and alopecia are rare.

6. Chlorambucil
  a. Chemistry. The R structure of chlorambucil is shown in Figure 11-5.
  b. Pharmacokinetics
   (1) Like melphalan, chlorambucil is well absorbed from the gastrointestinal tract.
   (2) It is completely metabolized.
   (3) It is the slowest-acting nitrogen mustard.
  c. Therapeutic uses
   (1) Chronic lymphocytic leukemia

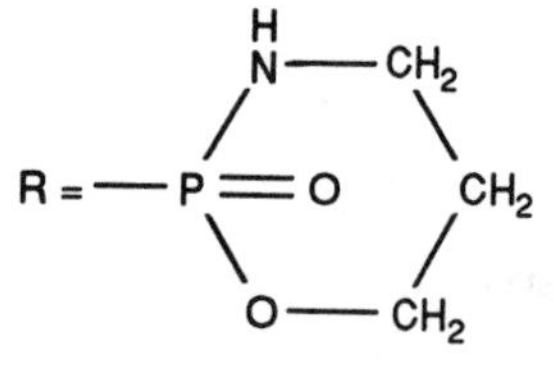

Figure 11-3. R structure of cyclophosphamide.

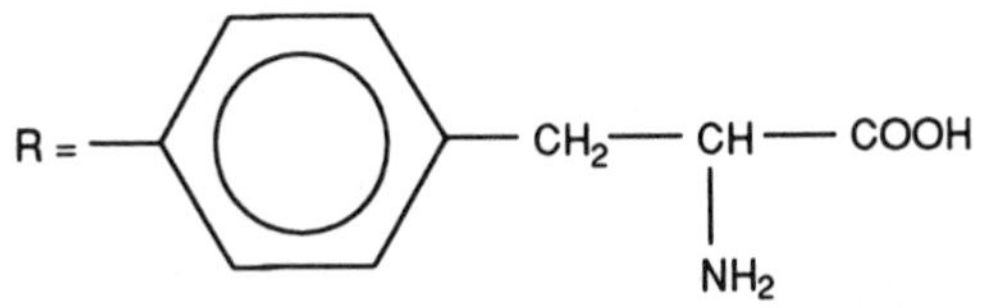

Figure 11-4. R structure of melphalan.

(2) Waldenström's macroglobulinemia
(3) Hodgkin's disease and non-Hodgkin's lymphomas
d. **Adverse effects**
(1) Myelosuppression
(2) Nausea
(3) Vomiting

C. Nitrosoureas

1. Chemistry
a. The basic structure is shown in Figure 11-6.
b. In general, the nitrosoureas are chemically unstable and decompose rapidly.
c. Acronyms derived from their chemical structures are commonly used.

2. Mechanism of action
a. In aqueous environments, the nitrosoureas decompose to alkylating and carbamylating intermediates.
b. The therapeutic and toxic effects of the nitrosoureas are due to both the alkylation of DNA and other nucleophiles and the carbamylation of lysine residues on proteins.
c. The consequences of DNA alkylation by the nitrosoureas are similar to those seen with other alkylating agents (see II A 3).
d. The **high lipid solubility** of some of the nitrosoureas allows penetration of the blood–brain barrier and are useful in the treatment of malignancies of the central nervous system (CNS).
e. The nitrosoureas are proliferation-independent.

3. Carmustine
a. **Chemistry**
(1) Carmustine is 1,3-bis(2-chloroethyl)-1-nitrosourea (BCNU).
(2) Both R_1 and R_2 in Figure 11-6 have the same structure: R_1 and R_2 = CH_2CH_2Cl.
b. **Pharmacokinetics**
(1) Carmustine is administered intravenously due to its rapid tissue uptake and metabolism.
(2) The plasma half-life is about 90 minutes.
(3) The major degradation and metabolic products are excreted in the urine.
c. **Therapeutic uses**
(1) Hodgkin's disease and non-Hodgkin's lymphomas
(2) Meningeal leukemia
(3) Tumors of the brain
(4) Multiple myeloma
(5) Malignant melanoma
d. **Adverse effects**
(1) Delayed hematopoietic depression
(2) Nausea and vomiting
(3) CNS toxicity
(4) Pulmonary fibrosis

4. Lomustine
a. **Chemistry**
(1) Lomustine is 1-(2-chloroethyl)-3-cyclohexyl-1-nitrosourea (CCNU).

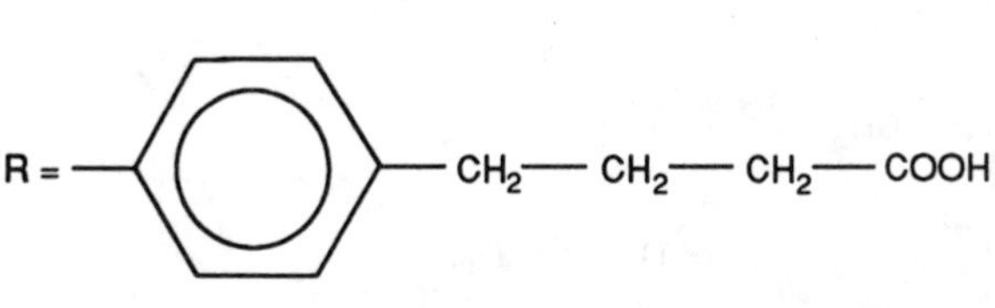

Figure 11-5. R structure of chlorambucil.

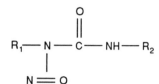

Figure 11-6. Basic structure of the nitrosoureas.

(2) The R structures are as follows:

$$R_1 = CH_2CH_2Cl$$

$$R_2 = $$

b. **Pharmacokinetics**
   (1) Lomustine, which is given orally, is rapidly absorbed from the gastrointestinal tract and metabolized.
   (2) The metabolites, however, have a long half-life (over 16 hours).
   (3) The metabolites can enter the cerebrospinal fluid (CSF).

c. **Therapeutic uses**
   (1) Hodgkin's disease and non-Hodgkin's lymphoma
   (2) Primary neoplastic disease of the brain, kidney, stomach, colon, and lung

d. **Adverse effects**
   (1) Myelosuppression
   (2) Nausea
   (3) Vomiting

D. Alkyl sulfonates

1. **Chemistry.** The prototypic agent is **busulfan**. Its bifunctional structure is shown in Figure 11-7.

2. **Mechanism of action.** Cleavage of the alkyl–oxygen bond in busulfan produces an electrophile, which forms intrastrand DNA cross-links.

3. **Pharmacokinetics**
   a. Busulfan is well absorbed after oral administration.
   b. Almost all of the drug is eliminated in the urine as methanesulfonic acid.

4. **Therapeutic uses**
   a. Chronic granulocytic leukemia
   b. Waldenström's macroglobulinemia

5. **Adverse effects**
   a. Myelosuppression is common.
   b. Endocrine dysfunction, including impotence, sterility, and amenorrhea, can occur.
   c. Hyperuricemia can result from rapid purine catabolism.
   d. Skin pigmentation and pulmonary fibrosis have been noted.

E. Triazenes

1. **Chemistry.** The prototype is **dacarbazine,** the chemical formula of which is 5-(3,3-dimethyl-1-triazeno)-imidazole-4-carboxamide (DTIC); its structure is shown in Figure 11-8.

2. **Mechanism of action**
   a. Dacarbazine is *N*-demethylated by liver microsomal enzymes and then functions as an alkylating agent.
   b. The active species has a methyl carbonium ion that can methylate DNA and RNA and inhibits the synthesis of DNA, RNA, and protein.

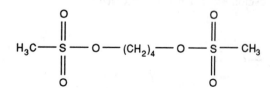

Figure 11-7. Busulfan.

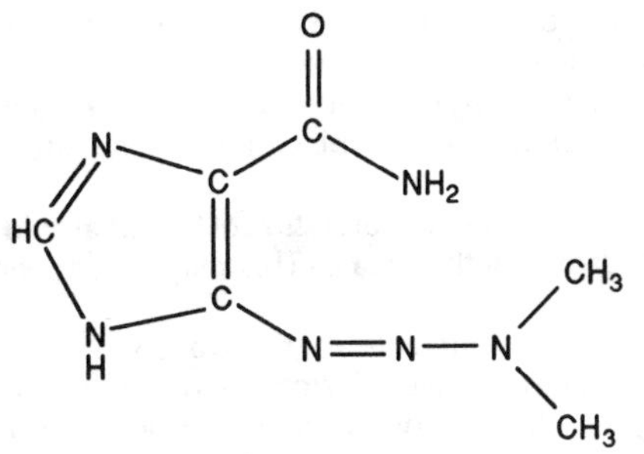

Figure 11-8. Dacarbazine.

3. Therapeutic uses
a. Dacarbazine is one of the most active agents against malignant melanoma.
b. It is also used for soft-tissue sarcomas and Hodgkin's disease.

4. Adverse effects
a. Nausea
b. Vomiting
c. Myelosuppression
d. Neurotoxicity

III. ANTIMETABOLITES

A. General considerations

1. Antimetabolites are compounds that bear a structural similarity to a naturally occurring substance, such as a vitamin, nucleoside, or amino acid.

2. The antimetabolite competes with the natural substrate for the active site on an essential enzyme or for an important receptor.

3. Some antimetabolites can be incorporated into DNA or RNA and, thus, can disrupt cellular function.

4. Most antimetabolites are phase-specific and act during DNA synthesis (the S phase; see Figure 11-1).

5. There are three major classes of antimetabolites:
a. Folic acid analogs (primarily methotrexate)
b. Pyrimidine analogs
c. Purine analogs and related inhibitors

B. Methotrexate

1. Mechanism of action
a. Methotrexate is a folic acid analog that competitively inhibits dihydrofolate reductase, the enzyme that catalyzes the formation of tetrahydrofolate from dihydrofolate.
(1) Normally, tetrahydrofolate is converted to a variety of coenzymes that are necessary for one-carbon transfer reactions involved in the synthesis of purines, thymidylate, methionine, and glycine.
(2) Therefore, methotrexate inhibits the formation of these coenzymes.
b. The primary cause of cell death is the blockade of the biosynthesis of thymidylate and purines required for DNA synthesis.
c. Thus, methotrexate kills cells in S phase.
d. Because methotrexate also inhibits RNA and protein synthesis, the drug slows the rate of entry of cells into S phase, and therefore, it is a **self-limiting** S-phase–specific drug.
e. The blockade caused by methotrexate can be circumvented.
(1) Substances such as **leucovorin** (also called citrovorum factor or folinic acid) and **thymidine** can be converted to the required tetrahydrofolate coenzymes or to thymidylate even in the presence of methotrexate.
(2) This allows the **"rescue"** of nonmalignant cells with a consequent reduction in toxicity from methotrexate.

2. Pharmacokinetics
a. Methotrexate is well absorbed after oral administration.

b. It is eliminated primarily by the kidneys without extensive metabolism and is approximately 50% bound to plasma proteins.
  (1) Weak acids, such as salicylates and sulfonamides, can increase methotrexate toxicity by inhibiting renal tubular secretion and displacing methotrexate from plasma proteins.
  (2) High doses of methotrexate can cause oversaturation of the renal acid secretory system with the formation of 7-hydroxy-methotrexate. This may be the etiology of nephrotoxicity (see III B 6 e).
c. Cellular uptake of the drug is by carrier-mediated active transport.
d. After an intravenous injection of methotrexate, plasma decay kinetics are triphasic with a half-life of 45 minutes for the first (distributional) phase, 3.5 hours for the second (renal clearance) phase, and 27 hours for the third (final excretion) phase.
e. Methotrexate does not penetrate the blood–brain barrier well, but it is one of a few agents that can be administered intrathecally for cerebral leukemia.

3. **Tumor cell resistance.** Tumor cells may become resistant to methotrexate because:
  a. Their cellular transport is impaired.
  b. An altered form of dihydrofolate reductase is formed.
  c. The tumor cells generate an increased concentration of dihydrofolate reductase through **gene amplification**. This is the major mechanism of tumor cell resistance.

4. **Therapeutic uses**
  a. Methotrexate is used in combination with other agents to treat acute lymphoblastic leukemia, Burkitt's lymphoma, trophoblastic choriocarcinoma, and carcinomas of the breast, cervix, lung, head, and neck.
  b. The drug is also useful in the treatment of mycosis fungoides and psoriasis.
  c. There is no good rationale for high-dose methotrexate therapy.
  d. At low, pulsed doses, this agent has been used experimentally in the treatment of rheumatoid arthritis.

5. **Route of administration.** Methotrexate can be administered intravenously, intra-arterially, intrathecally, or orally.

6. **Adverse effects**
  a. Myelosuppression is significant with leukopenia and thrombocytopenia occurring 1–2 weeks after drug administration.
  b. Gastrointestinal toxicity is manifested by ulcerative stomatitis and diarrhea and can disrupt therapy.
  c. Nausea and vomiting are common acute adverse effects.
  d. Prolonged low-dose methotrexate therapy can cause **hepatic dysfunction,** culminating in cirrhosis of the liver if drug treatment is not terminated.
  e. Renal failure can occur with high doses of methotrexate due to the precipitation of the drug in the renal tubules. Large volumes of alkaline urine must be maintained to prevent this toxicity. The drug is not administered to individuals with poor renal function.
  f. Methotrexate may cause dermatitis.
  g. There have been reports of necrotizing leukoencephalopathy when methotrexate was given with concomitant radiation therapy.

C. Purine analogs

1. **6-Mercaptopurine**
  a. Chemistry. 6-Mercaptopurine (Figure 11-9) is a structural analog of hypoxanthine.

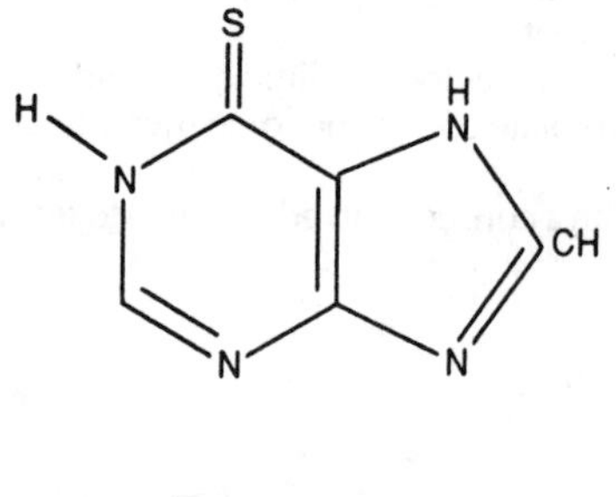

Figure 11-9. 6-Mercaptopurine.

b. Mechanism of action

   (1) 6-Mercaptopurine must be converted intracellularly to the nucleotide 6-mercapto-purine ribose phosphate by hypoxanthine–guanine phosphoribosyl transferase (HGPRT). 6-Mercaptopurine also can be converted to 6-methylmercaptopurine ribo-nucleotide.

   (2) 6-Mercaptopurine ribose phosphate and the methylated nucleotide are cytotoxic primarily because they inhibit de novo purine biosynthesis. Both block the aminotrans-ferase that is responsible for the first step in purine biosynthesis, namely, the formation of 5-phosphoribosylamine, by feedback inhibition.

   (3) In addition, 6-mercaptopurine ribose phosphate inhibits both adenylosuccinate syn-thetase, the enzyme that converts inosinic acid to adenylosuccinic acid, and inosinate dehydrogenase, the enzyme that converts inosinic acid to xanthylic acid.

c. Pharmacokinetics

   (1) 6-Mercaptopurine is well absorbed orally, and 50% is found in the urine in 24 hours, principally as 6-thiouric acid and inorganic sulfate.

   (2) After an intravenous injection, the plasma half-life is approximately 1 hour.

   (3) The drug is 20% bound to plasma protein and does not cross the blood–brain barrier.

   (4) 6-Mercaptopurine can be metabolically inactivated by desulfuration and by oxidation via xanthine oxidase to form 6-thiouric acid.

d. Tumor cell resistance. Tumor cells may become resistant to 6-mercaptopurine due to either a decreased drug activation by HGPRT or an increased inactivation by alkaline phos-phatase.

e. Therapeutic uses

   (1) 6-Mercaptopurine is used in the maintenance therapy of acute lymphocytic and acute lymphoblastic leukemia.

   (2) It is also useful in the treatment of acute and chronic myelogenous and granulocytic leukemia.

f. Route of administration. 6-Mercaptopurine is administered orally.

g. Adverse effects

   (1) 6-Mercaptopurine causes myelosuppression, but this is more gradual in onset than the suppression caused by methotrexate.

   (2) 6-Mercaptopurine also causes anorexia and nausea.

   (3) One-third of treated patients may develop jaundice associated with biliary stasis and hepatic necrosis. Discontinuation of therapy usually reverses this adverse effect.

   (4) Hyperuricemia and hyperuricosuria may occur with 6-mercaptopurine therapy.

      (a) This is due to the destruction of cells and the release of purines that are metab-olized by xanthine oxidase.

      (b) Allopurinol, an inhibitor of xanthine oxidase, can block the hyperuricemia and hyperuricosuria (see Chapter 9 IV E), but it also prevents the inactivation of 6-mercaptopurine.

      (c) Therefore, the dose of 6-mercaptopurine must be reduced when a patient is re-ceiving concurrent allopurinol to prevent significant toxicity.

2. 6-Thioguanine

   a. Chemistry. 6-Thioguanine (Figure 11-10) is a structural analog of guanine in which a sulf-hydryl replaces a hydroxyl group in the 6 position.

   b. Mechanism of action

      (1) Like 6-mercaptopurine, 6-thioguanine is converted by HGPRT to the nucleotide, in this case 6-thioguanine ribose phosphate.

      (2) The cytotoxicity of 6-thioguanine may be due to feedback inhibition of purine bio-synthesis by 6-thioguanine ribose phosphate.

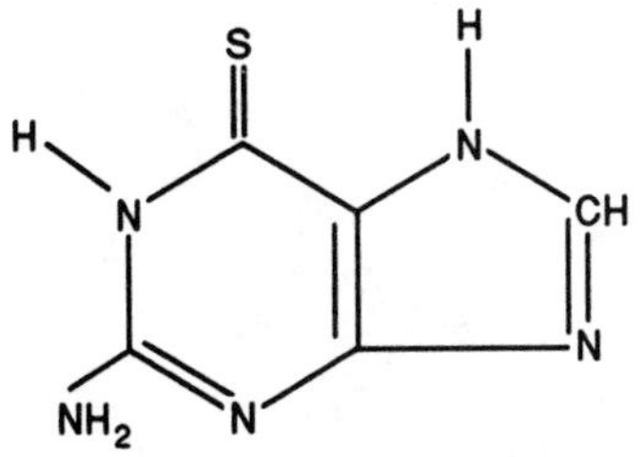

Figure 11-10. 6-Thioguanine.

(3) Alternatively, the cytotoxicity of 6-thioguanine may be due to conversion of 6-thioguanine to the deoxynucleoside triphosphate, which is incorporated into tumor cell DNA and RNA.

c. Pharmacokinetics

(1) 6-Thioguanine is only slowly absorbed orally, and less than 50% of the administered dose is found in the urine in 24 hours, all in the form of metabolites.

(2) 6-Thioguanine is not a good substrate for xanthine oxidase, in contrast to 6-mercaptopurine, and only small amounts of 6-thiouric acid are detected. Therefore, no dose reduction is required with concurrent allopurinol use.

d. Tumor cell resistance. The proposed mechanisms for tumor cell resistance to 6-thioguanine are the same as those for 6-mercaptopurine.

e. Therapeutic uses. 6-Thioguanine is used primarily in the treatment of acute myelogenous leukemia.

f. Route of administration. 6-Thioguanine is administered orally.

g. Adverse effects

(1) Myelosuppression is a common side effect.

(2) 6-Thioguanine causes mild nausea.

(3) Hepatotoxicity is less common with 6-thioguanine than with 6-mercaptopurine.

3. Pentostatin is a purine analog that is a potent inhibitor of adenosine deaminase. Pentostatin also interferes with the synthesis of nicotinamide adenine dinucleotide, resulting in DNA strand breakage. Pentostatin has been used for the treatment of hairy cell leukemia, mycosis fungoides, and chronic lymphocytic leukemia.

D. Pyrimidine analogs

1. 5-Fluorouracil

a. Chemistry. 5-Fluorouracil is a fluorine-substituted analog of uracil. Its structure is shown in Figure 11-11.

b. Mechanism of action

(1) Like the purine antimetabolites, 5-fluorouracil must be metabolically activated to a nucleotide, in this case 5-fluoro-2'-deoxyuridine-5'-monophosphate (FdUMP). There are three general pathways for FdUMP formation:

(a) 5-Fluorouracil can be metabolized to the deoxyribonucleoside with subsequent phosphorylation by thymidine kinase.

(b) 5-Fluorouracil can be converted to 5-fluorouridine-5'-phosphate by pyrimidine phosphoribosyltransferase and then to the deoxyribonucleoside by ribonucleotide reductase.

(c) FdUMP can also be formed by the conversion of 5-fluorouracil to fluorouridine, which is subsequently phosphorylated by uridine kinase to form 5-fluorouridine-5'-phosphate and ultimately FdUMP.

(2) The cytotoxicity of 5-fluorouracil is due primarily to inhibition of DNA synthesis caused by a FdUMP-produced blockage of thymidylate synthetase.

(3) Thymidylate synthetase normally transfers a methylene group from reduced folic acid to deoxyuridylate monophosphate (dUMP) to form thymidylate, which is essential for DNA synthesis.

(4) Cytotoxicity may also be due to incorporation of 5-fluorouridine triphosphate into RNA, which leads to "fraudulent" RNA formation.

(5) 5-Fluorouracil is **phase-nonspecific,** killing cells not only in S phase but throughout the cell cycle, perhaps due to its RNA actions.

c. Pharmacokinetics

(1) 5-Fluorouracil is administered intravenously and is catabolized by the liver.

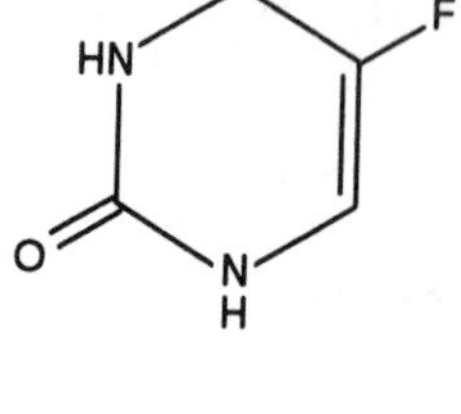

Figure 11-11. 5-Fluorouracil.

(2) The first, and rate-limiting, hepatic enzyme involved in 5-fluorouracil catabolism is dihydrouracil dehydrogenase. After cleavage of the pyrimidine ring, the final degradation products are ammonia, urea, 2-fluoro-3-alanine, and carbon dioxide.
(3) 5-Fluorouracil is distributed throughout the body, including the CSF.
d. Tumor cell resistance may result from any of several causes:
  (1) An increased synthesis of thymidylate synthetase
  (2) An altered affinity of thymidylate synthetase for FdUMP
  (3) An increased rate of 5-fluorouracil catabolism
  (4) The deletion of enzymes that convert 5-fluorouracil to the active nucleotide
  (5) An increase in the pool of deoxyuridylic acid
e. Therapeutic uses
  (1) 5-Fluorouracil is used in combination with other agents for the treatment of breast cancer.
  (2) It has palliative activity in gastrointestinal adenocarcinoma. Preliminary data suggest that adjuvant treatment with levamisole (an old antiparasitic drug) plus 5-fluorouracil may increase remissions and possibly prolong survival in some patients with resectable colon cancer.
  (3) It is also used to treat carcinomas of the cervix, bladder, and prostate.
  (4) Topical application of the drug has been useful for the treatment of premalignant keratoses of the skin and superficial basal cell carcinoma.
f. Route of administration. 5-Fluorouracil is usually administered intravenously.
g. Adverse effects
  (1) Myelosuppression, especially leukopenia, frequently occurs.
  (2) Stomatitis, diarrhea, nausea, and alopecia are seen.
  (3) Neurologic toxicity occurs in 1%–2% of treated patients.

2. Cytarabine (cytosine arabinoside, ara-C, 1-β-D-arabinofuranosylcytosine)
a. Chemistry
  (1) Cytarabine is an analog of cytidine in which the ribose moiety has been replaced with an arabinose.
  (2) Its structure is shown in Figure 11-12.
b. Mechanism of action
  (1) Cytarabine must be activated, by pyrimidine nucleoside kinase, to the nucleotide triphosphate, ara-cytosine triphosphate.
  (2) The nucleotide triphosphate competitively inhibits DNA polymerase and, thus, blocks DNA synthesis and causes cell death.
  (3) Cytarabine nucleotides can be incorporated into DNA and RNA, but the biologic significance of this remains to be established.
  (4) It is an S-phase–specific agent.
c. Pharmacokinetics
  (1) Cytarabine is poorly absorbed after oral administration.
  (2) It is rapidly metabolized in the liver and other tissues by cytidine deaminase.
  (3) It has an extremely short plasma half-life of 10 minutes.

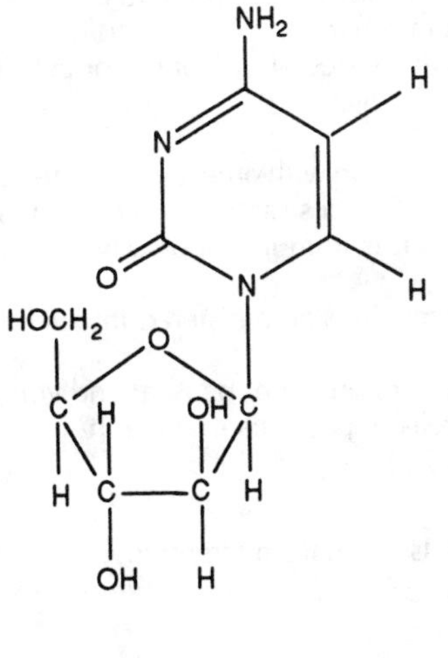

Figure 11-12. Cytarabine.

  d. Tumor cell resistance may be due to:

  (1) Depressed levels of the kinase required for activation

  (2) Enhanced levels of the deaminase that inactivates the drug

  e. Therapeutic uses. Cytarabine is used to treat acute myelogenous leukemia in combination with an anthracycline (see IV B 2) or 6-thioguanine. It is also used to treat acute granulocytic and acute lymphocytic leukemias.

  f. Route of administration

  (1) Cytarabine is given by intravenous, intramuscular, or subcutaneous injection.

  (2) Because it is a phase-specific agent and rapidly inactivated, continuous infusion is the preferred mode of administration.

  g. Adverse effects

  (1) Severe myelosuppression

  (2) Nausea

  (3) Mucosal inflammation

IV. NATURAL PRODUCTS

A. General considerations

1. Unlike the other classes of antitumor agents, membership in this group is determined by the source of the drug.

2. The natural products used in cancer chemotherapy are extracted from a variety of plants and lower organisms.

3. Most of the natural products have complex chemical structures and are not illustrated here.

4. The major classes of natural products are:

   a. Antibiotics

   b. Vinca alkaloids

   c. Enzymes

   d. Biologic response modifiers

   e. Epipodophyllotoxins

B. Antibiotics

1. **Dactinomycin (actinomycin D)**

   a. Chemistry

   (1) Dactinomycin is isolated from a *Streptomyces* species.

   (2) It contains two cyclic polypeptides that are linked by a chromophore moiety.

   b. Mechanism of action

   (1) Dactinomycin binds noncovalently to double-stranded DNA and inhibits DNA-directed RNA synthesis.

   (2) It is a phase-nonspecific agent.

   c. Pharmacokinetics

   (1) Dactinomycin is rapidly cleared from the plasma but is retained in the body for prolonged periods. Only 30% of the drug is recovered in the urine and stool after 7 days.

   (2) It does not cross the blood–brain barrier.

   d. Tumor cell resistance is due to a decreased ability of tumor cells to take up or retain the drug.

   e. Therapeutic uses

   (1) Dactinomycin is used in combination with other agents to treat Wilms' tumor, Ewing's sarcoma, rhabdomyosarcoma, Kaposi's sarcoma, and soft-tissue sarcomas.

   (2) Due to its lympholytic effects, it is immunosuppressive and has been used in renal transplantation.

   f. Route of administration. Dactinomycin is administered intravenously.

   g. Adverse effects

   (1) Dactinomycin produces myelosuppression, nausea, and vomiting.

   (2) Skin damage can occur in areas of previous irradiation.

2. **Anthracyclines**

   a. Chemistry

   (1) **Doxorubicin** is the prototype. Isolated from *Streptomyces,* it contains an amino sugar and an anthracycline ring.

    (2) Daunorubicin is structurally almost identical to doxorubicin, lacking only a hydroxyl moiety.

    (3) Mitoxantrone is a synthetic anthracene related to the anthracyclines.

b. Mechanism of action

    (1) The aglycone portion of the drug molecule intercalates with DNA and RNA.

    (2) The ionic sugar portion of the molecule bonds ionically to stabilize the intercalation.

    (3) As a result, DNA and RNA are distorted during synthesis.

    (4) This action is phase-nonspecific.

    (5) There may be some free radical production, which may play a role in tissue cytotoxicity. Mitoxantrone causes less free radical formation and lipid peroxidation than doxorubicin and theoretically should cause less cardiotoxicity.

c. Pharmacokinetics

    (1) Doxorubicin and daunorubicin are rapidly taken up by all tissues except the brain.

    (2) They are extensively bound to cellular components, which is responsible for their long plasma half-life.

    (3) Both drugs are metabolized primarily to hydroxylated and conjugated species.

    (4) Mitoxantrone is extensively bound to plasma proteins and tissues following intravenous administration. The plasma half-life is highly variable (3 hours to 12 days). The highest concentrations are found in the thyroid, liver, and heart. Mitoxantrone is metabolized in the liver.

d. Tumor cell resistance to doxorubicin or daunorubicin appears to result from reduced cellular uptake of the drug or a more rapid removal of the intracellular drug.

e. Therapeutic uses

    (1) Doxorubicin is one of the most effective agents against solid tumors. It is also effective against acute leukemias and malignant lymphoma.

    (2) Daunorubicin is most effective against acute lymphocytic and granulocytic leukemia. It has little activity against solid tumors.

    (3) Mitoxantrone appears to be as effective as daunorubicin but may be less toxic when combined with cytarabine for the initial treatment of acute nonlymphocytic leukemia. It may also be effective in some patients with advanced breast cancer.

f. Route of administration

    (1) Doxorubicin is administered intravenously. Because it causes severe tissue necrosis, doxorubicin *cannot* be injected subcutaneously or intramuscularly, and special care must be taken to avoid extravasation during intravenous infusions or injections.

    (2) Cumulative doses of doxorubicin appear to be important in the development of cardiac damage, and a maximum total dose of 550 mg/m^2 of body surface area is recommended to avoid cardiotoxicity.

    (3) Daunorubicin is administered similarly.

    (4) Mitoxantrone produces a lower frequency of severe local reactions after inadvertent extravasation compared to doxorubicin and daunorubicin.

g. Adverse effects

    (1) Doxorubicin, daunorubicin, and mitoxantrone cause both **acute** and **chronic cardiomyopathy**. The depression of cardiac function resulting from repeated doses limits the total amount of drug that can be administered.

    (2) Myelosuppression, especially leukopenia, occurs in most patients.

    (3) Alopecia is a common side effect.

    (4) Both drugs also cause nausea and vomiting.

    (5) Dermatitis at the site of previous irradiation can occur.

3. Bleomycin

a. Chemistry

    (1) Clinically used, bleomycin is a group of glycopeptides extracted from a *Streptomyces* species.

    (2) The mixture of glycopeptides found in this extract are referred to collectively as bleomycin.

    (3) Each individual bleomycin molecule has a planar end and an amine end. Different types of bleomycins differ in their terminal amine moieties.

b. Mechanism of action

    (1) The planar end of the bleomycin molecule intercalates with DNA.

    (2) The other end binds ferrous ion and facilitates its oxidation to ferric ion, thereby generating a free radical.

       (3) The free radical oxygen cleaves DNA, acting specifically at purine-guanosine-cytosine-pyrimidine sequences.

       (4) Cells in G_0 and G_2 phases are most sensitive.

  c. Pharmacokinetics

       (1) Bleomycin has a plasma half-life of approximately 1 hour.

       (2) More than half of the drug is eliminated unchanged in the urine within 24 hours.

       (3) Bleomycin is inactivated in most tissues, except skin and lungs, by an enzyme, bleomycin hydrolase. Toxicity in a specific organ occurs if the organ is lacking in enzyme activity.

  d. Tumor cell resistance

       (1) Tumor cells may fail to respond because of high levels of bleomycin hydrolase activity.

       (2) Tumor cells may mutate, altering the sequences that are sensitive to bleomycin intercalation.

       (3) Resistance may also be due to poor cellular accumulation of bleomycin or rapid drug removal.

  e. Therapeutic uses

       (1) Bleomycin is used only in combination with other agents.

       (2) It is effective with cisplatin and vinblastine for the treatment of testicular carcinoma.

       (3) It is also used for Hodgkin's disease and non-Hodgkin's lymphomas and for squamous cell carcinomas of the head and neck, cervix, and skin.

  f. Route of administration

       (1) Bleomycin is administered intravenously or intramuscularly.

       (2) It is sold in **units of activity**. The units are based upon the toxicity to bacteria; 1 unit equals approximately 1.7 mg.

       (3) A maximum total cumulative dose of 400 units is recommended to avoid pulmonary toxicity.

  g. Adverse effects

       (1) Bleomycin causes an age-related and cumulative-dose–related pulmonary toxicity. This consists of a pneumonitis, which can progress to fatal pulmonary fibrosis.

       (2) Bleomycin does *not* produce significant bone marrow toxicity.

4. Mitomycin (mitomycin C)

  a. Chemistry. Isolated from *Streptomyces,* mitomycin contains an aziridine ring as well as a urethane and a quinone moiety.

  b. Mechanism of action

       (1) Mitomycin is reduced intracellularly by a reduced nicotinamide adenine dinucleotide phosphate (NADPH)–dependent reductase, and then alkylates DNA. Thus, it can also be classified as an **alkylating agent**.

       (2) Because oxygen-derived free radicals can be formed, single-strand DNA lesions also can occur.

  c. Pharmacokinetics

       (1) After intravenous administration, mitomycin disappears rapidly from the blood.

       (2) Mitomycin does not penetrate the CNS.

       (3) It is extensively metabolized by the liver.

       (4) It is not absorbed through the bladder mucosa when given intravesically.

  d. Therapeutic uses

       (1) Mitomycin has limited use in the treatment of carcinomas of the stomach and cervix.

       (2) It is also used to treat superficial carcinoma of the bladder.

  e. Route of administration

       (1) Mitomycin is administered in a rapidly flowing intravenous infusion.

       (2) For superficial bladder carcinoma, it can also be given by intravesical infusion.

  f. Adverse effects

       (1) Myelosuppression is a major complication with intravenous administration.

       (2) Dermal, pulmonary, renal, and gastrointestinal toxicity may occur.

       (3) Extravasation can result in severe local injury.

       (4) Systemic side effects are lessened with intravesical administration.

C. Vinca alkaloids

  1. Chemistry

    a. The two prominent agents in this group, **vincristine** and **vinblastine** are derived from the periwinkle plant.

b. Both structurally complex compounds, vincristine differs from vinblastine only in having an aldehyde moiety.

c. Despite their similarity in chemical structure, the two alkaloids are quite different in their therapeutic applications and toxicities.

2. Mechanism of action

a. Both alkaloids bind to tubulin, thereby interfering with the assembly of spindle proteins during mitosis.

b. Both agents are M-phase–specific, blocking proliferating cells as they enter metaphase.

3. Pharmacokinetics

a. Both agents are extensively bound to tissue components. Less than 30% of a dose of vinblastine or its metabolites, for example, is recovered during a 6-day period after injection.

b. Only a small amount of either of these vinca alkaloids penetrates the brain or enters the CSF.

c. Both agents are metabolized by the liver and excreted in the bile.

4. Tumor cell resistance

a. It is currently believed that resistance to both agents is due to a reduced ability of tumor cells to retain the drugs.

b. Although cross-resistance between vinblastine and vincristine has been observed in experimental murine tumors, cross-resistance does *not* appear to occur in human tumors.

5. Therapeutic uses

a. Vinblastine is used in combination with bleomycin and cisplatin for the treatment of testicular carcinoma. It is also effective against lymphomas, neuroblastoma, and Letterer-Siwe disease.

b. Vincristine

(1) Vincristine is effective against acute lymphoblastic leukemia, Hodgkin's disease, and non-Hodgkin's lymphomas.

(2) It is also useful in the treatment of solid tumors in children and tumors of the breast, lung, and cervix in adults.

(3) Vincristine is less likely to cause myelosuppression and is preferred over vinblastine for use in combination with myelosuppressive agents in the therapy of lymphomas.

(4) Vincristine is used in combination with the corticosteroid prednisone, procarbazine, and an alkylating agent (e.g., mechlorethamine) in the MOPP regimen for treating Hodgkin's disease.

(5) The combination of vincristine with prednisone is considered the treatment of choice for inducing remission in childhood leukemia.

6. Route of administration

a. Vinblastine is administered intravenously with particular caution being taken not to produce subcutaneous extravasation.

b. Vincristine is also administered intravenously with avoidance of extravasation.

7. Adverse effects

a. Vinblastine causes leukopenia within 4–10 days after treatment. Minimal nausea, paresthesias, and jaw pain have been reported.

b. Vincristine is significantly neurotoxic with paresthesias and motor weakness being the most prominent effects. These neurologic manifestations are minimized by stopping or reducing the dose at the earliest onset of symptoms.

D. Biologic response modifiers are agents that act directly on tumor cells or indirectly by enhancing the immunologic response to neoplastic cells. Examples include:

1. Interleukin-2 (IL-2), which is a cytokine secreted by T cells that enhance natural killer cell activity. It is being tested alone and in combination for treatment of melanoma and renal cell cancer.

2. Interferons (alpha, beta, gamma). Alpha interferons have been approved for the treatment of hairy cell leukemia and Kaposi's sarcoma in patients with acquired immune deficiency syndrome (AIDS). Additionally, it is effective for condylomata acuminata.

E. Enzymes. L-Asparaginase catalyzes the hydrolysis of asparagine to aspartic acid and ammonia. Depriving the malignant cell of asparagine results in cessation of protein synthesis and cellular death. It has exhibited modest success in the treatment of acute lymphocytic leukemia.

F. Epipodophyllotoxins (etoposide and teniposide) are semisynthetic glycosides of the active podo-phyllotoxin (extracted from the mandrake plant) that show activity in several human neoplasms.

1. Mechanism of action

  a. At low concentrations, they block cells at the $S–G_2$ interface.

  b. At high concentration, they cause G_2 arrest.

  c. They stimulate DNA topoisomerase II to cleave DNA.

2. Pharmacokinetics

  a. Etoposide can be administered orally and intravenously. It has a terminal half-life of 8 hours. Forty percent is excreted in the urine.

  b. Teniposide is administered intravenously with a terminal half-life of 10–40 hours. As much as 80% is recovered as metabolite.

3. Therapeutic uses

  a. Etoposide is used for testicular tumors and in combination with cisplatin for small cell car-cinoma of the lung. It is active against a variety of other carcinomas, including non-Hodgkin's lymphoma, breast carcinoma, and AIDS-related Kaposi's sarcoma.

  b. Teniposide is being investigated for the treatment of refractory acute lymphoblastic leu-kemia.

4. Adverse effects

  a. Etoposide causes dose-limiting leukopenia.

  b. Teniposide causes myelosuppression.

V. HORMONES AND ANTAGONISTS

A. General considerations

1. Hormonal therapy relies upon the presence of receptors for endogenous hormones required for cell proliferation.

2. Unlike agents in the other classes of antineoplastic drugs, members of this class generally do not cause severe toxicity.

B. Tamoxifen

1. Chemistry. Tamoxifen is a nonsteroidal compound containing a triphenylethylene moiety (Figure 11-13).

2. Mechanism of action

  a. Some tumors, notably breast carcinomas, require estrogen for cell proliferation.

    (1) Estrogen binds to a cytoplasmic protein receptor, and the receptor–hormone complex translocates into the nucleus, inducing RNA synthesis.

    (2) Estrogen receptors are found in two-thirds of the breast tumors that occur in postmeno-pausal women.

  b. Tamoxifen, an estrogen receptor antagonist, is useful in women whose tumors contain es-trogen receptors.

    (1) Tamoxifen competes with estrogen for the cytoplasmic receptor, although it has little or no estrogenic activity.

    (2) The **antiestrogen action** of tamoxifen blocks the growth-promoting effects of estrogen in estrogen-dependent tumors.

3. Pharmacokinetics

  a. Tamoxifen is absorbed when given orally.

  b. It concentrates in tissues with estrogen receptors, such as the ovaries and breast tissue, as well as in tumors that contain these receptors.

  c. Tamoxifen undergoes extensive hepatic metabolism.

  d. It undergoes enterohepatic recirculation and then is found as metabolites in the stool.

4. Therapeutic uses. Tamoxifen is used for palliative treatment of advanced breast carcinoma in the postmenopausal woman.

  a. Although the response rate has been favorable in both estrogen receptor-rich and receptor-poor forms of breast carcinoma, the response is more favorable in the receptor-rich variant.

  b. The tumor reappears upon withdrawal of the drug.

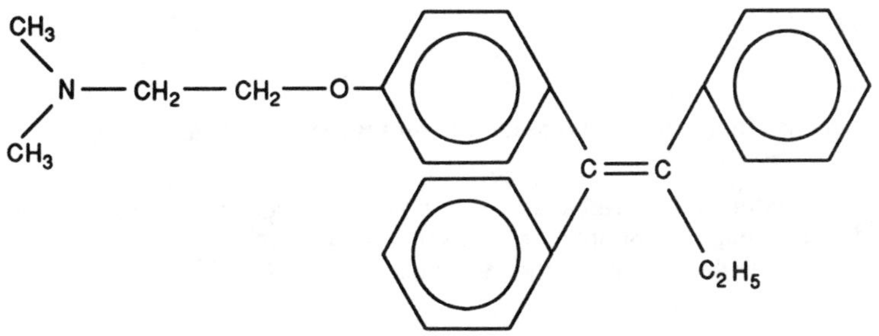

Figure 11-13. Tamoxifen.

5. Route of administration. Tamoxifen is administered orally.

6. Adverse effects
  a. Hot flashes, mild fluid retention, and nausea occur frequently.
  b. With high doses, corneal and retinal opacities have been observed.
  c. Hypercalcemia can occur.

C. Androgens and antiandrogens

  1. Androgens have been used in the treatment of breast carcinoma in postmenopausal women.
    a. The mechanism of action is not completely understood.
    b. A number of androgens are available, such as **fluoxymesterone, dromostanolone,** and **testosterone**. All are equally active and usually produce a response within 2 months.
    c. Common side effects are masculinization and fluid retention.

  2. Antiandrogens (flutamide)
    a. Flutamide is an oral antiandrogen used concurrently with an analog of luteinizing hormone-releasing hormone (LH-RH), such as leuprolide for the treatment of metastatic prostate cancer.
    b. Flutamide prevents adrenal androgens from binding to androgen receptors in the prostrate gland and in prostate cancer cells.
    c. Flutamide frequently causes gynecomastia and may cause hepatitis.

D. Adrenal corticosteroids

  1. Corticosteroids inhibit cellular protein synthesis and also attach to specific corticosteroid-binding proteins associated with leukemia cells. (See Chapter 10 III G for further information about their intracellular mechanism of action.)

  2. Prednisone, a glucocorticoid, has been used successfully in combination with cytotoxic agents in the treatment of lymphoblastic and chronic lymphocytic leukemia.

  3. Prednisone is also active in combination with other cytotoxic agents in the treatment of Hodgkin's disease (e.g., as a component of the MOPP regimen), non-Hodgkin's lymphomas, and multiple myeloma.

  4. Because of their ability to suppress androgen production by suppressing the adrenal cortex, corticosteroids (e.g., prednisolone) have also been used in the treatment of breast carcinoma.

E. Progestins

  1. Progestins bind to cytosolic progesterone receptors and cause maturation of the endometrium to a nonproliferating secretory state. Thus, progestins are sometimes used in the therapy of metastatic endometrial carcinoma that can no longer be treated with irradiation or surgery.

  2. The progestins most commonly used as antitumor agents are **medroxyprogesterone,** which is given intramuscularly, and **megestrol,** which is given orally.

  3. Progestins also have some limited use in the treatment of metastatic renal cell carcinoma. The mechanism of action in this tumor type is unclear.

  4. The progestins cause mild fluid retention and vaginal bleeding.

VI. MISCELLANEOUS AGENTS

A. Hydroxyurea

1. Chemistry. Hydroxyurea is a derivative of urea. Its structure is shown in Figure 11-14.

2. Mechanism of action

   a. Hydroxyurea inhibits ribonucleotide reductase. This enzyme is crucial to the biosynthesis of deoxyribonucleotides that are essential for the formation of DNA.

   b. Hydroxyurea is specific for the S phase of the cell cycle.

3. Pharmacokinetics

   a. Hydroxyurea is rapidly absorbed from the gastrointestinal tract.

   b. Twenty percent of a dose is metabolized in the liver, while the remainder is excreted via the kidney.

4. Therapeutic uses

   a. Hydroxyurea is an alternative to busulfan (see II D) in the treatment of chronic myelogenous leukemia.

   b. Hydroxyurea will reduce high white blood cell counts in patients with acute myelogenous leukemia.

   c. Other uses include polycythemia vera, essential thrombocytosis, and hypereosinophilic syndrome.

5. Route of administration

   a. Hydroxyurea can be administered orally or intravenously.

   b. Because of its renal elimination, administration in patients with impaired renal function must be conducted with caution.

6. Adverse effects

   a. Reversible myelosuppression is the major adverse effect.

   b. Gastrointestinal and cutaneous disturbances occasionally occur.

B. Procarbazine

1. Chemistry. Procarbazine (Figure 11-15) is a substituted hydrazine derivative with a structure similar to that of some monoamine oxidase (MAO) inhibitors.

2. Mechanism of action

   a. Procarbazine undergoes auto-oxidation and forms hydrogen peroxide, leading to the degradation of DNA.

   b. It also inhibits DNA, RNA, and protein synthesis.

   c. It also can transmethylate DNA at the 7-nitrogen position of guanine.

3. Pharmacokinetics

   a. Procarbazine is rapidly absorbed from the gastrointestinal tract.

   b. It readily equilibrates between the plasma and the CSF.

   c. It is rapidly metabolized, and about 40% is excreted in the urine within 24 hours, chiefly as a metabolite.

4. Therapeutic uses

   a. The major use of procarbazine is in the treatment of Hodgkin's disease, where it is used in combination with mechlorethamine, vincristine, and prednisone (i.e., in the MOPP regimen).

   b. Procarbazine also has some activity in the treatment of oat cell carcinomas.

5. Route of administration. Procarbazine is administered orally until the desired response occurs or limiting toxicity is seen.

6. Adverse effects

   a. Leukopenia and thrombocytopenia occur commonly.

   b. Gastrointestinal adverse effects as well as potentiation of other CNS-dependent drugs can occur.

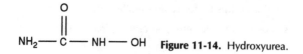

Figure 11-14. Hydroxyurea.

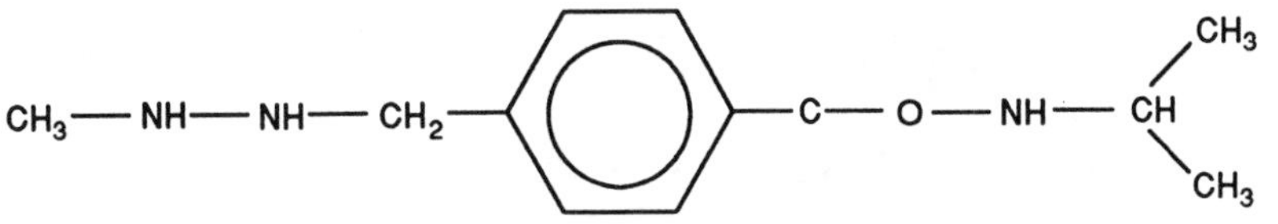

$$CH_3 — NH — NH — CH_2 — \bigcirc — C — O — NH — CH \begin{array}{c} CH_3 \\ CH_3 \end{array}$$

Figure 11-15. Procarbazine.

    c. Since procarbazine is a weak MAO inhibitor, hypertensive reactions can occur when sympathomimetics, tricyclic antidepressants, or foods with a high tyramine content are ingested concomitantly.

C. Mitotane (o,p′-DDD)

    1. Chemistry. Mitotane is a derivative of the insecticide DDT. Its structure is shown in Figure 11-16.

    2. Mechanism of action
        a. Mitotane selectively destroys normal and neoplastic adrenocortical cells by an unknown mechanism.
        b. It rapidly lowers adrenocorticosteroid levels.

    3. Pharmacokinetics
        a. Mitotane is partially (40%) absorbed from the gastrointestinal tract.
        b. Blood levels persist for up to 9 weeks after cessation of therapy.
        c. Mitotane is widely distributed with fat being the primary site of storage.

    4. Therapeutic uses. Mitotane is used as palliative treatment for inoperable adrenal carcinoma.

    5. Route of administration. Mitotane is administered orally.

    6. Adverse effects
        a. Gastrointestinal disturbances, lethargy, and dermatitis occur.
        b. If patients have Addison's disease, or if shock or trauma occur during mitotane therapy, adrenocorticosteroid replacement is indicated.

D. Cisplatin

    1. Chemistry. Cisplatin (*cis*-diamminedichloroplatinum) is an inorganic platinum coordination complex with a planar configuration (Figure 11-17). Only the *cis* isomer is active.

    2. Mechanism of action
        a. Cisplatin binds to DNA, causing both interstrand and intrastrand cross-linking similar to the actions of the bifunctional alkylating agents.
        b. It also binds extensively to nuclear and cytoplasmic proteins.
        c. Cisplatin is a phase-nonspecific agent.

    3. Pharmacokinetics
        a. After intravenous administration, 90% becomes protein-bound.
        b. Cisplatin has a long terminal half-life of greater than 2 days.
        c. It penetrates the CNS poorly.

    4. Therapeutic uses
        a. Cisplatin is one of the most effective agents against solid tumors.
        b. It is effective alone and in combination with bleomycin and vinblastine in the treatment of testicular tumors.
        c. Cisplatin is also very useful in the treatment of ovarian carcinoma.

    5. Route of administration. Cisplatin is administered intravenously with vigorous hydration and mannitol diuresis to avoid renal toxicity.

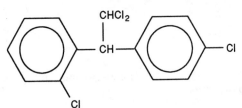

Figure 11-16. Mitotane.

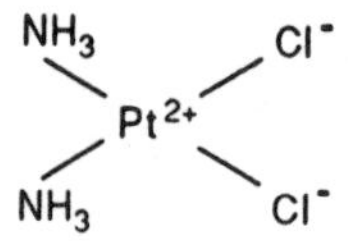

Figure 11-17. Cisplatin.

6. Adverse effects
a. Dose-dependent impairment of renal tubular function can occur, so that cisplatin should not be used in patients with impaired renal function.
b. High-frequency hearing loss can occur.
c. Severe nausea and vomiting are almost inevitable.
d. Anaphylaxis has occurred.

E. Carboplatin

1. **Chemistry.** Carboplatin is chemically related to cisplatin.

2. **Mechanism of action.** Like cisplatin, it binds to DNA and causes interstrand and intrastrand cross-links.

3. **Pharmacokinetics**
   a. The drug is eliminated primarily by the kidney.
   b. Sixty percent of a single dose is found in the urine within the first 24 hours.

4. **Therapeutic uses**
   a. Carboplatin can be used as a single agent in patients with persistent or recurrent ovarian cancer.
   b. The therapeutic response is slightly higher in patients not previously treated with cisplatin and much lower in those whose disease did not respond to cisplatin.

5. **Route of administration.** Carboplatin is also given by intravenous infusion, but unlike cisplatin, forced hydration or diuresis is not required.

6. **Adverse effects**
   a. Carboplatin induces less nausea and vomiting compared to cisplatin.
   b. There is less nephrotoxicity, neurotoxicity and ototoxicity seen compared to cisplatin.
   c. There is greater likelihood of dose-dependent bone marrow suppression, especially thrombocytopenia, compared to cisplatin.
   d. Allergic reactions have been reported.

F. Interleukin-2 (IL-2)

1. **Recombinant IL-2** is a lymphokine that stimulates growth of T lymphocytes. Its use is still considered experimental.

2. **Mechanism of action.** The incubation of peripheral T lymphocytes with IL-2 produces lymphocyte-activated killer cells that lyse several types of tumor cells in vitro. IL-2 plus the killer cells has caused regression of metastatic tumors in animals.

3. **Therapeutic uses.** IL-2 may offer some benefit to a small number of patients with metastatic renal cancer or melanoma.

4. **Route of administration.** IL-2 has been given by intravenous bolus or continuous infusion.

5. **Adverse effects**
   a. Fever
   b. Fluid retention leading to pulmonary edema
   c. Hypotension; capillary leak syndrome
   d. Cardiac arrhythmias
   e. Disorientation

VII. ANTIEMETICS FOR CANCER PATIENTS

A. General considerations

1. Chemotherapeutic agents may induce emesis by stimulating dopamine, serotonin, and opiate receptors in the vomiting center, the chemotrigger zone (CTZ).

2. **Effectiveness of the antiemetic agents** varies with:
   a. Route of administration
   b. Time of administration
   c. Anticancer agent used
   d. Dose of anticancer agent
   e. Mechanism of action

B. Nabilone

1. Nabilone is a synthetic cannabinoid that is chemically related to tetrahydrocannabinol.

2. It is rapidly absorbed and extensively metabolized in the liver.

3. It has a high potential for abuse.

4. **Adverse effects**
   a. Drowsiness
   b. Postural hypotension
   c. Ataxia
   d. Dry mouth
   e. Visual hallucinations

C. Dronabinol

1. Dronabinol is oral tetrahydrocannabinol.

2. Dronabinol and nabilone are equally effective antiemetics.

3. The potential for abuse and adverse effects are similar to nabilone.

D. Metoclopramide

1. Metoclopramide is a dopamine antagonist that can be administered intravenously or orally.

2. It should not be given concurrently with other dopamine antagonists, such as phenothiazines or butyrophenones, because they could precipitate acute dystonic reactions.

3. Somnolence and diarrhea are important adverse effects.

E. Phenothiazines and butyrophenones

1. Phenothiazines and butyrophenones (haloperidol) are effective when administered intravenously.

2. They can cause acute dystonic reactions, extrapyramidal symptoms, and hypotension.

F. Ondansetron

1. Ondansetron is a $5HT_3$ receptor antagonist acting on the afferent vagal nerve terminals in the upper gastrointestinal tract and in the CTZ.

2. Unlike metoclopramide or prochlorperazine, it does not have antidopaminergic activity and will not cause extrapyramidal effects.

3. It is metabolized in the liver, and the metabolites are excreted in the urine.

4. It is more effective than metoclopramide alone when given intravenously.

5. Adding dexamethasone increases the effectiveness of ondansetron.

G. Combinations

1. A variety of combinations have been used successfully to treat emesis.

2. Corticosteroids have been particularly synergistic in enhancing antiemetic activity when combined with metoclopramide or nabilone.

STUDY QUESTIONS

Directions: Each of the numbered items or incomplete statements in this section is followed by answers or by completions of the statement. Select the **one** lettered answer or completion that is **best** in each case.

1. All of the following drugs are components of the MOPP cancer chemotherapy regimen EXCEPT

(A) procarbazine
(B) vincristine
(C) mechlorethamine
(D) pentostatin
(E) prednisone

2. Proliferation-independent agents include all of the following EXCEPT

(A) vincristine
(B) carmustine
(C) cyclophosphamide
(D) mechlorethamine
(E) melphalan

3. All of the following adverse effects are commonly associated with cancer chemotherapy EXCEPT

(A) alopecia
(B) teratogenesis
(C) myelosuppression
(D) nausea
(E) exfoliative dermatitis

4. All of the following agents have been used for cancer chemotherapy EXCEPT

(A) alkylating agents
(B) antimetabolites
(C) vitamin D derivatives
(D) plant alkaloids
(E) hormonal agents

5. True statements regarding alkylating agents include all of the following EXCEPT

(A) they are phase-nonspecific
(B) they kill rapidly proliferating cells
(C) acquired resistance can occur
(D) they are structurally similar to naturally occurring endogenous substances
(E) they kill nonproliferating cells

6. Alkylating nitrogen mustards often produce all of the following side effects EXCEPT

(A) aplasia of the bone marrow
(B) renal toxicity
(C) alopecia
(D) menstrual irregularities
(E) nausea and vomiting

7. Cyclophosphamide can be used to treat all of the following neoplastic disorders EXCEPT

(A) Hodgkin's disease
(B) Burkitt's lymphoma
(C) choriocarcinoma
(D) ovarian carcinoma
(E) breast carcinoma

8. Characteristics of methotrexate include all of the following EXCEPT

(A) it can be used in the treatment of psoriasis
(B) it is eliminated by the kidneys
(C) it is a self-limiting S-phase–specific drug
(D) it penetrates the blood–brain barrier
(E) it competitively inhibits dihydrofolate reductase

9. All of the following statements about the purine analog 6-mercaptopurine are correct EXCEPT

(A) it is a structural analog of hypoxanthine
(B) it decreases the synthesis of 5-phosphoribosylamine
(C) it interferes with the formation of adenylosuccinic acid
(D) its metabolism is stimulated by allopurinol
(E) it is used in the maintenance therapy of acute lymphoblastic leukemia

1-D	4-C	7-C
2-A	5-D	8-D
3-E	6-B	9-D

10. All of the following statements regarding biologic response modifiers are true EXCEPT

(A) they can act directly on tumor cells
(B) they can act indirectly by enhancing the immunologic response to neoplastic cells
(C) IL-2 may have a role in the treatment of renal cell carcinoma
(D) they can deprive malignant cells of asparagene, resulting in the cessation of protein synthesis
(E) alpha interferon is useful for the treatment of hairy cell leukemia

11. All of the following statements about the epipodophyllotoxins, which show activity in several human neoplasms, are true EXCEPT

(A) at high concentrations, they cause G_2 arrest
(B) they stimulate RNA topoisomerase II
(C) etoposide can be used for testicular tumors
(D) etoposide can cause dose-limiting leukopenia
(E) teniposide is being investigated for the treatment of refractory acute lymphoblastic leukemia

12. Bleomycin is an antitumor agent that has all of the following characteristics EXCEPT

(A) it intercalates with DNA
(B) it acts by generating a free radical
(C) it requires ferrous ion for its action
(D) it kills cells in G_0 and G_2 phases
(E) it is a useful single agent for testicular carcinoma

13. Which of the following statements about the cancer chemotherapeutic agent mitomycin is true?

(A) It can be given orally
(B) It can be given intravesically
(C) It penetrates the CNS
(D) It is useful in treating breast cancer
(E) It is effective for the treatment of prostate carcinoma

14. A patient is placed on leuprolide plus flutamide, an oral antiandrogen. All of the following statements about flutamide are true EXCEPT that this agent

(A) prevents adrenal androgens from binding to androgen receptors in the prostate gland
(B) frequently causes gynecomastia
(C) can cause hepatitis
(D) plus leuprolide is effective against metastatic prostate cancer
(E) decreases plasma concentrations of luteinizing hormone and testosterone

10-D   13-B
11-B   14-E
12-E

Directions: Each item below contains four suggested answers of which **one or more** is correct. Choose the answer

A   if **1, 2, and 3** are correct
B   if **1 and 3** are correct
C   if **2 and 4** are correct
D   if **4** is correct
E   if **1, 2, 3, and 4** are correct

15. Characteristics of antineoplastic agents include which of the following?

(1) They frequently are self-limiting in their killing of cancer cells
(2) They kill a constant fraction of the tumor cells
(3) They are preferentially toxic to nonproliferating cells
(4) They are usually used in combination with each other

16. Nausea and alopecia are two of the most distressing consequences of cancer chemotherapy. These unwanted effects occur because

(1) anticancer drugs are most active during G_0 phase
(2) anticancer drugs are toxic to both tumor cells and normal tissues
(3) anticancer drugs kill a constant fraction of cells
(4) gastrointestinal mucosal cells and hair cells are rapidly proliferating cells

17. Drugs correctly matched with the drug category to which they belong include which of the following?

(1) Mechlorethamine—an alkylating agent
(2) Methotrexate—a natural product
(3) 5-Fluorouracil—a pyrimidine analog
(4) Vinblastine—a purine analog

15-C
16-C
17-B

Directions: The group of items in this section consists of lettered options followed by a set of numbered items. For each item, select the **one** lettered option that is most closely associated with it. Each lettered option may be selected once, more than once, or not at all.

Questions 18–21

Match each antiemetic agent with the statement that best describes it.

(A) Ondansetron
(B) Metoclopramide
(C) Nabilone
(D) Prochlorperazine
(E) Dexamethazone

18. This agent is a $5HT_3$ receptor antagonist.

19. This agent has a high potential for abuse.

20. This agent is a nonphenothiazine dopamine antagonist.

21. This agent when added to ondansetron increases its effectiveness.

18-A   21-E
19-C
20-B

ANSWERS AND EXPLANATIONS

1. The answer is D *[I B 1]*
The MOPP regimen combines mechlorethamine, vincristine (Oncovin), procarbazine, and prednisone. It is used primarily for the treatment of Hodgkin's disease. Cancer chemotherapy often employs a combination of drugs that have different mechanisms of action, chiefly because of the discovery that individual tumors are made up of heterogeneous subpopulations of neoplastic cells with differences that cause them to vary in their susceptibility to anticancer drugs. The aim is to destroy all of these cells by a multiple approach without an increase in toxic effects.

2. The answer is A *[I C 3; II A 2, B 3 b, 4, 5, C 2 e; IV C 2 b]*
Proliferation-independent agents are toxic to both proliferating and nonproliferating cells. Examples include carmustine, mechlorethamine, cyclophosphamide, melphalan, and irradiation. The vinca alkaloids, such as vincristine, bind to tubulin and are M-phase–specific, blocking cells as they enter metaphase.

3. The answer is E *[I D 2]*
Many cancer chemotherapeutic agents cause alopecia, induce bone marrow suppression, and are teratogenic. Gastrointestinal tract toxicity (i.e., nausea, diarrhea) is also common. Exfoliative dermatitis is not a common adverse effect of chemotherapy.

4. The answer is C *[I F]*
Vitamin D derivatives have not been effective as cancer chemotherapeutic agents. A good diet, of course, is always important for the patient. The alkylating agents, antimetabolites, plant alkaloids, and hormonal agents are major classes of antineoplastic agents available for clinical use.

5. The answer is D *[II A 2–4, B 2 d; III A 1]*
All alkylating agents are phase-nonspecific. In addition, cell death also occurs during interphase, and thus, they can be proliferation-independent. Both acquired resistance and cross-resistance can occur. They kill both rapidly proliferating and nonproliferating cells. Antimetabolites are substances with structural similarity to endogenous substances.

6. The answer is B *[II B 3 e, 4 e, 6 d]*
Nitrogen mustards can produce nausea, menstrual irregularities, alopecia, and myelosuppression. Renal toxicity is not a common problem with the alkylating agents but is a serious side effect of cisplatin.

7. The answer is C *[II B 4 c; III B 4 a]*
Cyclophosphamide is used alone or in combination for the treatment of Hodgkin's disease and Burkitt's lymphoma and for ovarian and breast carcinomas, but not for choriocarcinoma. The latter is most effectively treated with methotrexate. When used for lymphomas, cyclophosphamide is frequently used with vincristine and prednisone. Cyclophosphamide has also been used as an immunosuppressive agent during organ transplantation.

8. The answer is D *[III B 1 a, d, 2 b, e, 4 b]*
Methotrexate competitively inhibits dihydrofolate reductase and has been used in the treatment of psoriasis to suppress the proliferation of epidermal cells. It is a folic acid antagonist, which is eliminated unmetabolized, primarily via the kidneys. It slows the rate of entry of cells into S phase but kills cells in S phase. Thus, it can be labeled a self-limiting S-phase–specific drug. Methotrexate does not cross the blood–brain barrier well, but it can be administered intrathecally.

9. The answer is D *[III C 1]*
Allopurinol blocks rather than stimulates the metabolism of 6-mercaptopurine. Therefore, the dose of 6-mercaptopurine must be reduced when a patient is also receiving allopurinol, to prevent significant toxicity. Allopurinol is used in conjunction with 6-mercaptopurine because allopurinol blocks the formation of uric acid from hypoxanthine and xanthine. All of the other statements about 6-mercaptopurine in the question are correct.

10. The answer is D *[IV D 1, 2]*
All of the statements regarding biologic response modifiers are true except that it is the enzyme L-asparaginase that deprives the malignant cells of asparagene, which results in cell death. L-Asparaginase has exhibited modest success in the treatment of acute lymphocytic leukemia.

11. The answer is B *[IV F 1, 3, 4]*
Epipodophyllotoxins are semisynthetic glycosides of the active podophyllotoxin that show activity in several neoplasms. All of the statements in the question regarding epipodophyllotoxins are true except that they stimulate DNA (not RNA) topoisomerase II to cleave DNA.

12. The answer is E *[IV B 3 b, e].*
Bleomycin is a natural product that intercalates with DNA and generates a free radical, which cleaves DNA at purine-guanosine-cytosine-pyrimidine sequences. Ferrous ion is required to produce the free radicals necessary for the DNA strand breaks. The most sensitive cells are cells in G_0 and G_2 phases of the cell cycle. Bleomycin is used only in combination with other agents. It is effective for testicular carcinoma but only in combination with cisplatin and vinblastine.

13. The answer is B *[IV B 4 c–e]*
Mitomycin is not absorbed into the bloodstream through the bladder wall, and therefore, it can be given by intravesical infusion to treat superficial carcinoma of the bladder. Mitomycin is also used to treat carcinomas of the stomach and cervix for which it is given by intravenous infusion. It is not used to treat breast cancer or prostate carcinoma. Mitomycin cannot be given orally and does not penetrate the CNS.

14. The answer is E *[V C 2]*
The oral antiandrogen, flutamide, plus leuprolide is effective in treating metastatic prostate cancer. It prevents adrenal androgens from binding to androgen receptors in the prostate gland. It also blocks the inhibitory action of testosterone on luteinizing hormone (LH) production, resulting in increased plasma concentrations of LH and testosterone. Flutamide can cause gynecomastia and hepatitis.

15. The answer is C (2, 4) *[I B, C 3]*
Each dose of an antineoplastic agent kills a constant fraction of the tumor cells rather than a fixed number of cells. Many of the commonly used antineoplastic agents have been found to be much more effective when administered in combination with other antitumor drugs; the MOPP regimen, which combines mechlorethamine, vincristine (Oncovin), procarbazine, and prednisone, is an example. One reason combinations are effective is that the individual drugs may kill different tumor cell populations; moreover, because their toxic effects on the patient do not overlap, dose reductions of the individual drugs are not necessary. Although some drugs, such as methotrexate, are self-limiting, most agents are not. In general, antitumor agents are preferentially toxic to cells that are actively proliferating. Only a few of the antitumor agents (e.g., vincristine) act on cells in mitosis; most drugs that are phase-specific affect cells in other phases of the cell cycle.

16. The answer is C (2, 4) *[I C 3]*
Most anticancer drugs are chosen for their toxicity to proliferating cells, since this is a characteristic of tumors. Unfortunately, however, anticancer drugs are likely to be as toxic to normal proliferating cells as to tumor cells. Because the gastrointestinal epithelium and hair follicles are composed of highly proliferating cells, they are particularly affected by cancer chemotherapy; the same is true of the cells of the bone marrow, immune system, and the fetus. The G_0 phase is a resting phase in the cell cycle, when cells are not proliferating. Although anticancer drugs do kill a constant fraction of cells, rather than a fixed number of cells, this is not likely to play a major role in the occurrence of nausea or alopecia.

17. The answer is B (1, 3) *[II B 3; III B, D 1; IV C]*
Mechlorethamine, an alkylating agent, will produce DNA cross-linking, mispairing of bases, and depurination of DNA because of the highly reactive carbonium ion produced from mechlorethamine. This is true of all alkylating agents. Methotrexate is not a natural product but a folic acid antagonist and an antimetabolite. Vinblastine is a plant alkaloid, not a purine analog, while 5-fluorouracil is a flourine-substituted analog of uracil and, thus, a pyrimidine analog.

18–21. The answers are: 18-A *[VII F]*, **19-C** *[VII B]*, **20-B** *[VII D]*, **21-E** *[VII F 5]*
Ondansetron is a $5HT_3$ receptor antagonist that does not have antidopaminergic activity and will not cause extrapyramidal symptoms. It is more effective than metoclopromide alone when given intravenously.

Nabilone is a synthetic cannabinoid that is chemically related to tetrahydrocannabinol. It is rapidly absorbed and extensively metabolized in the liver. It has a high potential for abuse.

Metoclopramide is a dopamine antagonist, which can be administered intravenously or orally. It should not be given concurrently with other dopamine antagonists because they could precipitate acute dystonic reactions.

Dexamethasone enhances the antiemetic activity of metoclopramide, nabilone, and ondansetron.

I. INTRODUCTION

A. Definitions

1. **Antimicrobial agents** are chemical substances that can kill or suppress the growth of microorganisms.

2. **Antibiotics** are soluble compounds that are derived from certain microorganisms and that inhibit the growth of other microorganisms.

B. Types of infections and their treatment

1. **Bacterial infections** are readily treated in most instances by a wide variety of agents. Some antibacterial drugs are **bacteriostatic;** that is, they inhibit the growth of susceptible bacteria. Other antibacterials are truly **bactericidal;** that is, they kill susceptible bacteria.

2. **Fungal infections,** in contrast to bacterial infections, generally are quite resistant to chemotherapy, and the number of useful agents for these infections is somewhat restricted. Fungal infections often occur as **superinfections;** that is, secondary infections superimposed on the original infection as a result of changes in the host's flora (e.g., as a result of antibacterial therapy).

3. **Mycobacterial infections,** in the past, often required treatment in specialized centers; today this is no longer the case.
   a. **Tuberculosis** is one of the few diseases that requires a combination of antimicrobial drugs, which are used to prevent the appearance of resistant strains of the infecting organism.
   b. **Leprosy** is a disease whose course has been remarkably altered by chemotherapy.
   c. Infections with **atypical mycobacteria** (e. g., *Mycobacterium avium* complex), as well as tuberculosis, are seen in patients with acquired immune deficiency syndrome (AIDS).

4. **Helminthiasis** may now affect as many as 1 billion people each year, and its incidence is increasing with increased agricultural use of land and increased travel. With the advent of several new, highly selective anthelmintic drugs, older agents used to treat parasitic worm infections have become obsolete.

5. **Protozoal infections,** such as amebiasis and various trypanosomal infections, are treated by a wide variety of agents. Metronidazole is directly trichomonacidal and also is the agent of choice for several other protozoal infections.

6. **Viral infections** are difficult to treat because viruses are intracellular parasites, requiring the active participation of a host cell's metabolic processes, and few pharmacologic agents are selective enough to kill a virus without injuring the involved host cell.

C. General principles of anti-infective therapy

1. **Selection of an appropriate anti-infective agent**
   a. Identification of the infecting organism should precede antimicrobial therapy when possible.
      (1) The patient's condition may require empiric therapy before the infecting organism is known.

(2) In this case, "umbrella" therapy is often used. A broad-spectrum antimicrobial agent or a combination of agents is chosen that will be effective against the likeliest causative pathogens.

b. The organism's susceptibility to antimicrobial agents should be determined, if a suitable test exists.

c. Factors that influence the choice of an anti-infective agent or its dosage include:
  (1) The patient's age
  (2) The patient's renal and hepatic function
  (3) The patient's pregnancy status
  (4) The site of infection

2. Route of administration
  a. Oral administration is used for mild infections.
    (1) It is especially useful for outpatient therapy.
    (2) The agent must be orally absorbed.
    (3) Timing of administration is important if food impairs absorption.
  b. Parenteral administration is used for serious infections, especially when high serum levels are required.
  c. Intrathecal administration is used for meningeal infections when the appropriate agent does not cross the blood–brain barrier.

3. Antimicrobial combination therapy
  a. Therapy with two or more antimicrobial agents has several **purposes**:
    (1) To **provide broad coverage** (e.g., when infections are due to more than one organism)
    (2) For **initial (blind) therapy** when the patient is seriously ill and results of cultures are pending
    (3) To **provide synergism** when organisms are not effectively eradicated with a single agent alone; for example, in enterococcal endocarditis, both penicillin and an aminoglycoside are given because their combined effect is greater than the sum of their independent activities
    (4) To **prevent the emergence of resistance** in the treatment of tuberculosis
  b. Inappropriate use of combinations could result in:
    (1) Antagonism between the antimicrobial agents
    (2) An increase in the number or severity of adverse reactions
    (3) Increased cost

II. AGENTS USED FOR TREATMENT OF BACTERIAL INFECTIONS

A. Sulfonamides

  1. Chemistry
    a. The sulfonamides are derivatives of **sulfanilamide** (Figure 12-1).
    b. Derivatives are made by substitutions in the amide of the sulfonamide group.

  2. Mechanism of action
    a. Sulfonamides prevent the incorporation of para-aminobenzoic acid (PABA) into folic acid, which in the reduced form is necessary in purine biosynthesis for the transfer of one-carbon units.
    b. Susceptible bacteria are those that need PABA because they are incapable of using folic acid directly.
    c. Human cells use exogenous folic acid exclusively, and thus, a lack of PABA does not affect them.

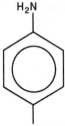

H_2N

SO_2NH_2 **Figure 12-1.** Sulfanilamide.

3. Pharmacokinetics
  a. Sulfonamides are absorbed within minutes following oral administration.
  b. They are distributed throughout the body water.
  c. They diffuse into cerebrospinal fluid.
  d. They are metabolized by acetylation of the para-NH_2, which negates the antibacterial activity but not the unwanted effects.
  e. Excretion is chiefly via the urine within 24 hours of administration. The urinary solubility of the various sulfonamides varies widely.

4. Pharmacologic effects
  a. Sulfonamides are effective against many gram-positive bacteria, including group A *Streptococcus pyogenes* and *Streptococcus pneumoniae.*
  b. Many gram-negative bacteria are resistant to sulfonamides, but some, such as *Hemophilus influenzae, Escherichia coli* (the organism most often suspect in acute urinary tract infections), *Shigella, Yersinia enterocolitica,* and *Proteus mirabilis,* often are sensitive.
  c. Other susceptible organisms include *Bacillus anthracis, Nocardia, Actinomyces,* and *Chlamydia trachomatis,* the agent responsible for trachoma, lymphogranuloma venereum, and inclusion conjunctivitis.

5. Therapeutic uses
  a. Sulfonamides are the preferred agents for treatment of:
    (1) Acute uncomplicated urinary tract infections
    (2) Nocardiosis
  b. They are effective for treatment of toxoplasmosis when used in combination with pyrimethamine.
  c. They are used in trachoma and inclusion conjunctivitis as an alternative to tetracycline.
  d. Aside from acute urinary tract infections, the use of sulfonamides alone in many infections has been replaced by more effective and safer drugs.

6. Preparations. Commonly used sulfonamides include:
  a. Trimethoprim–sulfamethoxazole
    (1) Sulfamethoxazole and trimethoprim inhibit two separate steps in folate metabolism.
    (2) Trimethoprim is a highly selective inhibitor of the dihydrofolate reductase of lower organisms.
    (3) In combination, the two drugs act synergistically.
    (4) The combination is useful for treating *Pneumocystis carinii* pneumonia, an opportunistic infection seen in patients with AIDS (see X B).
  b. Sulfisoxazole
  c. Sulfadiazine
    (1) Sulfadiazine is now used less often for urinary tract infections.
    (2) It is useful for treating nocardiosis.

7. Adverse effects
  a. About 75% of untoward effects involve the skin with sensitization often being responsible. Conditions produced include:
    (1) Exfoliative dermatitis
    (2) Stevens-Johnson syndrome (fever, malaise, erythema multiforme)
  b. Drug fever can occur and is probably due to sensitization.
  c. Blood dyscrasias are rare but can occur. Sulfonamide therapy is stopped immediately if any of the following hematologic conditions develop to a serious extent:
    (1) Acute hemolytic anemia, which is often, but not solely, due to an erythrocytic deficiency of glucose-6-phosphate dehydrogenase activity and is particularly likely to develop in blacks and children
    (2) Aplastic anemia
    (3) Agranulocytosis
    (4) Thrombocytopenia
  d. Eosinophilia may accompany other manifestations of hypersensitivity.
  e. Crystalluria is a condition that was seen with the older sulfonamides but rarely occurs with the newer, more soluble agents such as sulfisoxazole, although some renal damage is still possible.
  f. Hepatitis, causing focal or diffuse necrosis of the liver, occurs rarely and may be caused by either direct drug toxicity or sensitization.

g. Kernicterus can occur in the newborn because of displacement of bilirubin from plasma albumin.

B. Beta-lactam antibiotics

1. Overview

a. Chemistry

(1) A **beta-lactam ring** is a four-membered ring in which an amide linkage joins a carbonyl group and a nitrogen.

(2) The beta-lactam antibiotics have this ring as a key structural feature.

b. Classification. The beta-lactam antibiotics include:

(1) The penicillins

(2) The cephalosporins

(3) Imipenem

(4) Aztreonam

c. Mechanism of action. The beta-lactam antibiotics are **bactericidal**.

(1) The beta-lactam antibiotics inhibit key enzymes in bacterial cell wall synthesis.

(2) They also appear to activate one or more cell-wall autolytic enzymes, causing lysis of the bacterium.

d. Bacterial resistance

(1) **Beta-lactamases,** enzymes produced by many different bacteria, hydrolyze the beta-lactam ring, inactivating the antibiotic. **Penicillinase** (see II B 2 d) and **cephalosporinase** are beta-lactamases with narrow substrate specificities.

(2) Initially sensitive bacterial strains can become permanently resistant to a particular antibiotic by acquiring plasmids or R (resistance) factors carrying the genetic code for a beta-lactamase.

(3) The penicillins and the other beta-lactam antibiotics differ in their sensitivity to the beta-lactamases.

(4) Beta-lactamase inhibitors are substances that can irreversibly bind and, thus, inactivate bacterial beta-lactamases (see II B 2).

2. Penicillins

a. Chemistry

(1) The structure of the penicillins (Figure 12-2) consists of a thiazolidine ring connected to a beta-lactam ring, which is attached to a side chain.

(2) All penicillins are derived from 6-aminopenicillanic acid.

(3) The various penicillins differ in their side chain structure.

b. Classification of the penicillins is given in Table 12-1.

c. Mechanism of action

(1) Penicillins inhibit the synthesis of bacterial cell walls and are considered **bactericidal**.

(2) They combine with and inactivate transpeptidase, which normally is responsible for cross-linking the linear glycopeptide strands of bacterial cell walls. Loss of cell wall rigidity in the presence of normal high intracellular osmotic pressure causes lysis of the bacterial membrane.

d. Bacterial resistance (see II B 1 d)

(1) **Penicillinase** is a beta-lactamase that is produced by a number of bacteria. It can hydrolyze the beta-lactam ring of penicillin to form penicilloic acid, a substance that has no antibacterial activity.

(2) Microorganisms that are capable of producing penicillinase include:

(a) *Staphylococcus aureus*

(b) *Bacillus* species

(c) *Bacteroides* species

(d) *E. coli*

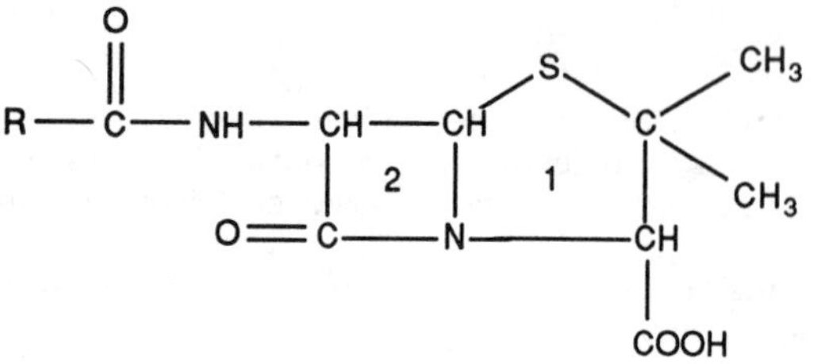

Figure 12-2. Structure of the penicillins. *R* = side chain; *1* = thiazolidine ring; *2* = beta-lactam ring.

Table 12-1. Classification of Penicillins

Penicillin G (benzylpenicillin)	"Antipseudomonas" penicillins
Penicillin V (phenoxymethyl penicillin)	Carbenicillin
Penicillinase-resistant penicillins	Carbenicillin indanyl
Methicillin	Ticarcillin
Oxacillin	Ureidopenicillins
Cloxacillin	Azlocillin
Nafcillin	Mezlocillin
Dicloxacillin	Piperacillin
"Broad-spectrum" penicillins	Combinations of penicillin and a beta-lactamase inhibitor
Ampicillin	Amoxicillin with clavulanic acid
Amoxicillin	Ampicillin with sulbactam
Bacampicillin	Ticarcillin with clavulanic acid
Cyclacillin	
Hetacillin	
Pivampicillin	

      (e) *Proteus* species
      (f) *Pseudomonas aeruginosa*
      (g) *Mycobacterium tuberculosis*
   e. Pharmacokinetics of penicillins G and V
     (1) Absorption
       (a) Oral administration
         (i) Because gastric acid inactivates **penicillin G,** only 30% of an oral dose is absorbed from the duodenum. **Penicillin V** is more stable in an acidic environment; an equivalent oral dose leads to plasma levels two to five times higher than those obtained with penicillin G.
         (ii) Because food interferes with absorption, penicillin G or V should be administered at least 1 hour before meals and at least 2–3 hours after meals.
         (iii) Peak plasma concentrations occur 30–60 minutes after administration.
       (b) Subcutaneous or intramuscular administration
         (i) Following injection of crystalline penicillin G, peak plasma concentrations occur in 15 minutes, then rapidly decline.
         (ii) The simultaneous administration of **probenecid** prolongs the duration of penicillin in the body because probenecid blocks the transport of penicillin in the proximal tubule. **Repository penicillin preparations** [see II B 2 h (2)] provide an alternative means for maintaining high plasma levels of penicillin.
     (2) Distribution
       (a) Penicillins G and V are distributed widely throughout the body with about 60% reversibly bound to plasma albumin.
       (b) They penetrate poorly into ocular, pericardial, and cerebrospinal fluids.
       (c) Significant amounts of the drug appear in the liver, intestine, and kidney, as well as in bile, semen, and lymph.
     (3) Excretion
       (a) From 60%–90% of an intramuscular dose of penicillin G is excreted within 1 hour.
       (b) Up to 99% of the dose is eliminated via the kidney; that is, about 90% by tubular secretion and 10% by glomerular filtration.
   f. Pharmacologic effects and therapeutic uses. The various types of penicillin differ in their spectrum of activity and in their degree of efficacy against particular species or strains. In general, microbial sensitivity should be verified whenever possible.
     (1) Gram-positive coccal (streptococcal and staphylococcal) infections. Penicillins G and V are highly effective against many strains of gram-positive cocci.
       (a) Infections due to *S. pneumoniae* (pneumococcal infections)
         (i) Penicillin G or V is the drug of first choice for treatment of pneumococcal pneumonia.
         (ii) For pneumococcal meningitis, penicillin G is usually administered intravenously. Intrathecal administration is sometimes used, but arachnoiditis and encephalopathy can complicate this form of therapy.

        (iii) Other pneumococcal infections for which penicillin G is the drug of first choice include suppurative arthritis, mastoiditis, endocarditis, pericarditis, and osteomyelitis.

    (b) Other streptococcal infections, especially those due to group A, *S. pyogenes,* are highly sensitive to penicillins G and V.

        (i) Streptococcal pharyngitis and scarlet fever both respond to oral penicillin V with rapid improvement occurring in 2–4 days.

        (ii) Otitis media due to *S. pyogenes* also responds to penicillin V.

        (iii) Other streptococcal infections responding favorably to penicillin G include endocarditis, arthritis, and meningitis.

        (iv) α-Hemolytic streptococci often are the cause of subacute endocarditis and, in this case, occasionally are resistant to penicillins G and V, necessitating the use of a semisynthetic penicillin such as nafcillin.

    (c) Staphylococcal infections that are sensitive to penicillin G should be treated with this form of the drug, since it is more active than the penicillinase-resistant penicillins.

        (i) Approximately 20% of strains of *S. aureus* are resistant, however, because of penicillinase activity.

        (ii) The penicillinase-resistant penicillins oxacillin, cloxacillin, dicloxacillin, methicillin, and nafcillin are highly effective for this type of infection.

(2) Gram-negative coccal (meningococcal, gonococcal) infections respond well to penicillins G and V.

    (a) For **gonococcal infections,** ceftriaxone is considered the drug of first choice because strains have become increasingly resistant to penicillin G.

    (b) In penicillin-resistant strains, procaine penicillin G, ampicillin, or amoxicillin is used, usually given with probenecid [see II B 2 e (1) (b) (ii)].

(3) Syphilis. Penicillin G is the most effective treatment for all stages of syphilis, since *Treponema pallidum* is very sensitive to penicillin G.

(4) Other microbial infections responding to penicillin G

    (a) Penicillin G is active against many oral anaerobes and is still widely used for oral, dental, pulmonary, and soft tissue infections caused by organisms normally found in the oral flora.

    (b) Penicillin G is also the drug of first choice in gas gangrene (usually due to *Clostridium*). However, subdiaphragmatic anaerobic infections (e.g., due to *Bacteroides fragilis*) are generally resistant to penicillins with the exception of the "antipseudomonas" penicillins [see Table 12-1 and II B 2 f (6)].

    (c) Most strains of *Corynebacterium diphtheriae* are sensitive to penicillin G, which is used in diphtheria to eliminate the acute and chronic carrier states. Specific antitoxin is used for treatment of diphtheria.

    (d) Penicillin G is also the drug of first choice in:

        (i) Anthrax (the majority of *B. anthracis* strains are sensitive)

        (ii) Actinomycosis

        (iii) *Listeria* infections

(5) The broad-spectrum penicillins—ampicillin, amoxicillin, and their various derivatives (e.g., bacampicillin, pivampicillin, hetacillin)—are effective against gram-positive organisms, some strains of *E. coli, H. influenzae, Salmonella,* and *Shigella,* and some *Proteus* species. When strains are sensitive, ampicillin and amoxicillin are used to treat:

    (a) Some forms of gonorrhea

    (b) Sinusitis and otitis media due to *H. influenzae,* pneumococci, or *S. pyogenes*

    (c) Urinary tract infections due to *E. coli* or *P. mirabilis*

    (d) Meningitis due to *H. influenzae,* meningococci, or pneumococci

(6) "Antipseudomonas" penicillins are chiefly used to treat serious infections (bacteremia, pneumonia, burn infections) due to gram-negative organisms, particularly *P. aeruginosa,* indole-positive *Proteus,* and *Enterobacter.*

    (a) Carbenicillin and **ticarcillin** have a spectrum of activity similar to that of ampicillin and, in addition, are effective against indole-positive *Proteus* and *Pseudomonas.*

        (i) Ticarcillin is two to four times more active against *P. aeruginosa* than carbenicillin is and may be preferable in serious *Pseudomonas* infections.

    (ii) The carbenicillin congener, **carbenicillin indanyl,** accumulates rapidly in the urine and, thus, provides effective therapy for urinary tract infections caused by indole-positive *Proteus* or *Pseudomonas.*

  (b) Azlocillin, mezlocillin, and **piperacillin** are known collectively as the **ureidopenicillins.**

    (i) Azlocillin and piperacillin are ten times more active than carbenicillin against *Pseudomonas* organisms.

    (ii) Mezlocillin and piperacillin are more active than carbenicillin against *Klebsiella.*

  (c) When a *Pseudomonas* infection is life-threatening, an antipseudomonas penicillin is often used in combination with gentamicin, amikacin, or tobramycin.

(7) Combinations of a penicillin and a beta-lactamase inhibitor

  (a) Clavulanic acid is a beta-lactamase inhibitor that is structurally related to the penicillins.

    (i) Clavulanic acid extends the antibacterial spectrum of beta-lactam antibiotics by irreversibly binding and, thus, inhibiting many bacterial beta-lactamases. It extends the **in vitro activity of amoxicillin** to include beta-lactamase–producing strains of *H. influenzae; E. coli; Proteus* species; *Klebsiella pneumoniae; Staphylococcus epidermidis* and *Staphylococcus saprophyticus,* as well as *S. aureus;* and *Branhamella catarrhalis.* It extends the **in vitro activity of ticarcillin** to include an extremely wide variety of gram-negative and gram-positive organisms and anaerobes.

    (ii) The combination of **amoxicillin and clavulanate** is used to treat infections caused by beta-lactamase–producing strains of *H. influenzae, B. catarrhalis, S. aureus, E. coli, Klebsiella,* and *Enterobacter.*

    (iii) The combination of **ticarcillin and clavulanate** is used to treat infections caused by beta-lactamase–producing strains of *Klebsiella, E. coli, S. aureus, Pseudomonas, H. influenzae, Citrobacter, Enterobacter cloacae,* and *Serratia marcescens.*

  (b) Sulbactam is a penicillanic acid sulfone with limited antibacterial activity. Its principal action is to inactivate bacterial beta-lactamases, thereby enhancing the antibacterial spectrum of ampicillin.

    (i) It extends the in vitro activity of **ampicillin** to include beta-lactamase–producing strains of *H. influenzae, E. coli, Proteus* species, *K. pneumoniae, S. aureus, S. epidermidis, B. catarrhalis, Enterobacter aerogenes, Acinetobacter calcoaceticus, Neisseria,* and several anaerobes, including *B. fragilis.*

    (ii) The combination of **ampicillin and sulbactam** has been useful in treating intra-abdominal and gynecologic infections.

g. Prophylactic uses. Penicillins G and V have been shown to be effective prophylactically in the following conditions:

(1) Streptococcal infections

(2) Rheumatic fever recurrences

(3) Gonorrheal ophthalmia in neonates for which conjunctival instillation of penicillin G solution is effective

(4) Surgical procedures in patients who have valvular heart disease

  (a) When undergoing dental extractions, tonsillectomy, or genitourinary or intestinal operations, such patients often receive penicillin prophylactically.

  (b) Bacteremia is not totally prevented by using prophylactic penicillin.

h. Preparations and administration

(1) Soluble forms of penicillins G and V

  (a) Penicillin G (benzylpenicillin) sodium and potassium salts are used intramuscularly, intravenously, and orally.

  (b) Penicillin V (phenoxymethyl penicillin) is a soluble form that is resistant to acid; it is used orally.

(2) Repository forms are insoluble salts that allow the slow absorption of penicillin from the site of injection, providing a duration of action lasting 12–24 hours. These forms are used intramuscularly only and include:

  (a) Procaine penicillin G

  (b) Benzathine penicillin G (This drug has a low solubility, and effective blood levels often are present for a week.)

    (3) Penicillinase-resistant penicillins
      (a) Methicillin
        (i) This drug has one-twentieth the potency of penicillin G.
        (ii) It is not administered orally because of poor absorption via this route.
      (b) Oxacillin
        (i) This drug is acid-stable and, therefore, can be given orally as well as intravenously and intramuscularly.
        (ii) It is highly protein-bound in the plasma.
        (iii) It is up to eight times as potent as methicillin.
      (c) Cloxacillin has pharmacologic and pharmacokinetic properties that are similar to those of oxacillin.
      (d) Nafcillin can be given orally, intravenously, or intramuscularly.
      (e) Dicloxacillin, because it is highly resistant to penicillinase and acid hydrolysis, is very effective when administered orally.
    (4) Broad-spectrum penicillins
      (a) Ampicillin is given orally, intravenously, or intramuscularly. It is acid-stable but not penicillinase-resistant.
      (b) Amoxicillin is given orally only.
        (i) It attains higher blood levels than ampicillin.
        (ii) It is thought to cause a lower incidence of diarrhea than ampicillin.
    (5) Antipseudomonas penicillins
      (a) Azlocillin is given intravenously.
      (b) Carbenicillin, ticarcillin, mezlocillin, and **piperacillin** are given intravenously or intramuscularly.
      (c) Carbenicillin indanyl is acid-stable and is administered orally.
    (6) Combinations of penicillin and a beta-lactamase inhibitor
      (a) Amoxicillin with clavulanate is given orally.
      (b) Ticarcillin with clavulanate is given intravenously.
      (c) Ampicillin with sulbactam is given intravenously or intramuscularly.
 i. Adverse effects
    (1) Hypersensitivity reactions to the penicillins occur in 5%–20% of patients receiving these drugs, and all forms of penicillin can cause hypersensitivity reactions. A reaction can occur in the absence of prior therapeutic penicillin administration.
      (a) The reaction can range from a mild rash to life-threatening anaphylaxis and may persist 1–2 weeks after discontinuation of therapy. Hypersensitivity reactions include:
        (i) Skin rashes of all types. In severe cases, the Stevens-Johnson syndrome can occur. The highest incidence of skin rash (about 9%) occurs after ampicillin administration.
        (ii) Fever, which disappears within 36 hours after termination of administration
        (iii) Eosinophilia
        (iv) Angioedema
        (v) Serum sickness
        (vi) Anaphylactic reactions. One in 50,000 patients treated with penicillin dies from this type of reaction, which is most common after parenteral administration, but it can occur after oral ingestion and with minute quantities of penicillin.
      (b) Recurrent reactions and cross-sensitivity
        (i) A hypersensitivity reaction to one form of penicillin places the affected patient at high risk of reaction to that form or to any other penicillin.
        (ii) The risk of cross-reactions with other beta-lactams is less clear. Penicillin-allergic individuals occasionally have allergic reactions to cephalosporins.
        (iii) In penicillin-allergic patients, serious infections due to gram-positive organisms are often treated with vancomycin. Alternatives for other infections include erythromycin, trimethoprim–sulfamethoxazole, aminoglycosides, and ciprofloxacin.
    (2) Other adverse effects
      (a) Gastrointestinal upset is more likely with orally administered preparations; an example is ampicillin-associated diarrhea.
      (b) Nephrotoxicity is very rare and usually occurs only in patients with compromised renal function.

      (c) Bone-marrow toxicity is uncommon.

         (i) Depression of bone marrow has been reported with methicillin administration.

         (ii) Agranulocytosis has been reported with ampicillin administration.

         (iii) Impairment of platelet aggregation has been reported with carbenicillin administration.

      (d) Superinfection results from alterations in intestinal flora.

         (i) A low incidence occurs with penicillin G administration.

         (ii) A higher incidence occurs with broad-spectrum penicillins, such as ampicillin and carbenicillin.

3. Cephalosporins

  a. Chemistry

    (1) The cephalosporins (Figure 12-3) are derivatives of 7-aminocephalosporanic acid and are closely related in structure to penicillin.

    (2) They have a six-membered sulfur-containing ring adjoining a beta-lactam ring.

    (3) They are relatively stable in dilute acid.

  b. Classification. The cephalosporins are typically classified by "generations" (Table 12-2), which roughly parallel their chronologic development and their antimicrobial spectrum.

  c. Mechanism of action. Cephalosporins, like the penicillins, inhibit bacterial cell wall synthesis and are considered **bactericidal**.

  d. Bacterial resistance

    (1) The cephalosporins are highly resistant to penicillinase.

    (2) Some bacteria elaborate a beta-lactamase called **cephalosporinase** that acts on the cephalosporin nucleus to destroy its antibacterial activity. However, many cephalosporins are resistant to the enzyme.

  e. Pharmacokinetics

    (1) Most cephalosporins are administered parenterally; some, however, are well absorbed from the gastrointestinal tract and can be given orally.

    (2) The cephalosporins become widely distributed throughout body tissues and fluids. The majority do not penetrate the blood–brain barrier and, thus, are not effective in the treatment of central nervous system (CNS) infections.

    (3) The half-life and the degree of serum protein binding vary widely from agent to agent.

    (4) Although some cephalosporins are excreted via the bile, most are excreted in the urine via renal tubular secretion. **Probenecid** blocks the tubular secretion of cephalosporins, often resulting in an increased half-life and elevated plasma concentration.

  f. Pharmacologic effects. All cephalosporins are active against most gram-positive cocci, including penicillinase-producing staphylococci and many strains of gram-negative bacilli. The cephalosporins are in general ineffective against enterococci.

  g. Therapeutic uses

    (1) Diseases produced by *S. aureus,* both penicillin-sensitive and penicillin-resistant, including skin infections, osteomyelitis, and endocarditis, respond favorably to the cephalosporins.

    (2) Cephalosporins are the drugs of first choice for *K. pneumoniae* infections.

    (3) These drugs are used successfully in the treatment of pneumococcal pneumonia and in infections caused by *S. pyogenes*.

    (4) Some of the parenteral cephalosporins are efficacious in the treatment of gonococcal disease that is resistant to other agents.

    (5) Diseases caused by a number of gram-negative bacteria, including respiratory and urinary tract infections, respond well.

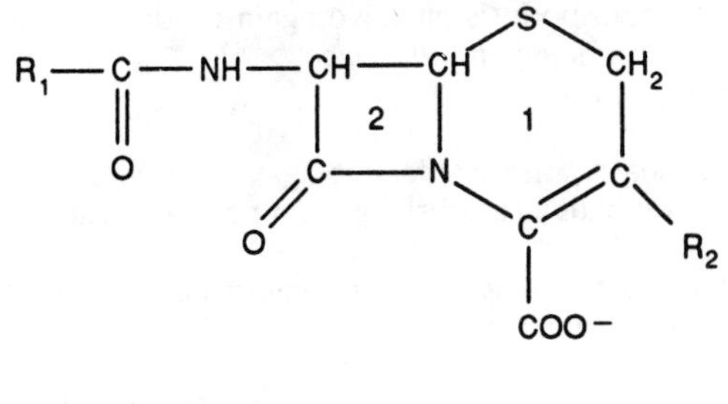

Figure 12-3. Structure of the cephalosporins. *1* = sulfur-containing ring; *2* = beta-lactam ring; R_1, R_2 = variable side chains.

Table 12-2. Classification of Cephalosporins

First-generation	Second-generation	Third-generation
Cephalothin	Cefamandole	Cefotaxime
Cephapirin	Cefoxitin	Ceftizoxime
Cefazolin	Cefaclor	Ceftriaxone
Cephalexin	Cefuroxime	Cefoperazone
Cephradine	Cefonicid	Ceftazidime
Cefadroxil	Cefotetan	Cefixime
Cephaloridine*	Ceforanide	Moxalactam*

*No longer used because of toxicity.

   (6) The expanded-spectrum of activity of the cephalosporins includes effectiveness against *Proteus, B. fragilis, Serratia, Enterobacter,* and some activity against *Pseudomonas.* These agents are effective for the treatment of meningitis caused by susceptible strains.
 h. **Prophylactic cephalosporin therapy** plays an important role in reducing perioperative infection.
 i. **Preparations and administration**
   (1) **First-generation cephalosporins** are *not* effective against indole-positive *Proteus, Pseudomonas, Serratia, Enterobacter,* or *B. fragilis.*
     (a) **Cephalothin**
        (i) It is not well absorbed from the gastrointestinal tract.
        (ii) It is usually given intravenously. Intramuscular injection is painful.
        (iii) It is excreted principally via renal tubular secretion.
     (b) **Cefazolin**
        (i) It is not well absorbed from the gastrointestinal tract and is administered intravenously or intramuscularly.
        (ii) Some 80% of the drug is reversibly bound to plasma proteins, substantially increasing its half-life.
        (iii) Cefazolin is eliminated primarily by renal glomerular filtration; renal tubular secretion and biliary secretion play secondary roles.
     (c) **Cephalexin**
        (i) It is well absorbed from the gastrointestinal tract because of its high acid stability.
        (ii) It is available in oral capsules, suspensions, and pediatric drops.
        (iii) More than 90% of this drug is excreted unchanged in the urine; it is also excreted into bile.
     (d) **Cephradine** is similar to cephalexin. It can be given orally, intravenously, or intramuscularly.
     (e) **Cefadroxil** is an orally active analog of cephalexin. It is used in the treatment of urinary tract infections.
   (2) **Second-generation cephalosporins**
     (a) **Cefamandole**
        (i) This expanded-spectrum cephalosporin is effective against indole-positive *Proteus* and beta-lactamase–producing *H. influenzae.*
        (ii) It is administered parenterally only.
     (b) **Cefoxitin**
        (i) This expanded-spectrum cephalosporin is effective against indole-positive *Proteus* and *B. fragilis.* It has less activity against the gram-positive organisms.
        (ii) It is given parenterally.
     (c) **Cefaclor** is similar to cephalexin but also is effective against beta-lactamase–producing *H. influenzae.* It is given orally.

(d) Cefonicid
    (i) Cefonicid has an antibacterial spectrum similar to that of cefamandole.
    (ii) Its extended half-life allows once-daily dosing; it is given parenterally.
(e) Cefuroxime is an expanded-spectrum cephalosporin that is useful for serious *H. influenzae* infections, particularly respiratory tract infections and otitis media. It is available for both parenteral and oral administration.
(f) Ceforanide is similar in structure to cefamandole but is less active against *H. influenzae*. It is given parenterally.
(g) Cefotetan has an in vitro spectrum similar to that of cefoxitin, but it is less active against some anaerobes. It is given parenterally.

(3) Third-generation cephalosporins
  (a) Cefotaxime, ceftizoxime, and ceftriaxone
    (i) These relatively new, semisynthetic cephalosporins are more potent than the parent drug.
    (ii) They are given parenterally.
    (iii) Ceftriaxone, because of its long half-life, can be administered once daily. It is particularly useful against penicillinase-producing strains of *Neisseria gonorrhoeae*.
  (b) Cefoperazone and ceftazidime have greater activity against *P. aeruginosa* than the other third-generation cephalosporins but lesser activity against some other organisms.
  (c) Cefixime is effective against beta-lactamase–producing strains of *H. influenzae*. It can be administered orally once a day.

j. Adverse effects
  (1) Hypersensitivity reactions occur in about 5% of patients receiving cephalosporin therapy.
    (a) Cephalosporins, like penicillins, elicit a spectrum of reactions that range from mild skin rash to anaphylaxis.
    (b) A **cross-sensitivity reaction** to the cephalosporins occasionally occurs in individuals who are allergic to penicillin.
    (c) Patients receiving large doses of a cephalosporin often have a positive direct Coombs' reaction.
  (2) Renal damage, although rare with normal doses of cephalosporins, can occur.
  (3) Local tissue reactions can occur with parenteral administration. Intravenous administration can cause thrombophlebitis.
  (4) Superinfections caused by gram-negative bacteria or yeasts can occur following administration of the cephalosporins.
  (5) Because moxalactam can induce a bleeding diathesis and cephaloridine is nephrotoxic, these drugs are no longer used clinically in the United States.

4. Imipenem is a beta-lactam antibiotic derived from thienamycin. Like other beta-lactam antibiotics, it acts by interfering with the synthesis of the bacterial cell wall and is bactericidal.
  a. Pharmacokinetics
    (1) Imipenem is given in combination with **cilastatin,** a dipeptidase inhibitor that inhibits the renal tubular metabolism of imipenem and prevents the formation of potentially nephrotoxic compounds.
    (2) The serum elimination half-life of both imipenem and cilastatin is 1 hour.
    (3) Imipenem is filtered and secreted by the kidney, and if given alone, it is inactivated by a dipeptidase enzyme in the kidney, which opens the beta-lactam ring.
  b. Pharmacologic effects. Imipenem has the broadest antimicrobial spectrum of all the beta-lactam antibiotics.
    (1) It is active against both gram-positive and gram-negative cocci (except methicillin-resistant staphylococci), Enterobacteriaceae, *P. aeruginosa,* and anaerobic bacteria, including *B. fragilis.*
    (2) Gonococci and *H. influenzae* strains that are resistant to both penicillin and ampicillin are susceptible to imipenem.
  c. Therapeutic uses
    (1) Use of imipenem is limited to the treatment of serious hospital-acquired infections due to susceptible organisms. It is given intravenously.
      (a) It is used in urinary tract, respiratory tract, skin, and soft tissue infections.

        (b) It is effective for the treatment of osteomyelitis, septic arthritis, bacteremia, and gynecologic and intra-abdominal infections.

    (2) Its usefulness in staphylococcal endocarditis has been established, but not in CNS infections.

  d. Adverse effects

    (1) *P. aeruginosa* may become resistant during imipenem therapy.

    (2) Allergic reactions may occur, as with other beta-lactam antibiotics. Patients allergic to penicillin should be considered allergic to imipenem.

    (3) Nausea, vomiting, and diarrhea have occurred.

5. Aztreonam

  a. Chemistry. Aztreonam, a monobactam, differs from penicillins and cephalosporins in having a monocyclic rather than a bicyclic beta-lactam nucleus.

  b. Mechanism of action

    (1) Like other beta-lactams, aztreonam interferes with the synthesis of the bacterial cell wall.

    (2) However, its action is due to a high affinity for bacterial penicillin-binding protein 3.

  c. Pharmacokinetics

    (1) The bioavailability of an intramuscular dose is 100%.

    (2) The serum elimination half-life is 1.7 hours.

    (3) Two-thirds of a dose appears in the urine within 24 hours.

  d. Pharmacologic effects

    (1) Aztreonam is highly resistant to beta-lactamases.

    (2) It is highly active against aerobic gram-negative bacteria, including *P. aeruginosa* and penicillinase-producing strains of *H. influenzae* and gonococci.

    (3) It shows poor activity against gram-positive cocci and anaerobic bacteria.

  e. Therapeutic uses

    (1) Aztreonam has substituted for aminoglycosides in the treatment of urinary tract, lower respiratory tract, and skin and soft tissue infections. Additionally, osteomyelitis, gonorrhea, and gynecologic and intra-abdominal infections due to susceptible pathogens have been successfully treated.

    (2) Because of its narrow spectrum, aztreonam is often used in combination with another antimicrobial agent.

    (3) Aztreonam is administered parenterally.

  f. Adverse effects

    (1) Colonization and superinfection with gram-positive cocci can occur.

    (2) Pseudomembranous colitis has been reported.

    (3) Aztreonam shows little or no immunologic cross-reactivity with other beta-lactams.

C. Aminoglycosides

1. Chemistry

  a. The aminoglycosides are compounds containing characteristic amino sugars joined to a hexose nucleus in glycosidic linkage.

  b. They are polycations, and their polarity accounts for their pharmacokinetic properties.

2. Mechanism of action

  a. The aminoglycosides inhibit protein biosynthesis by acting directly on the ribosome.

    (1) They interfere with the proper attachment of messenger RNA to ribosomes in the initiation of protein synthesis.

    (2) They also cause misreading of the genetic code and, hence, cause decreased or abnormal protein synthesis.

  b. The aminoglycosides also appear to disrupt the bacterial cytoplasmic membrane.

  c. The rapid **bactericidal** effect of the aminoglycosides is not, however, adequately explained by any of their known actions.

3. Pharmacokinetics

  a. All of the aminoglycosides are poorly absorbed after oral administration because of their polycationic structure.

  b. They are absorbed rapidly after intramuscular or subcutaneous administration.

    (1) They are distributed in all extracellular fluids, but tissue concentrations are low except in the kidney and ear.

(2) They cross the blood–brain barrier only if the meninges are inflamed.

(3) They are excreted by glomerular filtration.

c. All the aminoglycosides are more active in an alkaline environment.

4. Microbial resistance can result from several bacterial enzymes that inactivate the aminoglycoside molecule.

a. Plasmids and R (resistance) factors have spread the genetic codes for these enzymes, so that many initially sensitive microbes have become resistant to the aminoglycosides.

b. Synergism between beta-lactam antibiotics and aminoglycosides against enterococci can also be lost by this mechanism.

c. Cross-resistance between the aminoglycosides can occur.

d. Amikacin and netilmicin are not affected by most aminoglycoside-inactivating enzymes that cause bacterial resistance in some species.

5. Pharmacologic effects

a. Streptomycin

(1) High concentrations of streptomycin are bactericidal; low concentrations are bacteriostatic.

(2) Streptomycin is effective against the organisms that cause plague (*Yersinia pestis*) and tularemia (*Francisella tularensis*) and, in combination with penicillin [see II C 6 a (1)], against gram-positive enterococci and streptococci. In vivo, streptomycin suppresses tubercle bacilli.

b. Neomycin is effective against many gram-negative species and is also effective against several gram-positive bacteria (e.g., *S. aureus*). Streptococci are generally resistant to neomycin.

c. Gentamicin is bactericidal against a wide variety of gram-negative organisms, including indole-positive *Proteus, Pseudomonas,* and *Serratia* organisms. Some strains of *Staphylococcus* may be sensitive to gentamicin.

d. Tobramycin has a spectrum of activity similar to that of gentamicin but may be slightly more effective against *Pseudomonas*.

e. Amikacin also has a spectrum of activity similar to that of gentamicin but often is reserved for situations in which resistance to gentamicin has emerged.

f. Netilmicin has a spectrum of activity similar to that of amikacin and may be active against bacteria that are resistant to gentamicin.

g. Kanamycin has a more limited spectrum of activity than gentamicin has. It is ineffective against *Pseudomonas* and most gram-positive organisms.

h. Kanamycin, amikacin, streptomycin, and neomycin all have some activity against *M. tuberculosis*.

i. Anaerobic microorganisms are generally resistant to the aminoglycosides.

6. Therapeutic uses

a. Streptomycin

(1) Subacute bacterial endocarditis caused by the viridans group of streptococci or by enterococci is treated with streptomycin, usually in combination with penicillin G.

(2) Because of the frequent development of bacterial resistance (see II C 4), streptomycin is used alone to treat only two infections—tularemia and plague.

(3) Severe cases of brucellosis are treated with a combination of streptomycin and tetracycline.

(4) Urinary and respiratory tract infections, peritonitis, and bacterial meningitis may respond to streptomycin but are treated more effectively with other agents.

(5) Although streptomycin is no longer used alone in the treatment of pulmonary tuberculosis, it is often used in combination with other agents for the treatment of serious forms of tuberculosis (see IV F).

b. Gentamicin, tobramycin, amikacin, and netilmicin

(1) Many infections can be treated successfully with these agents, but their toxicity restricts their use to situations involving life-threatening infections caused by:

(a) *P. aeruginosa, Serratia, Enterobacter,* and *Klebsiella*

(b) Methicillin-resistant staphylococci that are sensitive to gentamicin

(2) These agents are sometimes used as part of an initial "blind therapy" for serious infections of unknown etiology, in which case a penicillinase-resistant penicillin or a cephalosporin is administered in combination with an aminoglycoside, such as gentamicin.

c. Neomycin, because of its serious toxic effects when absorbed systemically, is used most frequently in dermatologic and ophthalmic ointments. In addition, neomycin can be used orally as a bowel preparation for surgery or for the management of hepatic coma.

d. Kanamycin has also been largely superseded by less toxic, more effective agents.

7. Preparations and administration

a. Streptomycin
   (1) Intramuscular injection is the most common route of administration.
   (2) To avoid the development of bacterial resistance, streptomycin therapy rarely is extended beyond 10 days (except in tuberculosis and subacute bacterial endocarditis).

b. Gentamicin
   (1) This drug can be administered intramuscularly, intravenously, or as an ointment or cream.
   (2) When renal function is impaired, peak and trough serum concentrations of gentamicin are measured intermittently to allow optimal guidance for adjusting dosage, and renal function is monitored by means of the serum creatinine level.

c. Tobramycin, amikacin, and **netilmicin** can be given intramuscularly or intravenously.

d. Kanamycin can be given intramuscularly, intravenously, or orally.

e. Neomycin
   (1) This drug is available in the form of creams, ointments, and sprays, both alone and in combination with polymyxin, bacitracin, other antibiotics, and corticosteroids.
   (2) It is also available for oral and parenteral administration, although it is rarely used parenterally.

8. Adverse effects

a. All of the aminoglycosides have a narrow therapeutic index that limits their parenteral usage.

b. Ototoxicity and nephrotoxicity are the most serious side effects.
   (1) Ototoxicity. Both labyrinthine damage and vestibular disturbances can occur.
      (a) Permanent damage occurs in a small percentage of patients.
      (b) The incidence is directly related to daily dose and duration of therapy.
      (c) About 7% of patients receiving streptomycin for more than a week have a measurable decrease in hearing. The high-frequency sound range is first to be affected.
      (d) Ototoxicity occurs more commonly when renal failure is present.
      (e) The simultaneous administration of ethacrynic acid or furosemide increases the risk of ototoxicity.
   (2) Nephrotoxicity
      (a) Gentamicin is the most nephrotoxic of the aminoglycosides. It can produce acute renal insufficiency and tubular necrosis.
      (b) When renal failure of any degree is present, serum creatinine and aminoglycoside levels must be measured and drug dosage adjusted accordingly.
   (3) Animal studies suggest that netilmicin is less likely to produce ototoxicity and nephrotoxicity; however, this has not been proved in humans.

c. Dysfunction of the optic nerve can occur with streptomycin, producing scotomas.

d. Neuromuscular junction blockade may result when an aminoglycoside is given at high doses and in combination with curariform drugs. This apparently results from a decreased sensitivity of the postjunctional membrane to acetylcholine and decreased presynaptic release of the transmitter.

e. Hypersensitivity reactions can occur. Up to 8% of patients develop a skin rash when neomycin is applied topically.

f. Superinfection and intestinal malabsorption can occur following oral administration of neomycin.

D. Tetracyclines

1. Chemistry. Tetracycline (Figure 12-4) and its congeners are derivatives of the polycyclic naphthacenecarboxamide.

2. Mechanism of action

a. Tetracyclines are primarily **bacteriostatic,** inhibiting protein synthesis by binding to 30S ribosomes.

b. Tetracycline affects both eukaryotic and prokaryotic cells but apparently penetrates microbial membranes more readily due to the presence of active transport systems in microbes.

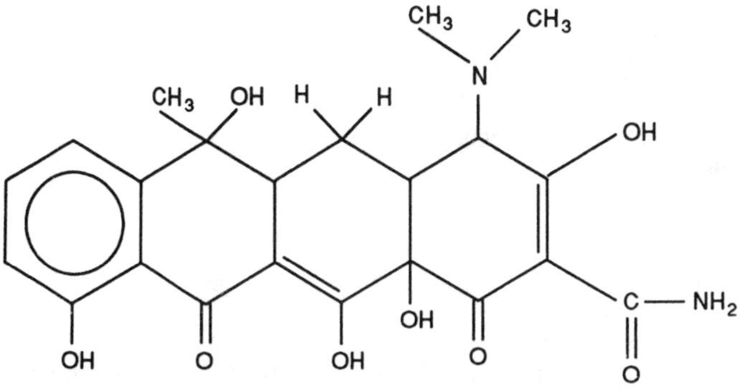

Figure 12-4. Tetracycline.

3. Pharmacokinetics
a. Tetracyclines are adequately but incompletely absorbed from the gastrointestinal tract, particularly from the stomach and upper small intestine.
  (1) Absorption is impaired by food, especially milk and milk products, by aluminum hydroxide gels, and by calcium and magnesium salts.
  (2) The cations in these substances chelate with tetracycline, preventing gastrointestinal absorption.
  (3) **Minocycline** and **doxycycline** are exceptions in that they chelate poorly with calcium, and food does not interfere with their absorption. However, like other tetracyclines, they do chelate with iron to form insoluble complexes.
b. The tetracyclines diffuse readily into body fluids and bind to plasma proteins to varying degrees, depending on the particular preparation. Concentrations in the cerebrospinal fluid are about 20% of serum levels unless the meninges are inflamed.
c. The tetracyclines are removed from the blood by the liver and are excreted into the intestine by way of the bile. They undergo enterohepatic circulation.
d. Excretion occurs primarily via the kidney, although there is some fecal excretion. Renal clearance of these drugs is by glomerular filtration.

4. Bacterial resistance
a. Gram-positive bacteria often become resistant to the tetracyclines, limiting the usefulness of these drugs.
b. Complete cross-resistance among the tetracycline preparations occurs.

5. Pharmacologic effects
a. Tetracyclines are effective against many gram-positive and gram-negative bacteria.
b. The tetracyclines are effective against *Mycoplasma, Borrelia, Chlamydia,* and rickettsial species.
c. They are useful secondary drugs against *Leptospira* and *Treponema* species.
d. In high concentrations, the tetracyclines inhibit the growth of the protozoan *Entamoeba histolytica.*

6. Therapeutic uses
a. The use of tetracyclines for treatment of infectious disease has declined because of increasing bacterial resistance and the development of newer, more effective antimicrobial agents.
b. Tetracyclines are useful in the treatment of the following conditions.
  (1) **Rickettsial infections.** Tetracyclines are the drugs of first choice for these diseases, which include:
    (a) Rocky Mountain spotted fever
    (b) Brill's disease
    (c) Murine and scrub typhus
    (d) Rickettsialpox
    (e) Q fever
  (2) **Chlamydial infections**
    (a) Lymphogranuloma venereum
    (b) Psittacosis
    (c) Inclusion conjunctivitis
    (d) Trachoma
  (3) **Mycoplasmal infections**

(4) Bacillary infections
    (a) Brucellosis
    (b) Tularemia
    (c) Cholera
    (d) Some *Shigella* and *Salmonella* infections
(5) Venereal infections
    (a) Gonorrhea
    (b) Syphilis
    (c) Chancroid
    (d) Granuloma inguinale
    (e) Chlamydial urethritis or cervicitis
(6) Amebiasis
c. Lyme disease, a multisystem inflammatory disorder, is caused by the spirochete *Borrelia burgdorferi,* which is transmitted by ticks. Oral tetracycline or doxycycline for 10–20 days shortens the duration of symptoms and often prevents the development of more serious sequelae.
d. Staphylococcal and streptococcal infections may respond to tetracyclines. However, the drugs are third-line agents against these infections.
e. In urinary tract infections, the use of tetracyclines is limited because of the increasing number of resistant microorganisms.
f. Tetracyclines may be beneficial in the treatment of acne.

7. Preparations and administration
a. Tetracyclines are available in formulations suitable for oral, intravenous, and intramuscular administration. They are also available for topical use, including ophthalmic solutions.
b. The various tetracyclines include:
    (1) Chlortetracycline
    (2) Oxytetracycline
    (3) Tetracycline
    (4) Demeclocycline. This drug has a greater acid and alkaline stability and slower rate of excretion than most tetracyclines; therefore, it produces higher and more prolonged blood levels.
    (5) Methacycline. This drug is absorbed rapidly.
    (6) Minocycline. Absorption of this drug is not impaired by food or calcium ion.
    (7) Doxycycline
        (a) Increased absorption of doxycycline allows once-daily administration after the first day.
        (b) As with minocycline, food and calcium ions do not affect absorption.
        (c) As opposed to the other tetracyclines, 90% of this drug is excreted in the feces; therefore, it does not accumulate in the blood of patients with compromised renal function. Thus, it is one of the safest tetracyclines for use against extrarenal infections in patients with renal dysfunction.

8. Adverse effects
a. Hypersensitivity reactions, including skin rash and drug fever, can occur. Cross-sensitivity among the various tetracyclines is common.
b. When tetracyclines are administered orally, gastrointestinal irritation is common.
c. The intravenous administration of tetracyclines often produces thrombophlebitis due to local irritation. Intramuscular injections are painful, cause local irritation, and result in poor absorption of the drugs.
d. Demeclocycline, and less often the other tetracyclines, can produce a phototoxic reaction, resulting in severe skin lesions in patients exposed to sunlight.
e. High doses of tetracyclines can produce hepatic dysfunction. This reaction is exacerbated during pregnancy.
f. Children receiving tetracycline may develop yellow-brown discoloration of the teeth and suffer depressed bone growth.
    (1) The drugs are deposited in the teeth and bones because of their chelating properties and form a tetracycline–calcium orthophosphate complex.
    (2) The tooth discoloration is related to the total dose and the time of ingestion.
        (a) The risk of discoloration is greatest when tetracyclines are given to infants prior to their first dentition.

        (b) Discoloration of the permanent teeth can result, however, from the administration of tetracycline at any time between the ages of 2 months and 7 years, the period of tooth calcification.

        (c) Tetracycline treatment during pregnancy can produce discoloration of the teeth in the offspring.

    g. The ingestion of outdated and degraded tetracycline can result in a form of the Fanconi syndrome (renal tubular dysfunction, which can lead to renal failure).

    h. Tetracyclines can cause increased intracranial pressure, especially in infants.

    i. Vestibular toxicity can occur following minocycline therapy.

    j. Superinfection by strains of resistant bacteria and yeasts is a significant problem that can result in staphylococcal enterocolitis, intestinal candidiasis, and pseudomembranous colitis.

E. Chloramphenicol

1. Chemistry. Chloramphenicol (Figure 12-5) is a nitrobenzene derivative.

2. Mechanism of action

    a. Chloramphenicol inhibits protein synthesis by acting on the 50S ribosomal subunit, a site of action shared with macrolide antibiotics and clindamycin.

    b. This drug is primarily **bacteriostatic,** although it may be bactericidal to some strains.

3. Pharmacokinetics

    a. Chloramphenicol is absorbed rapidly from the gastrointestinal tract.

    b. It is widely distributed in body fluids and reaches therapeutic levels in cerebrospinal fluid. It also is present in bile, milk, and aqueous humor.

    c. Chloramphenicol is metabolized in the liver by glucuronyl transferase.

    d. Its metabolites are excreted in the urine.

4. Pharmacologic effects

    a. Chloramphenicol has a fairly wide spectrum of antimicrobial activity, including:

        (1) Many gram-negative organisms (e.g., it is bactericidal for *H. influenzae*)

        (2) Anaerobic organisms, such as *Bacteroides* species (e.g., *B. fragilis*)

        (3) Some strains of *Streptococcus* and *Staphylococcus* (at a high antibiotic concentration)

        (4) Species of *Clostridium, Chlamydia,* and *Mycoplasma*

        (5) Rickettsiae, in which it suppresses growth

    b. *P. aeruginosa* is resistant.

5. Therapeutic uses. Potentially severe toxicity limits the use of chloramphenicol to those infections that cannot be treated effectively with other antibiotic agents. When another agent is as efficacious as chloramphenicol and potentially less toxic, the other agent should be used.

    a. Chloramphenicol is the drug of choice for typhoid fever.

    b. Bacterial meningitis caused by *H. influenzae* is effectively treated. When children are affected, the combination of ampicillin and chloramphenicol is recommended for initial therapy.

    c. Most anaerobic infections respond to chloramphenicol.

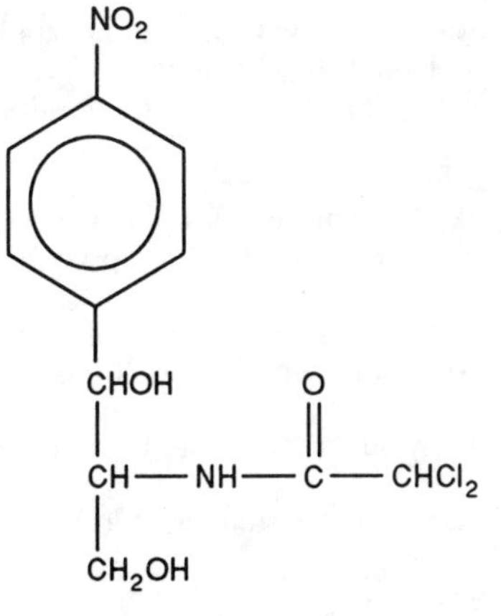

$$NO_2$$

$$CHOH$$
$$CH—NH—\overset{\overset{\displaystyle O}{\|}}{C}—CHCl_2$$
$$CH_2OH$$

Figure 12-5. Chloramphenicol.

d. Rickettsial diseases and brucellosis can be treated with chloramphenicol; however, tetracyclines are the preferred agents.

6. Preparations and administration

a. Chloramphenicol and its palmitate salt are given orally.

b. Chloramphenicol sodium succinate is given intravenously. It has no antibacterial activity until it has been hydrolyzed to chloramphenicol. Levels do not peak for 1 hour.

c. Ophthalmic solutions and ointments are also available.

7. Adverse effects

a. Hypersensitivity reactions can occur.

b. The most important effect, which may be related to hypersensitivity, is bone marrow depression, resulting in pancytopenia.

(1) The incidence of this reaction is not dose-related.

(2) It is usually associated with prolonged therapy and more than one episode of treatment with chloramphenicol.

(3) It occurs in 1 in 40,000 patients given chloramphenicol and often is fatal.

c. Dose-dependent, reversible blood dyscrasias may also occur.

d. Superinfections can occur, including oropharyngeal candidiasis and acute staphylococcal enterocolitis.

e. Gastrointestinal upset can occur, and, as with many of the other broad-spectrum antibiotics, the possibility of diarrhea due to superinfection must be differentiated from local irritation effects.

f. Gray-baby syndrome

(1) This condition is seen in neonates, especially premature infants, who have been given relatively large doses of chloramphenicol.

(2) Cyanosis, respiratory irregularities, vasomotor collapse, abdominal distention, loose green stools, and an ashen-gray color characterize this often fatal syndrome.

(3) The condition develops because of the immature hepatic conjugating mechanism and the inadequate mechanism for renal excretion in neonates.

F. Erythromycin, clindamycin, and vancomycin

1. Chemistry

a. Erythromycin is a macrolide antibiotic. Macrolides contain a lactone ring and one or more deoxy sugars.

b. Clindamycin is the 7-deoxy,7-chloro derivative of the parent drug, **lincomycin,** which it has essentially replaced.

c. Vancomycin is a complex glycopeptide.

2. Mechanism of action

a. Erythromycin and **clindamycin** inhibit bacterial protein synthesis by binding to 50S ribosomal subunits of sensitive microorganisms; they are usually **bacteriostatic** but can be bactericidal in certain situations.

b. Vancomycin inhibits synthesis of the bacterial cell wall. Thus, unlike erythromycin and clindamycin, vancomycin is clearly **bactericidal**.

3. Pharmacokinetics

a. Erythromycin

(1) All forms of erythromycin are absorbed following oral administration and diffuse into most body tissues and fluids except cerebrospinal fluid.

(a) The **base** is absorbed from the upper part of the small intestine. It is destroyed by gastric juice.

(b) The **estolate** is resistant to gastric inactivation.

(c) In children, the estolate appears to be more bioavailable than the ethylsuccinate.

(2) Erythromycin is concentrated in the liver and is excreted primarily in bile and feces.

b. Clindamycin

(1) Although it is well absorbed following oral administration, clindamycin most often is administered parenterally because pseudomembranous colitis is less likely to follow parenteral administration.

(2) The drug is widely distributed in body fluids and tissues but does not pass readily into cerebrospinal fluid.

(3) Most of the drug is metabolized to the inactive sulfoxide form, which then is excreted in the urine and bile.

   c. Vancomycin

       (1) This drug is absorbed poorly after oral administration, and intravenous administration is, therefore, preferred.

       (2) It is widely distributed and passes into the cerebrospinal fluid when the meninges are inflamed.

       (3) Most of the compound is excreted via the kidney.

4. Pharmacologic effects

  a. Erythromycin

    (1) This drug is effective against gram-positive organisms, including some strains of *S. aureus* that are penicillin G–resistant.

    (2) *Neisseria* species, some strains of *H. influenzae,* and *Bordetella, Legionella, Treponema,* and *Mycoplasma* species are sensitive to erythromycin.

    (3) In general, it is not very active against most gram-negative bacilli.

  b. Clindamycin

    (1) Clindamycin is effective against:

      (a) Gram-positive organisms, including anaerobic streptococci

      (b) Many other anaerobic bacteria, especially *B. fragilis*

    (2) It is not effective against gonococci, meningococci, or most aerobic gram-negative bacilli.

  c. Vancomycin is active primarily against gram-positive bacteria.

5. Therapeutic uses

  a. Erythromycin

    (1) This drug is useful for patients who are allergic to penicillin when the infecting organism is sensitive to erythromycin, particularly in cases of infection with group A *S. pyogenes* and *S. pneumoniae.*

    (2) Pneumonia due to *Mycoplasma* organisms is effectively treated.

    (3) Legionnaires' disease is treated with erythromycin.

    (4) Topical erythromycin preparations are used to treat acne.

  b. Clindamycin

    (1) Although this drug is effective against gram-positive organisms, its toxicity and the availability of more effective agents limit its systemic use to infections in which it is clearly superior.

    (2) Clindamycin is the drug of first choice against *Bacteroides,* especially *B. fragilis,* which often is the cause of anaerobic abdominal infections. Anaerobic infections of the brain are treated more effectively with chloramphenicol because clindamycin shows poor CNS penetration.

    (3) Topical clindamycin preparations are used to treat acne.

  c. Vancomycin

    (1) This antibiotic is very effective against penicillin-resistant staphylococci, streptococci of the viridans group, and serious enterococcal infections, such as staphylococcal enterocolitis and pseudomembranous colitis caused by *Clostridium difficile.*

    (2) Toxicity limits its use to serious infections.

6. Preparations and administration

  a. Erythromycin

    (1) Erythromycin base and several salts are available in various forms for oral administration.

    (2) Sterile erythromycin gluceptate is available for parenteral administration.

    (3) Erythromycin base is available in topical formulations.

  b. Clindamycin is available in oral, parenteral, and topical forms.

  c. Vancomycin

    (1) Because it is reserved for severe infections, vancomycin is most often administered intravenously.

    (2) Oral use is limited to the treatment of susceptible enteric infections.

7. Adverse effects

  a. Erythromycin has a very low incidence of serious side effects.

    (1) Cholestatic hepatitis has occurred in adults treated for a week or longer with the estolate form. Hepatitis can also occur with the ethylsuccinate and possibly with the stearate. The hepatitis is uncommon and is reversible.

    (2) Epigastric distress can occur.

(3) A high incidence of thrombophlebitis occurs when erythromycin is administered intravenously, even when the drug is dissolved in a large fluid volume.

(4) Superinfection can occur.

(5) Transient deafness has been reported, especially with high doses.

(6) Erythromycin can interfere with the hepatic metabolism of theophylline compounds, leading to toxic accumulation. It can also increase the effects and toxicity of oral anticoagulants, carbamazepine, and digoxin.

b. Clindamycin. Pseudomembranous colitis can occur, resulting in diarrhea, abdominal pain, fever, and mucus and blood in the stools. This potentially fatal condition, caused by *C. difficile,* can be treated with vancomycin.

c. Vancomycin

(1) Ototoxicity can lead to deafness.

(2) Nephrotoxicity can occur.

(3) Hypersensitivity reactions can occur.

(4) Thrombophlebitis is frequently observed following prolonged intravenous therapy.

G. Quinolones

1. **Chemistry. Norfloxacin** and **ciprofloxacin** are fluoroquinolones. These newer synthetic antimicrobials are structurally related to the older quinolone, **nalidixic acid** (Figure 12-6).

2. **Mechanism of action.** The quinolones act on DNA gyrase, an enzyme involved in DNA replication. They are rapidly bactericidal.

3. **Bacterial resistance.** Resistance to the fluoroquinolones does not develop rapidly as it does with nalidixic acid.

4. **Pharmacokinetics**
   a. Norfloxacin and ciprofloxacin are rapidly absorbed when given orally.
   b. Their serum elimination half-life is 3–4 hours.
   c. Both drugs are metabolized in the liver to some extent.
   d. They are excreted in the urine via glomerular filtration and tubular secretion.
   e. Both drugs are widely distributed throughout the body, but concentrations in the cerebrospinal fluid are low.

5. **Pharmacologic effects**
   a. Norfloxacin and ciprofloxacin are active against many gram-positive and gram-negative bacteria. Additionally, ciprofloxacin is active against some mycobacteria. They are highly active against gonococci.
   b. Norfloxacin, like ciprofloxacin, is active against virtually all urinary tract pathogens.
   c. Ciprofloxacin is highly active against bacteria that cause enteritis and against staphylococci, including strains resistant to methicillin.
   d. Both drugs are somewhat less active against *P. aeruginosa* and many streptococci, and they have poor activity against anaerobes.

6. **Therapeutic uses**
   a. Norfloxacin and ciprofloxacin are indicated for complicated and uncomplicated urinary tract infections.
   b. Ciprofloxacin is also indicated for serious infectious diarrhea; for infections of bones, joints, skin, and soft tissue; and for lower respiratory tract infections, including those in patients with cystic fibrosis.

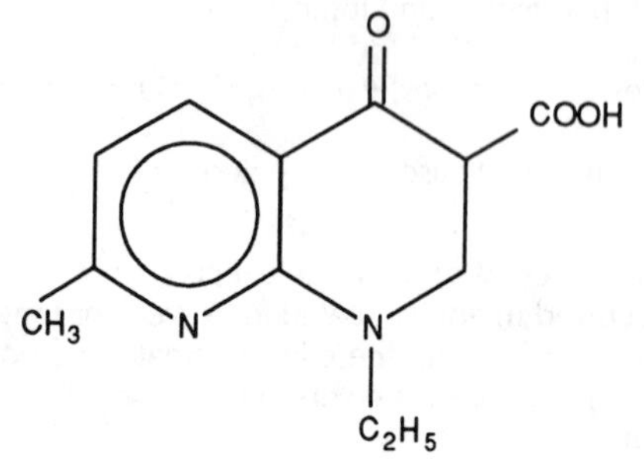

Figure 12-6. Nalidixic acid.

7. Preparations and administration. Norfloxacin and ciprofloxacin are administered orally with liberal fluid intake to avoid crystalluria.

8. Adverse effects
 a. Quinolones can cause arthropathy in young animals and are, therefore, not used in patients under age 17, during pregnancy, or in nursing mothers.
 b. Crystalluria has occurred rarely, particularly with alkaline urine.
 c. Fluoroquinolones are inhibitors of gamma-aminobutyric acid (GABA) and may cause seizures.
 d. Ciprofloxacin interferes with the hepatic metabolism of theophylline and coumadin and can increase their serum concentrations.
 e. Ciprofloxacin and norfloxacin have caused pseudomembranous colitis.

III. AGENTS USED FOR TREATMENT OF FUNGUS INFECTIONS

A. Nystatin

1. Chemistry. Nystatin is a polyene antibiotic.

2. Mechanism of action
 a. The drug is **fungistatic** and **fungicidal**.
 b. It binds to sterols, especially ergosterol, which is enriched in the membrane of fungi and yeasts. As a result of this binding, the drug appears to form channels in the membrane that allow small molecules to leak out of the cell.

3. Pharmacokinetics
 a. Nystatin is not absorbed appreciably from the gastrointestinal tract.
 b. It is not absorbed from the skin or mucous membranes.
 c. It is not employed parenterally.
 d. It is poorly soluble and decomposes rapidly in water.

4. Therapeutic uses
 a. Nystatin is used to treat *Candida* infections of the skin, mucous membranes, and intestinal tract.
 b. Thrush (oral candidiasis) and vaginitis are treated by topical application, whereas intestinal candidiasis is treated by oral administration.

5. Preparations. Nystatin is supplied as an ointment, oral suspension, oral tablets, drops, and powder.

6. Adverse effects. Occasional gastrointestinal disturbances occur with oral administration.

B. Amphotericin B

1. Chemistry. This drug is a polyene antibiotic.

2. Mechanism of action. The mechanism of action is the same for amphotericin B as for nystatin.

3. Pharmacokinetics
 a. Amphotericin B is absorbed poorly from the gastrointestinal tract.
 b. Intravenous administration results in a plasma half-life of about 24 hours.
 c. The drug is excreted very slowly in the urine.

4. Pharmacologic effects
 a. Amphotericin B is a broad-spectrum antifungal agent.
 b. *Histoplasma capsulatum, Cryptococcus neoformans, Coccidioides immitis, Candida* species, *Blastomyces dermatitidis,* and some strains of *Aspergillus* and *Sporotrichum* are sensitive.
 c. The concentration of amphotericin B determines whether it is fungistatic or fungicidal.

5. Therapeutic uses
 a. Amphotericin B is the most effective drug available for systemic fungal infections.
 b. It is frequently used for the treatment of life-threatening fungal infections in patients with impaired defense mechanisms (e.g., patients undergoing immunosuppressive therapy or cancer chemotherapy, and patients with AIDS).

    c. Amphotericin B is used in the treatment of the following infections:
       (1) Pulmonary, cutaneous, and disseminated forms of blastomycosis
       (2) Acute pulmonary coccidioidomycosis
       (3) Pulmonary histoplasmosis
       (4) *C. neoformans* infections—now the most common life-threatening fungal pathogen associated with AIDS
       (5) Candidiasis, including disseminated forms
    d. In addition, mucocutaneous lesions of parasitic American leishmaniasis may respond to amphotericin B therapy.
    e. Intrathecal infusion may be helpful in the treatment of fungal meningitis.

  6. Preparations
    a. Amphotericin B lyophilized powder is available for injection.
    b. Amphotericin B is also available in topical formulations for treating cutaneous and mucocutaneous candidiasis.

  7. Adverse effects. All patients receiving amphotericin B therapy should be hospitalized, at least during the initiation of therapy.
    a. Hypersensitivity reactions can occur, including anaphylaxis.
    b. Fever, chills, headache, and gastrointestinal disturbances are common with intravenous administration. Patients usually develop tolerance to these adverse effects with continuing administration of amphotericin B.
    c. Decreased renal function occurs in over 80% of patients treated with amphotericin B, necessitating close observation.
    d. Normochromic normocytic anemia can occur.
    e. Thrombophlebitis can occur.

C. Griseofulvin

  1. Chemistry. The drug is produced by *Penicillium griseofulvum*. It is poorly soluble in water.

  2. Mechanism of action
    a. Griseofulvin binds to polymerized microtubules, disrupting the mitotic spindle, but its exact mechanism of action is undetermined.
    b. It is fungistatic.

  3. Pharmacokinetics
    a. Griseofulvin is absorbed in the upper part of the small intestine following oral administration. Most of the drug is eliminated unchanged in the feces.
    b. Griseofulvin has a particular affinity for keratin.

  4. Pharmacologic effects. Griseofulvin is active against dermatophytes, including *Microsporum*, *Epidermophyton,* and *Trichophyton* species. It is ineffective against yeasts.

  5. Therapeutic uses. Because of its affinity for keratin, griseofulvin is useful for treating mycotic diseases of the skin, hair, and nails, such as tinea capitis, pedis (athlete's foot), cruris, corporis, and circinata. It is given orally; topical use has little effect.

  6. Preparations. Griseofulvin is available as tablets, capsules, and an oral suspension.

  7. Adverse effects
    a. Extensive clinical use of griseofulvin has revealed relatively low toxicity.
    b. Possible side effects include headache, neurologic alterations, hepatotoxicity, leukopenia, neutropenia, gastrointestinal distress, and skin reactions, including urticaria and photosensitivity.

D. Flucytosine

  1. Chemistry. This drug is a fluorinated pyrimidine.

  2. Mechanism of action. Flucytosine is converted within fungal cells (but not in the host's cells) to **5-fluorouracil** (see Chapter 11 III D 1), a metabolic antagonist that ultimately leads to inhibition of thymidylate synthetase.

  3. Pharmacokinetics
    a. Flucytosine is well absorbed from the gastrointestinal tract and is distributed widely throughout the body, including the cerebrospinal fluid.
    b. It is excreted in the urine, mainly in an unmetabolized form.

4. Pharmacologic effects
a. The drug is effective against *C. neoformans*.
b. It is effective against some strains of *Candida,* including some *Candida albicans* strains. However, *C. albicans* can become resistant to flucytosine during therapy.

5. Therapeutic uses
a. Although flucytosine is not as effective as amphotericin B, it is less toxic and can be administered orally.
b. It is used for systemic infections caused by *C. albicans* and *C. neoformans* (*Cryptococcus meningitidis*). It is most often used in combination with amphotericin B. Recently, the value of this combination has been challenged in patients with AIDS having cryptococcal meningitis because of its toxicity (see X B 5).

6. Preparations. Flucytosine is available as capsules for oral use.

7. Adverse effects have included:
a. Fatal bone marrow depression
b. Gastrointestinal upset
c. Skin rash
d. Hepatic dysfunction

E. Ketoconazole

1. Chemistry. Ketoconazole is a substituted imidazole derivative.

2. Mechanism of action. Ketoconazole alters membrane permeability by blocking the synthesis of ergosterol, the primary cellular sterol of fungi.

3. Pharmacokinetics
a. Ketoconazole is absorbed from the gastrointestinal tract.
b. Plasma levels peak in 1–2 hours after an oral dose.
c. Since the drug requires an acidic environment for dissolution, agents that increase pH, such as antacids or histamine H_2 blocking agents, can reduce its bioavailability.
d. Elimination is biphasic: The half-life is 2 hours during the first 10 hours after administration, and is 8 hours thereafter.

4. Pharmacologic effects and therapeutic uses
a. Ketoconazole is active in blastomycosis, coccidioidomycosis, histoplasmosis, paracoccidioidomycosis, chronic mucocutaneous candidiasis, and resistant dermatophyte infections.
b. Ketoconazole acts more slowly than the other available antifungal agents, requiring long periods of therapy and, thus, is less useful for severe or acute systemic infections.
c. Since it penetrates the cerebrospinal fluid poorly, it is not recommended for the treatment of fungal meningitis.

5. Preparations. Ketoconazole is available as tablets for oral use.

6. Adverse effects
a. Nausea and vomiting are the most common adverse reactions.
b. Hepatotoxicity, hypersensitivity reactions (including urticaria or anaphylaxis), and gynecomastia are less common untoward effects.
c. Ketoconazole transiently blocks testosterone synthesis and the adrenal response to corticotropin.
d. Ketoconazole blocks several cytochrome P-450–related enzyme steps and, therefore, has the potential to interact with drugs metabolized by the microsomal enzyme system (see Chapter 13 II D 5).

F. Fluconazole

1. Chemistry. This drug is a bis-triazole.

2. Mechanism of action. It inhibits cytochrome P-450–dependent enzymes, blocking the synthesis of ergosterol.

3. Pharmacokinetics
a. Fluconazole is more water-soluble than ketoconazole and is highly bioavailable.
b. Plasma levels peak in 1–2 hours, and $t_{1/2}$ is 30 hours.
c. It is excreted unchanged in the urine.

     d. Cerebrospinal fluid concentrations approach 50%–90% of simultaneous serum concentrations.

4. Pharmacologic effects and therapeutic uses

     a. Fluconazole is active against several systemic fungal pathogens, including *Aspergillus, B. dermatitides, C. albicans, C. neoformans, C. immitis,* and *H. capsulatum.*

     b. Fluconazole is effective against oropharyngeal and esophageal candidiasis, serious systemic candidal infections, and cryptococcal meningitis.

5. Preparations. Fluconazole can be administered orally or intravenously.

6. Adverse effects

     a. It is less toxic than amphotericin B or flucytosine and better tolerated than ketoconazole.

     b. Fluconazole should be discontinued in patients with progressive hepatic dysfunction.

     c. Though it has a lower binding affinity for cytochrome P-450 enzymes than ketoconazole, it may increase serum concentrations of phenytoin, cyclosporine, and oral hypoglycemic drugs and potentiate the effect of warfarin.

G. Naftifine

1. Chemistry. This synthetic antifungal agent is an allylamine.

2. Mechanism of action. Naftifine decreases the synthesis of ergosterol, an essential component of fungal cell membranes, by inhibiting the enzyme squalene epoxidase.

3. Pharmacologic effects and therapeutic uses

     a. In vitro, naftifine is fungicidal against dermatophytes and fungistatic against yeasts such as *C. albicans.*

     b. Clinically, it is used to treat tinea pedis, tinea cruris, and tinea corporis. It is not effective for fungal infections of the hair or nails.

4. Preparations and administration. Naftifine is available as a 1% cream, which is used topically.

5. Adverse effects. Burning, dryness, redness, and itching have been reported.

H. Miconazole and clotrimazole

1. These imidazole derivatives are used primarily as topical agents.

     a. They inhibit the growth of common dermatophytes and yeasts, including *Trichophyton* species, *Epidermophyton floccosum, C. albicans,* and *Malassezia furfur.*

     b. They are used for the treatment of ringworm and other skin infections caused by susceptible organisms, and for vulvovaginal candidiasis.

2. Miconazole is also available for parenteral administration in the treatment of severe systemic fungal infections, such as candidiasis, coccidioidomycosis, and cryptococcosis. However, toxicity and limited efficacy restrict its usefulness.

I. Haloprogin and tolnaftate

1. Haloprogin is fungicidal to *Epidermophyton, Pityrosporum, Microsporum, Trichophyton,* and *Candida.*

2. Tolnaftate is effective for the treatment of most cutaneous mycoses, such as *Trichophyton rubrum* and *Microsporum canis,* but is ineffective against *Candida.*

3. Unlike tolnaftate, which is free of toxic or allergic reactions, halprogin can cause irritation, pruritus, and burning sensations.

IV. AGENTS USED FOR TREATMENT OF TUBERCULOSIS

A. General considerations

1. Incidence. The incidence of tuberculosis has been increasing because the disease can occur in patients with AIDS.

2. Principles of treatment

     a. Drugs are used in combination because otherwise microbial resistance rapidly develops.

    b. Uncomplicated pulmonary tuberculosis is treated with isoniazid and rifampin daily for 6 months. Either pyrazinamide is added for the first 2 months of therapy, or therapy with isoniazid and rifampin is extended to 9 months.

    c. For **AIDS patients with tuberculosis,** three-drug therapy (isoniazid, rifampin, and either pyrazinamide or ethambutol) is sometimes extended beyond 9 months.

    d. Patients at risk of having **drug-resistant bacteria** and patients with **extensive or disseminated disease** (including tuberculous meningitis) are treated with four drugs: ethambutol or streptomycin is added to the treatment regimen.

    e. Prolonged bed rest in a specialized center is no longer required. Patients remain ambulatory with frequent checkups.

  3. Prophylaxis. Isoniazid prophylaxis is given to:

    a. Individuals in close contact with the tuberculosis patient, especially children

    b. Any person converting from a negative to a positive skin test

B. Isoniazid

  1. Chemistry. Isoniazid (Figure 12-7) is the hydrazide of isonicotinic acid and is a pyridine.

  2. Mechanism of action. Although this is not known, isoniazid probably interferes with cellular metabolism, especially the synthesis of mycolic acid, an important constituent of the mycobacterial cell wall.

  3. Pharmacokinetics

    a. The drug is well absorbed from the gastrointestinal tract and diffuses readily into all body tissues and body fluids, including cerebrospinal fluid.

    b. The plasma concentration and the metabolism of isoniazid are affected by whether a given patient is a **fast or a slow acetylator** of the drug, a genetically determined trait.

    c. Isoniazid is excreted mainly in the urine. Slow acetylators have a higher concentration of unchanged or free isoniazid than fast acetylators.

  4. Pharmacologic effects

    a. Isoniazid is effective against most tubercle bacilli.

    b. It is not effective against many atypical mycobacteria. To prevent mycobacterial resistance, isoniazid is used in conjunction with other agents in the treatment of tuberculosis.

  5. Therapeutic uses. Isoniazid is the most widely used agent in the treatment and prophylaxis of tuberculosis.

  6. Preparations. Isoniazid is available as tablets, as syrup, and in injectable form.

  7. Adverse effects

    a. Up to 20% of patients taking isoniazid develop elevated serum aminotransferase levels.

      (1) Severe hepatic injury occurs more frequently in patients over the age of 35, especially in those who drink alcohol daily.

      (2) Isoniazid is discontinued if symptoms of hepatitis develop or if the aminotransferase activity increases to more than three times normal.

    b. Peripheral and CNS toxicity occur.

      (1) This toxicity probably results from an increased excretion of pyridoxine induced by isoniazid, which produces a pyridoxine deficiency.

      (2) Peripheral neuritis, urinary retention, insomnia, and psychotic episodes can occur.

      (3) Concurrent pyridoxine administration with isoniazid prevents most of these complications.

    c. Isoniazid can also exacerbate pyridoxine-deficiency anemia and can produce blood dyscrasias.

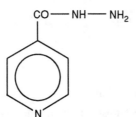

Figure 12-7. Isoniazid.

d. Isoniazid can reduce the metabolism of phenytoin, enhancing its toxicity.

e. Hypersensitivity reactions (i.e., fever, various rashes) can occur.

C. Rifampin

1. Chemistry

a. Rifampin belongs to the group of complex macrocyclic antibiotics.

b. It is zwitterionic and is soluble in water at low pH.

2. Mechanism of action. Rifampin inhibits RNA synthesis in bacteria and chlamydiae by binding to DNA-dependent RNA polymerase.

3. Pharmacokinetics

a. Rifampin is well absorbed from the gastrointestinal tract.

b. It is widely distributed in tissues and is excreted mainly through the liver.

4. Pharmacologic effects

a. Most gram-positive and many gram-negative microorganisms are sensitive to rifampin.

b. Prolonged administration of the drug as the single therapeutic agent promotes the emergence of highly resistant organisms.

5. Therapeutic uses

a. Rifampin is used in the treatment of:

  (1) Tuberculosis (in combination with other agents, often isoniazid, pyrazinamide, or ethambutol)

  (2) Atypical mycobacterial infections

  (3) Leprosy

b. Rifampin is not used for minor infections because of the emergence of rifampin-resistant bacteria.

6. Preparations. Rifampin is available as capsules for oral use.

7. Adverse effects

a. Urine, sweat, tears, and contact lenses may take on an orange color because of rifampin administration; this effect is harmless.

b. Light-chain proteinuria and impaired antibody response may occur.

c. Rifampin induces hepatic microsomal enzymes and, therefore, affects the half-life of a number of drugs. For example, a decrease in the effect of some anticoagulants and increased metabolism of methadone occur when these agents are administered concomitantly with rifampin. Methadone withdrawal symptoms may be induced.

d. Rashes, gastrointestinal disturbances, and renal damage have been reported.

e. Jaundice and severe hepatic dysfunction are occasionally produced.

D. Pyrazinamide

1. Chemistry. Pyrazinamide is the pyrazine analog of nicotinamide.

2. Mechanism of action. This is unknown.

3. Pharmacokinetics

a. Pyrazinamide is distributed throughout the body after oral administration.

b. It is excreted mainly by glomerular filtration.

4. Therapeutic uses. Pyrazinamide is now widely used in multiagent short-term therapy of uncomplicated pulmonary tuberculosis.

5. Preparations. Pyrazinamide is available as tablets for oral use.

6. Adverse effects

a. Liver function studies are performed before and during therapy, because liver damage can occur.

b. Hyperuricemia and gout can occur.

E. Ethambutol

1. Chemistry. The structural formula of ethambutol is shown in Figure 12-8.

2. Mechanism of action. Ethambutol's mechanism of action is unknown. Resistance to the drug occurs rapidly when it is used alone.

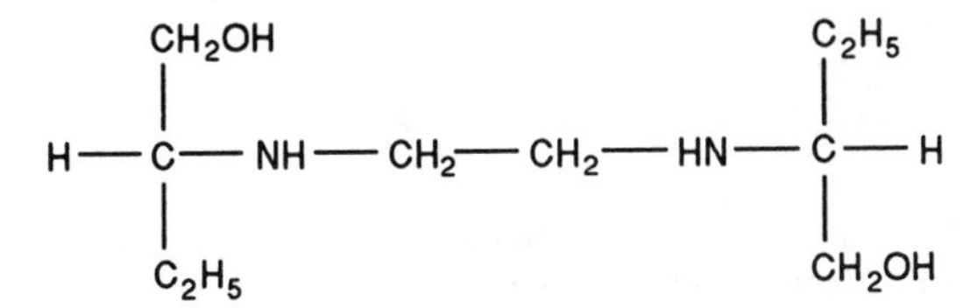

Figure 12-8. Ethambutol.

3. **Pharmacokinetics**
   a. Ethambutol is well absorbed from the gastrointestinal tract.
   b. It is widely distributed in the body, including the cerebrospinal fluid.
   c. Most of an ingested dose is excreted unchanged in urine and feces.

4. **Pharmacologic effects and therapeutic use.** Ethambutol inhibits many strains of *M. tuberculosis*. It is used in combination with other agents for the treatment of tuberculosis.

5. **Preparations.** Ethambutol hydrochloride is available in tablet form for oral use.

6. **Adverse effects**
   a. Visual disturbances, including optic neuritis and red–green color-blindness, can occur but are reversible.
   b. Hypersensitivity occurs occasionally, resulting in rash or drug fever.

F. **Streptomycin** (see II C 6 a)

1. The use of streptomycin in the treatment of tuberculosis has been declining ever since more effective agents became available.

2. When a three-agent combination is used to treat severe forms of tuberculosis (e.g., disseminated or meningeal), streptomycin may be one of the drugs used.

V. AGENTS USED FOR TREATMENT OF LEPROSY

A. **Sulfones**

1. **Chemistry**
   a. The sulfones, the principal class of agents used to treat leprosy, are chemically related to the sulfonamides.
   b. The most important derivatives come from **dapsone** (Figure 12-9).

2. **Mechanism of action**
   a. Dapsone is bacteriostatic for *Mycobacterium leprae*.
   b. Its mechanism of action is similar to that of the sulfonamides (see II A).

3. **Pharmacokinetics**
   a. Dapsone is slowly but completely absorbed from the gastrointestinal tract.
   b. It undergoes intestinal reabsorption from the bile, resulting in a sustained level of the drug in the circulation.
   c. It is principally excreted in the urine.

4. **Pharmacologic effects**
   a. Dapsone is effective against *M. leprae,* although resistance to the drug can develop.
   b. It is bacteriostatic for *M. tuberculosis* in vitro.

5. **Therapeutic uses.** Dapsone is the most important drug in the treatment of leprosy. Because of recent resistance to dapsone, it is now usually given with rifampin, with clofazimine, or with both.

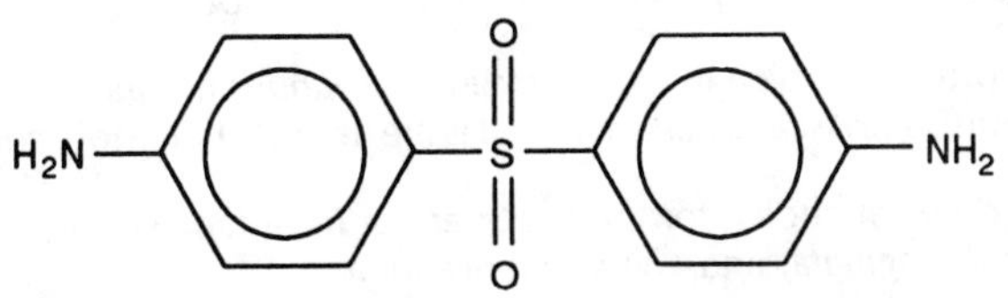

Figure 12-9. Dapsone.

6. Preparations and administration
   a. Dapsone is administered orally.
   b. Therapy usually is continued for a minimum of 2 years.

7. Adverse effects
   a. The most common untoward effects include hemolysis, methemoglobinemia, nausea, vomiting, rash, transient headache, and anorexia.
   b. The sulfones can cause an exacerbation of lepromatous leprosy.
   c. A fatal infectious mononucleosis–like syndrome has been reported.

B. Clofazimine

1. Chemistry. Clofazimine is a phenazine congener.

2. Mechanism of action. Clofazimine binds to mycobacteria DNA, thereby inhibiting template function.

3. Pharmacokinetics
   a. Clofazimine is absorbed slowly from the gastrointestinal tract; 50% of an oral dose reaches the systemic circulation.
   b. It is lipophilic and can accumulate in adipose tissue and reticuloendothelial cells.
   c. The elimination half-life after repeated oral dosing is 70 days.

4. Pharmacologic effects
   a. Clofazimine exerts a slow bactericidal effect on *M. leprae.*
   b. It is also active in vitro against other mycobacteria, including the *Mycobacterium avium* complex, which can cause disseminated infection in AIDS patients.
   c. It is not active against microorganisms other than mycobacteria.

5. Therapeutic uses
   a. Clofazimine is used in combination with dapsone and rifampin in multibacillary leprosy to prevent the emergence of resistance.
   b. Clofazimine in combination with rifampin is effective in treating dapsone-resistant infections.
   c. Clofazimine has an anti-inflammatory effect in erythema nodosum leprosum reactions.

6. Preparations and administration
   a. For multibacillary disease, clofazimine is administered orally as part of a three-agent combination for a minimum of 2 years.
   b. For dapsone-resistant leprosy, clofazimine is given first in combination with one or more other agents for 3 years, and then alone.

7. Adverse effects
   a. Dose-related abdominal symptoms include pain, nausea, and vomiting.
   b. A reddish to dark brown discoloration of the skin, cornea, and all body fluids can occur. This pigmentation may take months or years to disappear after the drug is discontinued.
   c. Anticholinergic symptoms can occur.

VI. ANTHELMINTICS. These drugs are used to treat parasitic infections due to flatworms and roundworms. The major target is usually the nongrowing adult stage of the parasite's life cycle.

A. Diethylcarbamazine is the drug of choice for filaria worms. It effectively treats *Wuchereria bancrofti, Wuchereria malayi, Loa loa,* and *Onchocerca volvulus.*

B. Praziquantel is a broad-spectrum anthelmintic that is considered one of the drugs of choice for tapeworm infections and the drug of choice for the treatment of schistosomiasis and other fluke infections.

C. Metrifonate and niridazole are effective against *Schistosoma haematobium.*

D. Mebendazole is one of the drugs of choice in the treatment of *Trichuris trichiura* (whipworm) infestation, hookworm, pinworm, and *Ascaris* infestations; it is the drug of choice for echinococcosis.

E. Niclosamide is one of the drugs of choice for the treatment of most tapeworms, including *Diphyllobothrium latum, Taenia saginata,* and *Hymenolepis nana.*

F. Pyrantel pamoate is one of the drugs of choice for the treatment of ascariasis, hookworm, and pinworm. It produces persistent nicotinic activation, resulting in spastic paralysis of the worms.

G. Piperazine is an alternative drug for the treatment of ascariasis and pinworms. This agent is thought to block the response of *Ascaris* muscle cells to acetylcholine; the flaccid worm can then be expelled by peristalsis.

H. Thiabendazole is very effective against cutaneous and visceral larva migrans and strongyloidiasis. It is also used in trichinosis.

I. Ivermectin, although still an investigational drug, has become the drug of choice for onchocerciasis (river blindness).

VII. AGENTS USED FOR TREATMENT OF PROTOZOAL INFECTIONS AND MALARIA

A. Metronidazole

1. This drug is very active in protozoal infections, including trichomoniasis, *Giardia lamblia* infestation, and *E. histolytica* amebiasis.

2. It is also effective in the treatment of anaerobic bacterial infections (e.g., caused by *Bacteroides* species).

3. A disulfiram-like (Antabuse-like) reaction (see Chapter 13 II D 4 c) can occur when metronidazole is taken in combination with an alcoholic beverage.

B. Diloxanide furoate is amebicidal. It is used for the treatment of asymptomatic passers of amebic cysts.

C. Suramin is a nonmetallic polyanionic compound employed in the treatment of African trypanosomiasis in both the early and late stages of the disease. It is also highly effective in onchocerciasis but has largely been superseded by the less toxic ivermectin.

D. Nifurtimox is the drug of choice in South American trypanosomiasis.

E. Stibogluconate, an antimonial, is the drug of choice for leishmaniasis.

F. Pentamidine isethionate

1. Although antimonials are considered to be the drugs of choice for the treatment of leishmaniasis, pentamidine can be highly effective in patients who do not respond to antimonial therapy.

2. Pentamidine is effective against early cases of African trypanosomiasis and in the prophylaxis and treatment of *P. carinii* pneumonia. The latter is an opportunistic infection associated with AIDS (see X B 1).

G. Chloroquine is the drug of choice for the treatment of uncomplicated acute malaria due to any of the *Plasmodium* organisms (except resistant forms) and for prophylaxis during residence in an endemic area.

H. Primaquine is used to cure and prevent relapses of *Plasmodium vivax* and *Plasmodium ovale* malaria after departure from endemic areas. It is given in combination with chloroquine or another schizontocide.

I. Pyrimethamine and **sulfadoxine** are used concurrently for prophylaxis and treatment of chloroquine-resistant strains of *Plasmodium falciparum*.

J. Quinine

1. Quinine sulfate, given orally, is effective in the treatment of acute uncomplicated malarial attacks due to chloroquine-resistant *P. falciparum*.

2. Quinine dihydrochloride, administered parenterally, is used in the treatment of severe illness caused by chloroquine-resistant *P. falciparum*.

VIII. AGENTS USED FOR TREATMENT OF VIRUS INFECTIONS. Viruses are obligate intracellular parasites that require the active participation of the metabolic processes of the invaded cell to survive. Thus, agents that are able to kill viruses often injure host cells as well. Despite this interrelationship, there are a growing number of drugs that have substantial therapeutic merit in the treatment of viral infections. Zidovudine (azidothymidine, AZT), used to treat AIDS, is discussed in section X; other antiviral agents are discussed here.

A. Amantadine

1. **Chemistry.** Amantadine is a synthetic tricyclic amine with a structure unrelated to that of any other antimicrobial agent.

2. **Mechanism of action.** This is unknown. Amantadine may block either the assembly of influenza A virus or the release of viral nucleic acid in the host cell.

3. **Pharmacokinetics.** The drug is well absorbed from the gastrointestinal tract, is not metabolized, and is excreted via the kidney.

4. **Therapeutic uses**
   a. **Antiviral use**
      (1) The major anti-infective use for amantadine is for prophylaxis during influenza A virus epidemics at which time unvaccinated patients of all ages who are at high risk are advised to receive the drug.
         (a) Amantadine does not alter the immune response to influenza A vaccine; thus, vaccination can be given concurrently with the drug.
         (b) Amantadine can help to protect immunodeficient patients and those on dialysis, who may have a poor antibody response to the vaccine.
      (2) Amantadine may also be useful in shortening the duration of symptoms when administered after the onset of illness.
   b. The use of amantadine in parkinsonism is discussed in Chapter 3 IV C.

5. **Adverse effects**
   a. These are dose-related and include confusion, hallucinations, seizures, and coma.
   b. Patients with psychiatric disorders or a history of epilepsy require close monitoring when receiving the drug.

B. Vidarabine (adenine arabinoside, ara-A)

1. **Chemistry.** Vidarabine is an adenosine analog.

2. **Mechanism of action.** Vidarabine acts by inhibiting viral DNA polymerase. Mammalian DNA synthesis is affected to a lesser extent.

3. **Therapeutic uses**
   a. Vidarabine is used in the treatment of serious herpes simplex infections, including encephalitis, keratoconjunctivitis, and neonatal infections.
   b. It is also effective in the treatment of herpes zoster and varicella infections in immunocompromised patients.

4. **Preparations and administration**
   a. Vidarabine is available for intravenous use in the treatment of systemic herpes infections.
   b. For herpes simplex keratoconjunctivitis, vidarabine is administered as an ophthalmic ointment.

5. **Adverse effects**
   a. Gastrointestinal disturbances and dose-related CNS toxicity are relatively infrequent.
   b. Vidarabine may be carcinogenic and should not be used to treat insignificant infections.

C. Idoxuridine

1. **Chemistry.** Idoxuridine resembles thymidine in structure, being a halogenated pyrimidine.

2. **Mechanism of action.** Idoxuridine is incorporated into both viral and mammalian DNA, producing DNA that is more susceptible to breakage, and ultimately causing production of altered proteins.

3. **Therapeutic uses**
   a. Idoxuridine is used in the treatment of herpes simplex keratitis.
   b. Herpes simplex virus type 2 does not respond to idoxuridine.

4. **Preparations and administration.** Idoxuridine is available as an ophthalmic solution or ointment. Since it is incorporated into host DNA, idoxuridine cannot be used systemically.

5. **Adverse effects.** The drug may cause ocular itching, painful irritation, and photophobia.

D. Trifluridine

1. **Chemistry.** Like idoxuridine, trifluridine is a halogenated pyrimidine and resembles thymidine in structure.

2. **Mechanism of action.** As with idoxuridine, trifluridine is phosphorylated to the triphosphate and, as such, competes with thymidine triphosphate for incorporation into viral DNA.

3. **Therapeutic uses.** Trifluridine is approved for the treatment of herpetic keratitis.

4. **Preparations and administration.** Trifluridine is applied topically. Since it is incorporated into the DNA of uninfected cells, it cannot be used systemically.

E. Acyclovir

1. **Chemistry.** Acyclovir is a synthetic purine nucleoside analog with an acyclic side chain.

2. **Mechanism of action**
   a. After being converted in vivo to the triphosphate form, acyclovir inhibits herpes virus DNA synthesis by two means.
      (1) It interferes with viral DNA polymerase and inhibits viral DNA replication.
      (2) It is incorporated into DNA and leads to premature chain termination.
   b. The drug is several hundred times more toxic for the herpes viruses than for mammalian cells due to an enhanced affinity of the viral enzyme thymidine kinase for acyclovir.

3. **Pharmacologic effects.** Acyclovir has inhibitory activity in vitro against herpes simplex virus types 1 and 2, varicella-zoster virus, Epstein-Barr virus, and cytomegalovirus.

4. **Therapeutic uses**
   a. The drug is indicated for primary and recurrent mucocutaneous herpes simplex infections in immunocompromised patients.
   b. It is also useful in herpes genitalis infections.
      (1) Oral therapy can shorten the duration of initial genital herpes infections, but it does not cure genital herpes.
      (2) It is only marginally effective for the treatment of recurrent episodes. Infections recur when the drug is stopped.
      (3) If taken continuously, oral acyclovir can decrease the frequency of recurrences, but such use should be limited to those patients with severe recurrences.

5. **Preparations and administration.** Acyclovir is available in topical, oral, and intravenous forms for the treatment of herpes simplex virus infections.

6. **Adverse effects**
   a. Topical applications can cause local discomfort and pruritus.
   b. With oral therapy, nausea, vomiting, diarrhea, and headache are the most common unwanted effects.
   c. Intravenous therapy can cause nephrotoxicity, neurologic reactions, local phlebitis, rash, and hives.
   d. Orally, acyclovir is well tolerated. Intravenously, encephalopathy develops in 1% of patients.

F. Ganciclovir

1. **Chemistry.** Ganciclovir is a synthetic nucleoside analog of 2'-deoxyguanosine.

2. **Mechanism of action.** Ganciclovir inhibits viral DNA synthesis in a manner much like that of acyclovir.

3. **Pharmacologic effects**
   a. Ganciclovir inhibits replication of herpes simplex virus types 1 and 2, cytomegalovirus, Epstein-Barr virus, and varicella-zoster virus.
   b. Ganciclovir is more active against cytomegalovirus, in vitro, than is acyclovir, but resistant strains can develop.

4. **Therapeutic uses.** Ganciclovir is indicated for the treatment of cytomegalovirus retinitis in immunocompromised individuals, including patients with AIDS. However, relapse is common, even with continued treatment.

5. **Preparations and administration.** Ganciclovir is available for intravenous injection. It has also been injected directly into the eye.

6. **Adverse effects**
   a. When administered intramuscularly or subcutaneously, ganciclovir may cause severe tissue irritation.
   b. Granulocytopenia occurs in 40% and thrombocytopenia in 20% of patients treated. These are generally reversible on discontinuation of treatment.
   c. CNS effects, from headache to psychosis, convulsions, or coma, can occur in 5%--15% of patients.
   d. Anemia, fever, rash, and abnormal liver function values can occur.
   e. Ganciclovir is teratogenic and mutagenic in animals.

G. Ribavirin

1. **Chemistry.** Ribavirin is a synthetic purine nucleoside analog.

2. **Mechanism of action.** This appears to be multiple:
   a. Ribavirin monophosphate inhibits enzymes needed for the synthesis of guanine nucleotides.
   b. Ribavirin triphosphate inhibits viral RNA polymerase by competing for substrate sites.
   c. The triphosphate also interferes with the formation of viral messenger RNA.

3. **Pharmacologic effects.** Ribavirin is active in vitro against several DNA and RNA viruses, including herpes simplex, influenza A and B, and respiratory syncytial virus (RSV). High concentrations inhibit replication of the virus that causes AIDS.

4. **Therapeutic uses and administration.** Ribavirin in aerosol form may decrease morbidity from severe RSV infection in infants and young children. It must be administered via a specific small-particle aerosol generator.

5. **Adverse effects**
   a. Ribavirin is contraindicated for patients requiring mechanical ventilation because the small aerosol particles precipitate on the respirator valves and tubing, causing malfunction that can be lethal.
   b. Rash and conjunctivitis have occurred with aerosol use.
   c. Ribavirin is mutagenic, teratogenic, and possibly carcinogenic.

H. Human interferon

1. **Chemistry**
   a. Interferons are naturally occurring glycoproteins that can be produced by almost any mammalian cell type, including lymphocytes and fibroblasts, when the cells are stimulated in the inflammatory process.
   b. Interferons are of three major classes; those used clinically are alpha interferons.

2. **Mechanism of action**
   a. The antiviral and antitumor effects of interferons are thought to be due to the induction of enzymes that inhibit the synthesis of protein and DNA.
      (1) Interferon-treated cells develop the ability to block viral replication.
      (2) Interferon is able to suppress cell proliferation.
      (3) Interferon also has immunomodulating effects.
         (a) It enhances phagocytosis by macrophages.
         (b) It increases the target-cell-specific cytotoxicity exerted by lymphocytes.
   b. The antiviral state takes several hours to develop after interferon treatment.

3. **Therapeutic uses**
   a. Interferon preparations are currently used for the treatment of:
      (1) Hairy-cell leukemia
      (2) AIDS-related Kaposi's sarcoma
      (3) Genital (venereal) warts (condylomata acuminata)
   b. In patients with lymphoma, early treatment of a herpes zoster infection with interferon appears to prevent the spread of infection.

    c. Interferon alpha has also been applied topically in herpes keratoconjunctivitis in combination with acyclovir and trifluridine.

    d. Interferon alpha has also shown some promise in chronic hepatitis B infections, in laryngeal papillomatosis, and in prophylaxis (but not therapy) of the common (rhinoviral) cold.

4. Preparations and administration

    a. Two recombinantly produced products are available: interferon alfa-2a and interferon alfa-2b; they differ by only one amino acid residue.

    b. Administration is by the intramuscular or subcutaneous route, or intralesionally into genital warts.

5. Adverse effects

    a. Influenza-like symptoms (i.e., fever, chills, myalgias) occur minutes to hours after parenteral administration; they are self-limited.

    b. Progressive fatigue is the most common dose-limiting adverse effect when administered chronically.

    c. Interferon in high doses acts as an abortifacient in primates.

    d. Bone marrow suppression with granulocytopenia and thrombocytopenia is common.

    e. The plasma concentration of hepatic enzymes increases.

    f. The metabolism of other drugs can be reduced by interferon's action on the cytochrome P-450 system.

IX. VACCINES AND TOXOIDS. The information given here concerns the use of these agents in adults. Routine immunization of infants and children is not considered here.

A. Viral vaccines

1. Measles virus vaccine

    a. Chemistry. Measles (rubeola) vaccine is made from an attenuated live virus grown in chick fibroblasts.

    b. Therapeutic uses and administration

        (1) Persons born before 1956 presumably have had measles and can be considered immune.

        (2) Persons born after 1956 who did not have measles and were never vaccinated can be considered candidates for immunization.

        (3) The risks associated with revaccination are nil.

            (a) Persons who were vaccinated before age 12 months may require revaccination.

            (b) Revaccination appears safe for immunosuppressed patients.

        (4) Vaccination is not recommended during pregnancy.

    c. Adverse effects. Transient rash occurs in 5% of those vaccinated, and a low-grade fever is not uncommon.

2. Rubella virus vaccine

    a. Chemistry. Rubella (German measles) vaccine is made from an attenuated live virus grown in human diploid cells.

    b. Therapeutic uses and administration. Immunization of adults is recommended, especially for unimmunized women of childbearing age. The goal is to prevent fetal rubella infection and consequent fetal damage, which can occur during both the first and second trimesters of pregnancy.

    c. Adverse effects. Adults often experience joint pain after vaccination. Low-grade fever, rash, and lymphadenopathy can also occur.

3. Influenza vaccine

    a. Chemistry

        (1) Influenza vaccine is made from inactivated whole virus or viral subunits grown in chick embryo cells.

        (2) The United States Public Health Service establishes the formulation to be used for each influenza season.

    b. Therapeutic uses and administration

        (1) Immunization decreases morbidity and mortality due to influenza, especially in the elderly.

        (2) Influenza usually does not occur before December and peaks in January and February. November is the best time to vaccinate.

(3) Annual immunization is recommended for:
  (a) Persons with metabolic diseases, severe anemia, cardiopulmonary disorders, or renal disease
  (b) Immunosuppressed patients
  (c) Persons older than 65 years of age
  (d) Health personnel who may have contact with high-risk patients
(4) Influenza vaccine is contraindicated in patients allergic to egg products.
  c. Adverse effects
  (1) Fever, chills, myalgia, and malaise occasionally occur.
  (2) Local redness and soreness at the injection site last a day or two.

4. Hepatitis B vaccine
  a. Chemistry. Two types are available.
    (1) The earlier vaccine is made from chemically inactivated hepatitis B surface antigen particles.
    (2) A recombinant hepatitis B vaccine is also currently available.
  b. Therapeutic uses and administration. Immunization is recommended for persons at increased risk of developing hepatitis B. Among these are:
    (1) Susceptible male homosexuals
    (2) Household and sexual contacts of hepatitis B carriers
    (3) Intravenous drug abusers
    (4) Recipients of clotting factors VIII or IX
    (5) Dialysis patients
    (6) Hospital personnel exposed to blood or blood products
    (7) The staff of institutions for the mentally handicapped
  c. Adverse effects
    (1) Soreness at the injection site is the most common untoward effect.
    (2) The most frequent systemic complaints include fatigue, headache, fever, and malaise.

5. Other viral vaccines
  a. Vaccines for **poliomyelitis, pertussis** (whooping cough), and **mumps** are available for routine immunization of infants and children.
  b. Vaccines for immunization against **rabies, yellow fever, equine encephalitis,** and other less common viral diseases are available for use in special high-risk situations.

B. Bacterial vaccines and toxoids

1. Tetanus and diphtheria toxoids
  a. Chemistry. These are prepared by detoxifying the toxins produced by *C. diphtheriae* and *Clostridium tetani.*
  b. Therapeutic uses and administration
    (1) The toxoids induce levels of antitoxin that are thought to be protective for at least 10 years.
    (2) Primary immunization with these toxoids is often combined with **pertussis vaccine,** but the latter is not recommended for routine use in adults.
    (3) A tetanus–diphtheria toxoid booster should be administered every 10 years.
  c. Adverse effects. These include local pain and swelling.

2. Pneumococcal vaccine
  a. Chemistry. This vaccine contains purified capsular polysaccharides from the 23 types of *S. pneumoniae* that are responsible for 90% of all pneumococcal infections.
  b. Therapeutic uses and administration
    (1) Adult candidates for immunization are quite similar to those for influenza vaccine.
      (a) Adults should not be revaccinated with pneumococcal vaccine, since this may increase the incidence and severity of adverse reactions.
      (b) Although the vaccine is quite effective in people with normal immune systems, severely immunocompromised patients are not protected.
    (2) The duration of protective antibody titers is not yet known, but titers are expected to persist for up to 5 years.
  c. Adverse effects. Erythema and pain at the injection site are the most common untoward effects.

3. Other bacterial vaccines
  a. Meningococcal polysaccharide vaccine is available for use in epidemics.

b. **Typhoid vaccine** is given to exposed persons and to those traveling to epidemic areas, but it is no longer given to travelers in endemic areas. Protection is incomplete, and carefulness in the choice of food and drink is probably more effective.

c. **Cholera vaccine** is used in endemic areas. It gives only partial protection, and a booster dose is needed every 6 months.

X. AGENTS USED FOR TREATMENT OF AIDS AND RELATED OPPORTUNISTIC INFECTIONS

A. Antiviral agents

1. **General considerations**
   a. AIDS is caused by a retrovirus; specifically, the human immunodeficiency virus (HIV), a member of the lentivirus family. Two subtypes, HIV-1 and HIV-2, have been recovered from patients with AIDS.
   b. A large number of human cells can be infected by HIV, including macrophages and glial cells. However, the virus preferentially replicates in $CD4^+$ helper T lymphocytes.

2. **Zidovudine**
   a. **Chemistry.** Zidovudine is a synthetic thymidine analog.
   b. **Mechanism of action**
      (1) Zidovudine, as the triphosphate, inhibits the DNA polymerase (reverse transcriptase) of HIV. HIV reverse transcriptase is 100 times more susceptible to inhibition by zidovudine than is the DNA polymerase of mammalian cells.
      (2) Zidovudine triphosphate is incorporated into viral DNA and terminates chain growth during DNA synthesis.
   c. **Pharmacokinetics**
      (1) Zidovudine is well absorbed from the gastrointestinal tract.
      (2) It is cleared rapidly from the blood ($t_{1/2} = 1$ hour), metabolized in the liver, and excreted by the kidneys.
      (3) Zidovudine penetrates readily into the cerebrospinal fluid.
   d. **Therapeutic uses.** Zidovudine is used in adults with AIDS or with symptomatic advanced AIDS-related complex (ARC).
      (1) Clinical trials with zidovudine indicate that the drug significantly reduces mortality in patients with ARC or with AIDS of recent onset.
      (2) Patients had fewer opportunistic infections and had increased T4 lymphocyte counts while on therapy. Neuropsychiatric function also improved.
   e. **Preparations and administration.** Zidovudine is administered orally every 4 hours around the clock. When anemia develops, therapy is either interrupted or the dose is reduced or the hematocrit is maintained with transfusions.
   f. **Adverse effects**
      (1) **Hematologic toxicity**
         (a) Severe anemia, often with a megaloblastic bone marrow, is the main toxic effect.
         (b) Neutropenia is fairly common, especially in patients with AIDS.
         (c) Anemia, granulocytopenia, and thrombocytopenia are usually reversible when the dosage is decreased or the drug is stopped.
      (2) **Neurotoxicity**
         (a) Severe headaches and insomnia are common but are less severe after the first week of therapy.
         (b) Seizures and Wernicke's encephalopathy have been reported.
      (3) **Other adverse effects.** Nausea and myalgias occur often at the start of therapy.
      (4) **Drug interactions**
         (a) Ribavirin interferes with the antiviral effect of zidovudine.
         (b) Probenecid slows the metabolism and excretion of zidovudine increasing the risk of hematotoxicity.
         (c) Acetaminophen interferes with glucuronidation of zidovudine in the liver.

3. **Other antiviral agents**
   a. Ribavirin in high doses inhibits HIV replication and may give transient clinical benefits. However, ribavirin and zidovudine are antagonistic and cannot be used concurrently.
   b. Acyclovir, interferon, and various experimental antiviral agents are being tested.

B. Treatment of AIDS-related opportunistic infections

1. *P. carinii* pneumonia

a. General considerations. This infection occurs in 80% of patients with AIDS. Episodes occur when the CD4$^+$ lymphocyte count is less than 200 cells/mm^3.

b. Therapeutic regimens

(1) Intravenous trimethoprim–sulfamethoxazole and intravenous pentamidine isethionate have been used, but severe adverse effects have been limiting. Lower dose, oral therapy with trimethoprim–sulfamethoxazole has been used successfully in AIDS patients with less severe pneumonia.

(2) Pneumocystis prophylaxis is recommended for HIV-positive patients with low CD4$^+$ lymphocyte counts and for those who have had *Pneumocystis* pneumonia.

(3) Pentamidine aerosol administered once a month has been effective in preventing both initial episodes and recurrences of *Pneumocystis* pneumonia in AIDS patients.

(a) Plasma concentrations of inhaled pentamidine are less than 10% of those seen with intravenous administration.

(b) Adverse effects

(i) Atypical *Pneumocystis* pneumonia and disseminated infection have occurred in patients taking pentamidine aerosol prophylactically.

(ii) Other untoward effects have included transient cough, acute pancreatitis, and cutaneous eruptions.

2. Mycobacterial infections

a. General considerations. Both tuberculosis and atypical mycobacterial disease (caused by *M. avium* complex) occur in the course of HIV-induced immunosuppression.

(1) Although the tuberculosis responds excellently to chemotherapy, AIDS patients infected with tuberculosis have a high mortality.

(2) *M. avium* complex is acquired orally or is inhaled as a saprophyte. It progresses to a continuous bacteremia, infecting multiple organs. Concurrent infections with *Cryptosporidium* can occur; they present as gastrointestinal symptoms.

b. Therapeutic regimens. New regimens are being developed that involve administering existing antimycobacterial agents via new drug delivery systems (e.g., liposome encapsulation).

3. Cytomegalovirus infections

a. General considerations. These are also common superinfections in patients with AIDS. Retinitis is a frequent manifestation.

b. Therapeutic regimens. Ganciclovir (see VIII F) has been used in therapy.

4. Toxoplasmosis

a. General considerations. The protozoan *Toxoplasma gondii* produces most intracranial mass lesions in AIDS patients; the lesions present as a global encephalitis.

b. Therapeutic regimens. The most effective available treatment is pyrimethamine plus sulfadiazine. However, the tissue–cyst form is resistant to these and other currently available agents.

5. Cryptococcosis

a. General considerations. *C. neoformans,* a fungus, is acquired by inhaling the organism. However, 80% of AIDS patients with cryptococcal disease develop cryptococcal meningitis.

b. Therapeutic regimens

(1) Amphotericin B is currently the treatment of choice.

(2) Patients *without* AIDS are also given flucytosine, but the toxicity of this combination precludes its use in AIDS patients who are already immunosuppressed.

c. Adverse effects

(1) Amphotericin B decreases renal function.

(2) Dose-dependent leukopenia can occur with increased levels of amphotericin B caused by decreased renal function.

STUDY QUESTIONS

Directions: Each of the numbered items or incomplete statements in this section is followed by answers or by completions of the statement. Select the **one** lettered answer or completion that is **best** in each case.

1. All of the following statements concerning anti-infective agents and their proposed mechanisms of action are true EXCEPT

(A) sulfadiazine prevents the incorporation of PABA into folic acid
(B) ampicillin inactivates transpeptidase
(C) gentamicin interferes with the function of messenger RNA and ribosomes
(D) ganciclovir inhibits viral RNA polymerase by competing for substrate sites
(E) zidovudine inhibits the reverse transcriptase of HIV

2. Correct statements about the beta-lactam antibiotic imipenem include all of the following EXCEPT

(A) its value in meningitis has not been established
(B) it is effective against both gram-positive and gram-negative cocci
(C) it is given in combination with cilastatin to extend its spectrum
(D) its use is limited to serious hospital-acquired infections
(E) patients allergic to penicillin should be considered allergic to imipenem

3. All of the following statements about aminoglycoside therapy are true EXCEPT

(A) aminoglycosides are generally less potent in an acidic environment
(B) cross-resistance between the aminoglycosides can occur
(C) as an antibiotic group, aminoglycosides have a large therapeutic index
(D) kanamycin has poor activity against *Pseudomonas* species
(E) amikacin is effective against *Serratia* species

4. All of the following statements about the effects of orally administered tetracyclines are true EXCEPT

(A) tetracyclines produce frequent gastrointestinal irritation
(B) tetracycline therapy can shorten the duration of symptoms of Lyme disease
(C) the ingestion of outdated tetracycline can result in a form of the Fanconi syndrome
(D) tetracycline therapy has no effect on teeth or bones
(E) staphylococcal enterocolitis may follow tetracycline administration

5. All of the following statements about antifungal agents are true EXCEPT

(A) miconazole is primarily used as a topical agent
(B) clotrimazole is effective for ringworm
(C) ketoconazole does not penetrate the cerebrospinal fluid
(D) amphotericin B is effective when given orally
(E) nystatin is effective for vulvovaginal candidiasis

6. Which of the following agents is used to treat tapeworm infestations?

(A) Niclosamide
(B) Niridazole
(C) Piperazine
(D) Diloxanide
(E) Pentamidine

1-D	4-D
2-C	5-D
3-C	6-A

7. All of the following statements about antiviral agents are true EXCEPT

(A) acyclovir may be given orally for initial genital herpes infections

(B) ribavirin may be given by aerosol for respiratory syncytial virus infections

(C) amantadine may be given orally in conjunction with influenza vaccine

(D) relapse is common with continued treatment with ganciclovir for cytomegalovirus retinitis in AIDS patients

(E) idoxuridine may be applied topically for type 2 herpes simplex genital infections

8. Correct statements about vaccines include all of the following EXCEPT

(A) individuals vaccinated before age 12 months may require measles revaccination

(B) rubella vaccine is recommended for women of childbearing age

(C) influenza vaccine decreases influenza mortality among the elderly

(D) pneumococcal vaccine is recommended for people who are severely immunocompromised

(E) hepatitis B vaccine is recommended for individuals at high risk for hepatitis B (i.e., homosexuals, intravenous drug abusers)

Questions 9–11

A 27-year-old intravenous drug abuser is diagnosed as being positive for human immunodeficiency virus. The patient's CD4$^+$ lymphocyte count was 150 cells/mm^3. At this time, the patient did not have *Pneumocystis carinii* pneumonia.

9. Zidovudine is prescribed. Common dose-related adverse effects include all of the following EXCEPT

(A) severe anemia

(B) neutropenia

(C) severe nephrotoxicity

(D) neurotoxicity

(E) myalgias

10. Which of the following agents should be considered for prophylactic administration?

(A) Ganciclovir

(B) Fluconazole

(C) Human interferon

(D) Pentamidine

(E) Rubella vaccine

11. Three months later, the patient develops oropharyngeal and esophageal candidiasis. The treatment of choice would be

(A) griseofulvin

(B) fluconazole

(C) miconazole

(D) clotrimazole

(E) naftifine

7-E 10-D
8-D 11-B
9-C

Directions: Each question below contains four suggested answers of which **one or more** is correct. Choose the answer

  A   if **1, 2, and 3** are correct
  B   if **1 and 3** are correct
  C   if **2 and 4** are correct
  D   if **4** is correct
  E   if **1, 2, 3, and 4** are correct

Questions 12–14

A 57-year-old man with known diverticulitis presents with severe abdominal pain. Examination reveals a "board-like" abdomen, while abdominal x-ray films demonstrate free air under the left diaphragm. The surgeon considers an operation to be mandatory.

12. Correct initial antimicrobial therapy could include

(1) gentamicin
(2) ciprofloxacin
(3) clindamycin
(4) nafcillin

13. Postoperatively, the patient develops severe abdominal pain, bloody diarrhea, and fever. Perforation is ruled out. Antimicrobial agents capable of producing this clinical picture include

(1) vancomycin
(2) gentamicin
(3) erythromycin
(4) clindamycin

14. Culture of a stool sample from the patient confirms *Clostridium difficile*. Correct therapy would now include

(1) discontinuation of the clindamycin
(2) instituting erythromycin therapy
(3) instituting vancomycin therapy
(4) discontinuation of the gentamicin

15. Clavulanic acid is given in combination with amoxicillin in order to

(1) reduce the risk of allergic reactions
(2) prolong amoxicillin's half-life
(3) reduce the severity of diarrhea
(4) extend amoxicillin's antibacterial spectrum

Directions: The group of items in this section consists of lettered options followed by a set of numbered items. For each item, select the **one** lettered option that is most closely associated with it. Each lettered option may be selected once, more than once, or not at all.

Questions 16–18

For each illness presented below, select the best combination therapy.

(A) Clofazimine plus dapsone plus rifampin
(B) Nafcillin plus gentamicin
(C) Isoniazid plus rifampin plus pyrazinamide or ethambutol
(D) Flucytosine plus amphotericin B
(E) Pentamidine plus amantadine

16. A neutropenic patient is hospitalized with a fever of 104° F; blood cultures are drawn

17. A patient is diagnosed as having multibacillary leprosy

18. An AIDS patient who is currently receiving zidovudine develops a severe cough, and tubercle bacilli are isolated from the sputum

12-B	15-D	18-C
13-D	16-B	
14-B	17-A	

ANSWERS AND EXPLANATIONS

1. The answer is D *[II A 2 a, B 2 c (2); II C 2 a (1); VIII F 2; X A 2 b (1)]*
Ganciclovir interferes with DNA polymerase and inhibits viral DNA replication. The proposed mechanisms of action for sulfadiazine, ampicillin, gentamicin, and zidovudine are correct as stated in the question.

2. The answer is C *[II B 4 a–d]*
Imipenem has one of the broadest antimicrobial spectrums of all the beta-lactam antibiotics. Its spectrum of activity includes gram-positive and gram-negative cocci (except methicillin-resistant staphylococci), enteric and anaerobic bacteria, and *Pseudomonas aeruginosa*, although this organism may become resistant during therapy. Imipenem is given with cilastatin, but this is to inhibit renal enzymatic degradation and nephrotoxicity, not to expand imipenem's spectrum of activity. Imipenem is used to treat serious hospital-acquired infections, including staphylococcal endocarditis, but its value in meningitis has not been established.

3. The answer is C *[II C 3 c, 4 c, 5 e, g, 8 a]*
All of the aminoglycosides have a narrow therapeutic index and are similar in their potential for causing adverse effects. The most serious of these are ototoxicity and nephrotoxicity.

4. The answer is D *[II D 6 c, 8 b, f, g, j]*
Children receiving either short-term or long-term tetracycline therapy may develop yellow-brown discoloration of the teeth. Tetracyclines are deposited into developing teeth and bones due to their chelating properties and the formation of a tetracycline–calcium orthophosphate complex.

5. The answer is D *[III A 4, B 3 a, 6, E 4 c, H 1]*
Miconazole is primarily used as a topical agent because of its systemic toxicity. Clotrimazole is used topically for the treatment of ringworm and other superficial fungal infections. Ketoconazole is not used for fungal meningitis because it penetrates the cerebrospinal fluid poorly. Amphotericin B is a broad-spectrum antifungal agent that must be administered parenterally for systemic fungal infections. Nystatin, amphotericin B, miconazole, and clotrimazole are all effective for the topical treatment of vulvovaginal candidiasis.

6. The answer is A *[VI C, E, G; VII B, F]*
Niclosamide is the drug of choice for the treatment of most tapeworms. Niridazole is used to treat schistosomiasis. Piperazine is used to treat ascariasis and pinworms. Diloxanide is an amebicide. Pentamidine is used in leishmaniasis and trypanosomiasis. Pentamidine is also used to treat *Pneumocystis carinii* pneumonia, which occurs in AIDS patients and in other immunosuppressed patients.

7. The answer is E *[VIII A 3, 4 a, C 3 b, E 5, 6 d, F 4, G 4]*
Acyclovir has an enhanced affinity for the viral enzyme thymidine kinase, which makes it several hundred-fold more toxic to herpes viruses than to mammalian cells. Acyclovir is effective against both type 1 and type 2 herpes simplex viruses. Ribavirin decreases morbidity from severe respiratory syncytical virus infections. It is given in aerosol form. Amantadine is given orally for prophylaxis of influenza A; it does not alter the immune response to influenza A vaccine and, therefore, can be given concurrently. Ganciclovir is indicated for the treatment of cytomegalovirus retinitis in AIDS patients; however, relapse has been reported with continued treatment. Idoxuridine is used in the treatment of herpes simplex keratitis, which is caused by type 1 herpes simplex, but it is not effective against herpes simplex type 2, the cause of genital herpes infections.

8. The answer is D *[IX A 1 b (3) (a), 2 b, 3 b (1), 4 b, B 2 b (1) (b)]*
Individuals born before 1956 are likely to be immune to measles and, thus, would not need the vaccine. However, revaccination is recommended for individuals vaccinated before age 12 months. Immunization with rubella vaccine is recommended for unimmunized women of childbearing age, since the aim is to prevent rubella infection in the fetus. Influenza vaccine decreases morbidity and mortality in the elderly. Pneumococcal vaccine is most effective in individuals with normal immune systems; it does not protect severely immunocompromised patients. Hepatitis B vaccine is now made chemically via recombinant technology. Homosexuals, hemophiliacs, intravenous drug abusers, and dialysis patients are all at high risk, and immunization is recommended.

9–11. The answers are: 9-C *[X A 2 f]*, **10-D** *[X B 1 b (3)]*, **11-B** *[III F 4 b]*
Severe anemia, often with a megaloblastic bone marrow, is the main toxic effect of zidovudine admin-istration. Neutropenia is also fairly common. Neurotoxicity, including severe headache and insomnia are common but are less severe after the first week of therapy. Nausea and myalgias occur often at the start of therapy. Nephrotoxicity is rare. Pentamidine aerosol administered once a month has been effective in preventing both initial episodes and recurrences of *Pneumocystis* pneumonia in AIDS patients. Gan-ciclovir is used for the treatment of cytomegalovirus. Fluconazole is useful in treating systemic viral in-fections. Human interferon may be useful in AIDS-related Kaposi's sarcoma. Rubella vaccination is es-pecially useful for the immunization of unimmunized women of childbearing age.

Fluconazole is emerging as the treatment of choice for oropharyngeal and esophageal candidiasis. Mi-conazole and clotrimazole are used for the treatment of ringworm and vulvovaginal candidiasis. Naftifine is used to treat tinea pedis, cruris, and corporis. Griseofulvin is useful for treating mycotic diseases of the skin, hair, and nails.

12–14. The answers are: 12-B (1, 3) *[II C 5 c, 6 b (1), F 4 b]*, **13-D (4)** *[II F 7 b]*, **14-B (1, 3)** *[II F 5 c (1)]*
Gentamicin provides excellent gram-negative coverage while clindamycin is excellent against *Bacter-oides fragilis*, a likely offending pathogen. Ciprofloxacin can only be administered orally and, therefore, is not indicated as initial therapy. Nafcillin has a gram-positive spectrum and is inactive against gram-negative and anaerobic organisms.

Clindamycin is capable of producing pseudomembranous colitis due to superinfection. Vancomycin is effective in the treatment of the causative organism of this syndrome, namely *Clostridium difficile*.

15. The answer is D (4) *[II B 2 f (7) (a) (i)]*
Clavulanic acid extends the antibacterial spectrum of beta-lactam antibiotics by irreversibly binding many bacterial beta-lactamase enzymes. Clavulanic acid does not alter the half-life or untoward effects of the antibiotic.

16–18. The answers are: 16-B *[I C 3 a (2)]*, **17-A** *[V B 4 a, 5 a]*, **18-C** *[IV A 2 c]*
Initial (blind) therapy, using nafcillin and gentamicin, should be administered to a seriously ill individual after blood cultures are taken. This will provide complete gram-positive and gram-negative coverage.

Clofazimine exerts a slow bactericidal effect on *Mycobacterium leprae*. It is used in combination with dapsone and rifampin in multibacillary leprosy to prevent the emergence of resistance.

For AIDS patients with tuberculosis, new drug regimens are being developed. Currently, three-drug therapy (i.e., isoniazid, rifampin, and either pyrazinamide or ethambutol) is given.

13

Principles of Drug Interactions

I. INTRODUCTION

A. Definition. A **drug interaction** occurs whenever the pharmacologic action of a drug is altered by a second substance. Theoretically, this change may be related to:

1. **Pharmacokinetic interactions**—that is, differences in the **plasma levels** of a drug achieved with a given dose of that drug

2. **Pharmacodynamic interactions**—that is, differences in **effects** produced by a given plasma level of a drug

B. General considerations

1. Although many examples of drug interactions are known, many are *not* clinically important. Clinically important changes often are seen with agents having a low therapeutic index (e.g., cardiac glycosides) or a poorly defined therapeutic endpoint (e.g., antipsychotic agents).

2. Often drug interactions can be avoided by using a different drug, which has the desired pharmacologic effect, but not the unwanted interaction.

II. PHARMACOKINETIC INTERACTIONS

A. General considerations

1. The duration and intensity of a drug's action are a function of the plasma level of the drug, which is related directly to the drug's rates of absorption, distribution, metabolism, and excretion. One or more of these rates may be altered by the following:
   a. Concomitant or previous drug therapy
   b. Dietary factors
   c. Exposure to environmental chemicals; that is, to chemicals not used for therapeutic purposes

2. Physical factors, such as the ambient temperature, and effects of disease (e.g., fever) can also alter the pharmacokinetic properties of drugs but will not be considered here.

B. Interactions affecting systemic delivery of drugs

1. **Drug interactions in vitro.** Some drugs are **incompatible** with intravenous infusion fluids.
   a. Ampicillin, ascorbic acid, chlorpromazine, barbiturates, and promethazine react with dextran solutions. The drugs break down or form chemical complexes.
   b. Benzylpenicillin (penicillin G), chlorpromazine, erythromycin, gentamicin, hydrocortisone, kanamycin, methicillin, promazine, streptomycin, and tetracyclines react with heparin solutions. Chemical complexes form.

2. **Drug absorption interactions in vivo**
   a. **Altered parenteral absorption** is not common but can occur.
      (1) For example, a subcutaneous or intramuscular injection of epinephrine or methacholine given concomitantly with another drug will alter the entry of the other drug into nearby capillaries.
      (2) This occurs because of the vasoconstricting or vasodilating effects of the accompanying adrenergic or cholinergic agonist.

b. Altered absorption after oral administration is more commonly observed.
   (1) Complexes can be formed. For example:
      (a) Tetracycline and cations, such as calcium (e.g., in milk and some antacids) or aluminum ion (e.g., in some antacids), combine to produce an insoluble salt, which results in very poor and erratic tetracycline blood levels.
      (b) Cholestyramine binds acidic compounds, cardiac glycosides, and thyroxine, blocking their absorption.
   (2) Intestinal motility can be altered. The ultimate effect on drug absorption in this case depends upon the site at which the drug is primarily absorbed (small intestine, stomach).
      (a) For example, anticholinergic agents (e.g., atropine) and opiate-like agents delay gastric emptying and slow the absorption of some drugs, such as acetaminophen, which are absorbed in the intestine.
      (b) Stimulation of gastrointestinal motility can reduce drug absorption. For example, metoclopramide decreases absorption of cimetidine, which is absorbed primarily in the stomach.
   (3) Absorption can be blocked. For example:
      (a) Phenytoin and oral contraceptives inhibit the hydrolysis of folic acid (to the monoglutamate) in the gut, and thus, they reduce its absorption.
      (b) Colchicine produces malabsorption of vitamin B_{12}.
   (4) Diet may influence drug absorption.
      (a) The presence of food in the stomach may exert a nonspecific effect in reducing or slowing the absorption of some drugs.
      (b) A fatty meal will increase the absorption of lipid-soluble drugs (e.g., griseofulvin).
   (5) Changes in gastric pH can alter absorption.
      (a) Weak acids, such as salicylates, are not absorbed well when the gastric pH is elevated with antacids.
      (b) Ketoconazole is poorly absorbed in the absence of gastric acidity.
c. Monoamine oxidase (MAO) inhibitors block oxidative deamination of naturally occurring monoamines, including tyramine.
   (1) Many fermented foods contain tyramine, which is formed as a bacterial breakdown product of tyrosine.
   (2) Exogenous tyramine can result in the release of norepinephrine and epinephrine, resulting in severe headache and hypertensive crisis.

C. Interactions affecting drug distribution

1. Competition for plasma protein–binding sites. Many drugs, especially acidic ones, bind to plasma proteins. Drugs, and also other substances, can compete for plasma protein–binding sites.
   a. The effect is often to release more free drug and, thus, enhance its pharmacologic effect.
   b. This is especially important when a high percentage of the drug (over 90%) is normally protein-bound, as is the case with coumarin anticoagulants, sulfonamides, salicylates, indomethacin, and most other nonsteroidal anti-inflammatory agents. For example:
      (1) Sulfisoxazole in premature infants increases the likelihood of fatal kernicterus because the sulfonamide displaces bilirubin from protein-binding sites.
      (2) Phenylbutazone potentiates the anticoagulant actions of warfarin by this mechanism and may cause excessive bleeding.

2. Displacement of a plasma protein–bound drug can result in complex changes in the pharmacologic effects of the drug that can be difficult to predict.
   a. There is a transient rise in the plasma levels of free drug, but the plasma half-life is frequently reduced.
   b. A marked increase in the pharmacologic effect can occur if the normal route of drug elimination is impaired due to disease (e.g., cirrhosis) or to saturation of metabolizing enzymes required for drug elimination.

D. Interactions affecting drug metabolism

1. Rate of biotransformation. The most common and most important cause for differences in plasma levels of a drug is a change in the rate of biotransformation of the drug.

2. Rate of first-pass metabolism. Variations in a person's plasma drug levels are more common with drugs that undergo extensive gastrointestinal metabolism or first-pass hepatic metabolism (e.g., propranolol).

3. Inhibition of metabolism. Many drugs that are inactivated by biotransformation can have a prolonged duration of action if their metabolism is inhibited by other agents.

4. Inhibition of nonmicrosomal enzymes [see Chapter 1 II D 2 a (2)]
   a. Drugs that can inhibit MAO, such as the antitumor agent procarbazine and the antidepressant tranylcypromine, can retard the metabolism of various drugs, such as barbiturates and benzodiazepines, and of amines, such as serotonin and norepinephrine.
   b. Because 6-mercaptopurine is inactivated in part by xanthine oxidase, the concurrent administration of the xanthine oxidase inhibitor, allopurinol, can result in an accumulation of 6-mercaptopurine with a consequent increase in bone marrow depression.
   c. Disulfiram inhibits acetaldehyde dehydrogenase and, thus, prevents acetaldehyde, the oxidation product of ethanol, from being further metabolized. The resulting accumulation of acetaldehyde causes flushing, nausea, vomiting, and tachycardia.

5. Induction or inhibition of microsomal enzymes (mixed-function oxygenases, or the cytochrome P-450 system) can also affect drug metabolism [see Chapter 1 II D 2 a (1)].
   a. Inducers. More than 200 drugs and a large number of dietary and environmental chemicals are known inducers of this enzyme system.
      (1) Induction of mixed-function oxygenases results in an accelerated metabolism of substrates.
      (2) The induction is due to new protein synthesis. The pattern of the newly synthesized proteins and the rate of appearance of new mixed-function oxygenase activities differ with different inducers.
      (3) Some inducers of mixed-function oxygenases are:
         (a) Barbiturates, glutethimide, phenytoin
         (b) Polycyclic aromatic hydrocarbons, such as benzo[a]pyrene
         (c) Halogenated hydrocarbon insecticides (e.g., DDT)
         (d) Nicotine
         (e) Ethanol, when ingested chronically
      (4) Some inducers stimulate their own metabolism.
   b. Inhibitors. There are also a number of inhibitors of mixed-function oxygenases, including:
      (1) Organophosphorus insecticides
      (2) Carbon tetrachloride
      (3) Ozone
      (4) Carbon monoxide
      (5) Cimetidine

E. Interactions affecting drug excretion
   1. Reduction in urinary elimination. Many weak organic acids (e.g., aspirin, penicillin, methotrexate) are excreted by a common **transport system** in the proximal tubules. Competition for this transport system by weak acids can result in a reduction in the urinary elimination of the competing drugs. (Comparable interactions between weak organic bases have not been well characterized in humans.) For example:
      a. Probenecid can block the excretion of penicillin, indomethacin, cefazolin, and methotrexate.
      b. Aspirin can block the excretion of methotrexate and, thus, cause serious adverse effects.

   2. Changes in urinary pH can influence the elimination of weak acids and bases since their passive reabsorption requires that they be un-ionized. This can be important in the treatment of overdoses of weak acids and bases (e.g., aspirin or amphetamines).
      a. Agents that alkalinize the urine (e.g., acetazolamide or sodium bicarbonate) will increase the excretion of weak acids.
      b. Agents that acidify the urine (e.g., ammonium chloride) will enhance the elimination of weak bases.

   3. Changes in urinary volume, such as with diuretics, often can reduce the renal toxicity of chemicals and drugs, presumably by reducing the tubular concentration of the toxin. For example, mannitol reduces cisplatin toxicity.

   4. Stimulation of biliary excretion by some drugs can alter the elimination of other drugs.
      a. For example, phenobarbital enhances the biliary excretion of many drugs by increasing both bile flow and the synthesis of proteins that function in the biliary conjugation–excretion mechanism.

b. Activated charcoal and cholestyramine increase the excretion of drugs that undergo extensive enterohepatic recirculation by binding to them in the gastrointestinal tract.

III. PHARMACODYNAMIC INTERACTIONS

A. Receptor interactions. Drug interactions can occur at the level of the **drug receptor**. For example, the H_2-receptor antagonist cimetidine blocks the action of histamine-like agonists, such as betazole, by this mechanism.

B. Physiologic interactions. Agents can **reduce** the effect of other drugs by acting via different cellular mechanisms (**physiologic antagonism**). For example, acetylcholine and norepinephrine have opposing effects on heart rate (see Chapter 1 III A 1 b, D 4).

C. Drug interactions

1. Agents can **enhance** the actions of other drugs although they act via different cellular mechanisms. For example, ethanol can enhance the central nervous system depression caused by opioids or tranquilizers.

2. The action of one drug can be influenced by **changes in the intracellular or extracellular environment** that are caused by another drug. For example, diuretic-induced hypokalemia can increase the possibility of digitalis-induced cardiac toxicity.

3. **Chemical inactivation** can occur systemically to reduce a drug's action. For example, protamine binds to heparin, thereby neutralizing it.

STUDY QUESTIONS

Directions: Each of the numbered items or incomplete statements in this section is followed by answers or by completions of the statement. Select the **one** lettered answer or completion that is **best** in each case.

1. Pharmacokinetic drug interactions can result from all of the following EXCEPT

(A) impaired absorption
(B) induction of the drug microsomal enzyme metabolizing system
(C) inhibition of the drug microsomal enzyme metabolizing system
(D) inhibition of renal excretion
(E) the combination of a bacteriostatic antibiotic and a bactericidal antibiotic

2. All of the following are drug interactions that affect absorption EXCEPT

(A) tetracycline—milk
(B) tetracycline—antacids containing aluminum
(C) tetracycline—cimetidine
(D) cholestyramine—cardiac glycosides
(E) cholestyramine—thyroxine

3. Drinking beer after taking disulfiram causes flushing, nausea, and tachycardia. This occurs because disulfiram inhibits the

(A) accumulation of acetaldehyde
(B) metabolism of acetaldehyde
(C) excretion of acetaldehyde
(D) intestinal transport of acetaldehyde
(E) protein binding of acetaldehyde

4. All of the following agents would be capable of inducing the cytochrome P-450 metabolizing system EXCEPT

(A) barbiturates
(B) cimetidine
(C) DDT
(D) glutethimide
(E) phenytoin

5. A classic example of the inhibition of renal secretion of a drug is the interaction between probenecid and

(A) streptomycin
(B) chloramphenicol
(C) chlortetracycline
(D) penicillin G
(E) neomycin

1-E	4-B
2-C	5-D
3-B	

Directions: Each item below contains four suggested answers of which **one or more** is correct. Choose the answer

A   if **1, 2, and 3** are correct
B   if **1 and 3** are correct
C   if **2 and 4** are correct
D   if **4** is correct
E   if **1, 2, 3, and 4** are correct

6. The concomitant administration of antacids with tetracycline will reduce the effectiveness of the antibiotic because

(1) antacids inhibit the absorption of tetracycline
(2) antacids stimulate the drug microsomal metabolizing system, so that the tetracycline is metabolized more rapidly
(3) ions in antacids chelate the tetracycline
(4) antacids enhance the renal excretion of tetracycline

7. Displacement of a drug from plasma protein–binding sites might cause which of the following effects?

(1) Increased plasma levels of free drug
(2) Prolonged plasma half-life of the drug
(3) An increase in unwanted effects
(4) A decrease in desired effects

Directions: The group of items in this section consists of lettered options followed by a set of numbered items. For each item, select the **one** lettered option that is most closely associated with it. Each lettered option may be selected once, more than once, or not at all.

Questions 8–12

Barbiturates can be involved in drug interactions with many other drugs. For each drug listed below, select the mechanism that is the most likely cause of an interaction with a barbiturate.

(A) Incompatibility in vitro
(B) Induction of microsomal enzymes
(C) Inhibition of nonmicrosomal enzymes
(D) Enhancement of pharmacologic effects
(E) Interference with renal excretion

8. Warfarin

9. Dextran

10. Tranylcypromine

11. Digitoxin

12. Phenothiazines

ANSWERS AND EXPLANATIONS

1. The answer is E *[II A 1, B 2, D 5, E]*
Pharmacokinetic drug interactions are those that involve altered plasma levels of a drug. All of the factors in the question can result in altered plasma levels of a drug after its administration except for the combination of a bacteriostatic antibiotic with a bactericidal one. The latter is a pharmacodynamic type of drug interaction since plasma drug levels are not altered. Instead, the bacteriostatic agent can block the desirable actions of the bactericidal antibiotic by preventing cell replication.

2. The answer is C *[II B 2 b (1)]*
Tetracyclines do not interact with the H_2-receptor antagonist cimetidine. Tetracyclines do form insoluble complexes with cations, such as the calcium in milk and aluminum in antacids. The anion-exchange resin, cholestyramine, binds both cardiac glycosides and thyroxine, thus blocking their absorption.

3. The answer is B *[II D 4 c]*
Disulfiram inhibits the enzyme acetaldehyde dehydrogenase and consequently inhibits the metabolism of acetaldehyde, the oxidation product of ethanol. The resulting accumulation of acetaldehyde causes flushing, nausea, and tachycardia.

4. The answer is B *[II D 5 a]*
Barbiturates, glutethimide, phenytoin, and DDT are capable of inducing the cytochrome P-450 metabolizing system, so that they all would enhance the metabolism of other agents degraded by this system. The induction of mixed-function oxygenases results from new protein synthesis. Cimetidine inhibits the activity of cytochrome P-450, thereby slowing the metabolism of many drugs that are substrates for hepatic mixed-function oxidases.

5. The answer is D *[II E 1 a]*
Probenecid is capable of blocking the renal tubular excretion of penicillin G, thereby prolonging its half-life. In fact, probenecid was originally developed for this purpose, in the days when penicillin was in short supply. Probenecid also blocks the renal excretion of many other drugs. However, the renal excretion of streptomycin, chloramphenicol, chlortetracycline, oxytetracycline, or neomycin would not be significantly affected by the coadministration of probenecid.

6. The answer is B (1, 3) *[II B 2 b]*
Antacids inhibit the absorption of tetracycline because ions, such as calcium and aluminum, in the antacids can chelate the tetracycline. Antacids do not stimulate or inhibit the drug microsomal metabolizing system, nor do they enhance the renal excretion of tetracycline.

7. The answer is B (1, 3) *[II C]*
Drugs can compete with one another and also with endogenous substances, for plasma protein–binding sites. When one drug causes displacement of another drug from these binding sites, the results can be complex. The displaced, unbound drug is not free to carry out its pharmacologic effects, both desired and unwanted; however, it is now also available for metabolism and excretion. Hence, plasma levels of free drug are increased at first with a resulting increase in both wanted and unwanted effects, but the plasma half-life will probably be shortened because of increased metabolism of the drug.

8–12. The answers are: 8-B *[Ch 3 II A 5 g]*, **9-A** *[Ch 13 II B 1 a]*, **10-C** *[Ch 13 II D 4 a]*, **11-B** *[Ch 3 II A 5 g]*, **12-D** *[Ch 3 II A 5 a]*
Most drug interactions involving the barbiturates result from induction of hepatic microsomal enzymes by the barbiturate; this causes accelerated metabolism of the other drug (e.g., warfarin, digitoxin, corticosteroids, and β blockers, to name only a few). However, other mechanisms can also be involved. Thus, a barbiturate plus another CNS depressant (e.g., a phenothiazine, ethanol, or an antihistamine) can cause marked depression. Tranylcypromine is an inhibitor of MAO, a nonmicrosomal enzyme, and this can retard the metabolism of a barbiturate. Dextran solutions are incompatible with various drugs, including barbiturates. Barbiturates can also interfere with the absorption of some drugs (e.g., dicumarol and griseofulvin), and some barbiturates compete with other drugs (e.g., aspirin) for plasma protein–binding sites.

14

Poisons and Antidotes

I. INTRODUCTION

A. Definition. Toxicology is the study of poisons, including their actions, adverse effects, and treatment of the conditions that they produce. These poisons include household, environmental, industrial, or pharmacologic substances.

B. Subdivisions of toxicology

1. **Experimental toxicology** involves the investigation of the toxic effects of chemicals on biologic systems.

2. **Clinical toxicology** involves the diagnosis and treatment of poisonings.

3. **Environmental toxicology** involves the identification and elimination of environmental poisons.

C. Poisons and their antidotes

1. A variety of industrial solvents, heavy metals, gases, and common household chemicals can be dangerous poisons. Drugs that are used clinically may also be poisons in high doses.

2. Acute exposure to a toxic substance is likely to produce different symptoms than symptoms produced by chronic exposure to lower concentrations.

3. Antidotes have been developed for some poisons. These act either by preventing absorption or by inactivating or antagonizing the actions of the poisons.

D. Quantitative toxicity

1. **Median lethal dose (LD$_{50}$)** is the smallest dose of a given chemical that will kill 50% of a test group of animals. The LD$_{50}$ is used to extrapolate the toxic potential of a compound to the human. It is used with all routes of poisoning except inhalation.

2. **Median lethal concentration (LC$_{50}$)** is the smallest concentration of a given chemical that will kill 50% of a test group of animals. It is applicable to chemicals that are inhaled. The LC$_{50}$ is expressed relative to the duration of exposure.

3. **Threshold limit value (TLV)** is the maximal amount of a chemical that is considered safe. Industrial and governmental hygienists provide an official listing of the TLV levels of airborne poisons to which workers may safely be exposed for an 8-hour period.

II. SPECIFIC POISONS

A. Gaseous poisons

1. **Simple asphyxiants** are usually inert industrial gases, such as **nitrogen** (N_2), **carbon dioxide** (CO_2), and **methane** (CH_4). Asphyxiants decrease the oxygen available to the lungs and cause hypoxia.

2. **Irritants** that affect the respiratory tract can cause asphyxia.
   a. **Water-soluble irritants** affect the eyes and upper respiratory tract. They can affect the lungs and can be corrosive. Examples include **hydrochloric acid** (HCl), **hydrofluoric acid** (HF), **sulfur dioxide** (SO_2), and **ammonia** (NH_3).

b. Water-insoluble irritants can be trapped in nasopharyngeal secretions and can descend into the alveoli, causing pneumonitis and pulmonary edema. Examples include **chlorine gas** and **ozone**.

3. **Systemic toxicants** are absorbed by inhalation or percutaneously.
   a. **Cyanide** (hydrocyanic acid, HCN) is one of the most rapidly acting poisons.
      (1) **Mechanism of action.** Cyanide anions form complexes with ferric ions of the cytochrome oxidase system, interfering with electron transfer in the **cytochrome a–a$_3$ complex**. This leads to a blockage in oxygen transfer to tissues and causes a cytotoxic hypoxia.
      (2) **Diagnosis.** The patient's breath will have the characteristic odor of oil of bitter almond, which should assist in diagnosis.
      (3) **Treatment** must be rapid and is designed to prevent or reverse the cyanide–ferric ion binding in the cytochrome oxidase system.
         (a) **Amyl nitrite** is administered by inhalation, accompanied by **intravenous sodium nitrite**.
            (i) Nitrite oxidizes a limited amount of hemoglobin to methemoglobin, which has a greater affinity for cyanide ion than does cytochrome a–a$_3$.
            (ii) The cyanide–cytochrome complex, therefore, dissociates, and normal oxidative metabolism resumes.
         (b) A mitochondrial trans-sulfurase can convert cyanide to thiocyanate, which is relatively nontoxic. This detoxification can be increased by the intravenous administration of thiosulfate.
         (c) If the cyanide has been ingested, gastric lavage should follow the above-mentioned treatment procedures.
   b. **Carbon monoxide** is the most common cause of accidental and suicidal poisoning.
      (1) **General considerations**
         (a) Carbon monoxide is an odorless, colorless, and tasteless gas.
         (b) Two common sources of carbon monoxide are houses with inadequate ventilation and automobile exhaust systems.
      (2) **Pharmacokinetics and mechanism of action**
         (a) The affinity of hemoglobin for carbon monoxide is about 220 times greater than its affinity for oxygen.
         (b) Carbon monoxide is absorbed and excreted by the lungs.
         (c) Exposure to very high ambient concentrations of carbon monoxide can result in rapid death with no premonitory signs.
         (d) Exposure to lower concentrations of carbon monoxide will cause unconsciousness, then coma, followed by convulsions and death.
      (3) **Diagnosis.** Usually the circumstances surrounding acute carbon monoxide poisoning, such as a running automobile engine, combined with the patient's "cherry red" cyanosis, will make the diagnosis obvious.
      (4) **Treatment**
         (a) The patient should be removed from the air containing carbon monoxide and may require resuscitation.
         (b) Oxygen (100%) should be administered, which reduces the half-life of carboxyhemoglobin from 5 hours to 1 hour.
         (c) When the poisoning is severe, hypobaric oxygen therapy at a pressure of 2–3 atm is recommended, which reduces the half-life of carboxyhemoglobin to 20 minutes.
         (d) Oxygen should be given until the level of carboxyhemoglobin decreases to at least 10%.
         (e) Patients may also require treatment for resultant hypotension, metabolic acidosis, and cardiac effects.

4. **Organic solvents**
   a. **General considerations**
      (1) Organic solvents have an appreciable vapor pressure, are volatile, and can become an inhalation hazard, especially in an industrial environment.
      (2) They are fat-soluble and can be absorbed through the skin, accumulating in both fat and nervous tissue.
   b. **Classification.** Classes of toxic organic solvents include:
      (1) Saturated hydrocarbons, such as pentane, hexane, heptane, and octane

(2) Unsaturated hydrocarbons, such as kerosene

(3) Aromatic compounds, such as benzene and toluene

(4) Halogenated hydrocarbons, such as methylene dichloride, dichloromethane, chloroform, and carbon tetrachloride

  c. Adverse effects. The toxic manifestations of organic solvents vary with the individual substance.

  d. Treatment. In general, the best and only therapy is to remove the individual from the exposure to the solvent.

B. Heavy metal intoxication

1. Mechanism of action

  a. All of the heavy metals bind to a wide variety of macromolecules in membranes and the cytosol. Since heavy metals are not metabolized, they may accumulate in the body.

  b. The heavy metals can inactivate important enzyme activities and disrupt membranes.

  c. Because of the diverse affinities for the multiple organic ligands, it has been difficult to identify a single molecular target for the toxicity of these substances.

2. Specific intoxicants

  a. Arsenic poisoning can be produced by absorption from lungs, gastrointestinal tract, and skin.

    (1) Pharmacokinetics and mechanism of action

      (a) Arsenic is often used in household plant-spray pesticides as lead arsenate.

      (b) The trivalent form (As^{3-}) is toxic and binds to thiol groups of enzymes and other proteins in tissue.

      (c) Tolerance to chronic arsenic poisoning can develop.

    (2) Adverse effects

      (a) Acute poisoning causes hypotension, capillary transudation, muscle spasms, vertigo, delirium, and interference with kidney function.

      (b) Chronic poisoning results in persistent capillary dilation, malaise, and fatigue. Encephalopathy, peripheral neuritis, and sensory loss can occur.

    (3) Diagnosis. Sulfhydryl-rich tissues—namely, nails and hair—take up arsenic, and pale bands appear in the fingernails and toenails that are useful in diagnosis.

    (4) Treatment. The **antidote** for arsenic poisoning is dimercaprol (see II B 3 a). Dimercaprol contains sulfhydryl groups, which compete with sulfhydryl moieties on proteins for the arsenic.

  b. Lead is the most common cause of heavy metal poisoning, especially in large urban areas.

    (1) Pharmacokinetics and mechanism of action

      (a) Acute poisoning is rare. Exposure has been markedly reduced because of stringent regulations on the use of lead in paints and other products. The most common routes of absorption of lead are the gastrointestinal tract and respiratory system.

      (b) Organic lead poisoning

        (i) This is rare, except among "gasoline sniffers."

        (ii) Tetraethyl lead is found in some gasoline and can be absorbed when inhaled.

        (iii) Penetration can also occur via the skin because tetraethyl lead is fat-soluble.

        (iv) Eventually, the organic lead is converted in the body to inorganic lead, producing the symptoms of chronic lead poisoning.

    (2) Diagnosis

      (a) Wristdrop and to a lesser extent footdrop occur as a result of degenerative changes in motor neurons.

      (b) An abdominal syndrome, consisting of constipation, anorexia, and a persistent metallic taste, appears early in the course of lead poisoning.

      (c) A black "lead line" can occur on the gums but may be absent if the intoxicated person practices good dental hygiene.

      (d) Since the distribution of lead is similar to that of calcium, lead is deposited in and mobilized from bone.

      (e) Lead is a potent inhibitor of hemoglobin synthesis and produces a normocytic hypochromic anemia. A reticulocytosis can also occur.

      (f) A characteristic basophilic stippling of red blood cells often occurs.

      (g) Increased coproporphyrin and δ-aminolevulinic acid levels are found in the urine.

      (h) The most serious manifestation is **lead encephalopathy**.

        (i) The patient will often demonstrate clumsiness, irritability, vertigo, and projectile vomiting.

        (ii) The condition must be differentiated from meningitis.

        (iii) A fatality rate as high as 25% has been reported. In addition, 40% of the survivors demonstrate various neurologic abnormalities, including seizures, cerebral palsy, optic atrophy, and mental retardation.

    (3) Treatment consists of intravenous infusions of calcium disodium ethylenediamine tetraacetic acid (edetate calcium disodium, $CaNa_2EDTA$; see II B 3 b).

      (a) Initially (for 3–5 days), $CaNa_2EDTA$ is given in combination with dimercaprol.

      (b) Oral penicillamine, which is a good chelator of lead, can be given as long-term therapy (for 3–6 months) after the initial dimercaprol and $CaNa_2EDTA$ therapy.

  c. Mercury

    (1) Pharmacokinetics and mechanism of action

      (a) Toxicity can occur by inhalation, skin penetration, or ingestion of substances containing mercury.

        (i) Mercurial fungicides are present in some latex paints and can be inhaled.

        (ii) Dermal application of methylmercury ointments can result in absorption through the skin.

        (iii) Inorganic mercury preparations can be ingested, resulting in acute poisoning, in contrast to the two instances above, which usually produce chronic poisoning.

      (b) Mercurous (Hg^+) salts are less toxic than mercuric (Hg^{2+}) salts because they are less soluble, resulting in decreased skin penetration.

      (c) Mercury is capable of attaching to sulfhydryl groups of enzymes and other proteins. In addition, it concentrates in the kidney.

    (2) Diagnosis

      (a) Acute intoxication can result in cardiovascular collapse and anuria.

      (b) Chronic intoxication due to inhalation or skin penetration can result in:

        (i) Neurologic manifestations, including irritability, tremors, and psychosis

        (ii) Mercuria lentis, a brown discoloration of the anterior portion of the optic lens

        (iii) Gingivitis and stomatitis

        (iv) Progressive renal damage

    (3) Treatment. Dimercaprol is used in the treatment of mercury poisoning. Diaphoresis can be used adjunctively.

  d. Other metals

    (1) Antimony produces effects similar to those of arsenic. Chronic poisoning can result in myocardial damage.

    (2) Gold produces effects similar to those of arsenic.

    (3) Nickel is a sensitizing agent and causes a dermatitis known as "nickel itch."

    (4) Beryllium is an industrial hazard capable of causing a chronic granulomatous condition somewhat similar to sarcoidosis. In some instances, lung carcinoma can occur.

    (5) Zinc intoxication can occur from inhalation of fresh fumes in smelting, causing a condition known as "metal-fume fever." Delayed chills with fever lasting up to 36 hours can occur. Tolerance develops with chronic exposure.

3. Chelating agents as antidotes

  a. Dimercaprol (2,3-dimercaptopropanol, British antilewisite, **BAL**)

    (1) Mechanism of action. Dimercaprol forms stable chelates, enhancing their excretion.

    (2) Preparations and administration. Dimercaprol cannot be administered orally. It is administered intramuscularly as a 10% solution of dimercaprol in oil. It is most effective when administered within 1–2 hours after toxic ingestion.

    (3) Therapeutic uses. Dimercaprol is indicated for the treatment of arsenic, antimony, gold, lead, and mercury poisoning.

    (4) Adverse effects include a dose-related rise in blood pressure and tachycardia. Nausea, vomiting, and headache, as well as a burning sensation of the lips and mouth, have been reported. The drug is potentially nephrotoxic.

  b. $CaNa_2EDTA$

    (1) Mechanism of action. It forms stable, soluble metal chelates.

    (2) Preparations and administration

      (a) The calcium disodium derivative of EDTA ($CaNa_2EDTA$) is recommended rather than Na_2EDTA because $CaNa_2EDTA$ is less likely to cause hypocalcemia tetany.

(b) Because of poor oral absorption, it is administered intramuscularly. Pain occurs at the site of intramuscular injection.

(c) It is not metabolized and is rapidly excreted.

(3) Therapeutic uses. CaNa$_2$EDTA is used principally for lead poisoning but has been used for iron, copper, and zinc poisoning as well.

(4) Adverse effects. Hydropic degeneration of the proximal tubule has been reported, but generally CaNa$_2$EDTA has a low toxicity potential.

c. Penicillamine and *N*-acetylpenicillamine

(1) Mechanism of action. It forms stable, soluble metal chelates.

(2) Preparations. The *l* isomer is a pyridoxine antagonist.

(3) Therapeutic uses. These orally administered agents are used for the treatment of heavy-metal poisoning. It is particularly effective in chelating copper.

(4) Adverse effects. *d*-Penicillamine has caused serious allergic, hematologic, and renal toxicity.

d. Deferoxamine

(1) Mechanism of action

(a) Deferoxamine exhibits a high affinity for the ferric ion.

(b) It competes with the iron of ferritin and hemosiderin, while the iron of transferrin and of cytochromes is not affected.

(2) Preparations and administration. Since oral absorption of deferoxamine is poor, it is given parenterally to chelate iron that has been absorbed.

(3) Therapeutic uses. Deferoxamine is used to treat acute iron poisoning.

(4) Adverse effects include hypotension and allergic reactions. Anuria, renal disease, and pregnancy are contraindications.

C. Commonly occurring overdoses

1. Ethanol accounts for approximately one-fourth of all drug poisonings each year.

a. The lethal blood level of ethanol is considered to be 0.5 g/dl; however, it varies from patient to patient.

b. A microdiffusion test is a simple screening test for the presence of blood ethanol.

c. Gas chromatography, a procedure used to separate out volatile substances, allows one to differentiate between ethanol and methanol. In addition, blood ethanol concentrations can be determined.

d. Treatment of ethanol overdosage consists of intensive supportive care with special attention to preventing hypoglycemia and ketoacidosis.

2. Barbiturate overdosage is a common form of poisoning in adults.

a. The treatment of barbiturate overdosage is mainly supportive. Maintenance of cardiopulmonary stability is of prime importance.

b. Lavage or emesis can be attempted if proper precaution has been taken to avoid aspiration. Gastric lavage is contraindicated in the comatose patient.

c. Since most barbiturates are acidic, alkalinization of the urine and the promotion of diuresis is often beneficial.

d. Hemodialysis is the most effective means of treating severe barbiturate overdosage. It tends to be more effective in removing short-acting barbiturates rather than long-acting ones because the degree of protein binding is considerably less.

e. Analeptic agents are contraindicated.

3. Salicylate intoxication

a. Poisoning primarily occurs in children.

b. For the frequently observed signs and symptoms of salicylate intoxication, see Chapter 9 II A 6.

c. Plasma salicylate levels are often good indicators of the severity of salicylate poisoning.

(1) Plasma levels below 50 mg/dl produce no major symptoms, and treatment is to induce emesis or administer gastric lavage.

(2) With plasma levels between 50 and 100 mg/dl, the patient often presents with hyperpnea due to salicylate stimulation of the respiratory center. Increased blood glucose levels and hyperpyrexia may be seen.

(a) Treatment is by inducing emesis or using gastric lavage.

(b) The administration of sodium bicarbonate to alkalinize the urine may be advisable, but must be performed with caution.

(c) Correction of hyperthermia with ice blankets is often needed.

(d) The blood salicylate level is rechecked within a few hours.

(3) With plasma levels over 110 mg/dl, the same procedures as above are performed; however, hemodialysis or peritoneal dialysis may be needed.

(4) Plasma levels over 160 mg/dl are usually lethal, death being due to respiratory arrest.

4. Acetaminophen overdose can result in liver toxicity (see Chapter 9 II B 6 b).

5. Acids (e.g., hydrochloric, nitric, sulfuric, sodium bisulfate) are found in home products, such as cleaning agents and automobile batteries.

    a. If swallowed, severe mucous membrane burns can occur. Respiratory distress due to epiglottal edema and gastrointestinal scarring can result.

    b. Emetics and lavages are **contraindicated**.

    c. Dilution or therapy with water or milk following ingestion is the treatment of choice.

6. Alkalies (e.g., sodium hypochlorite, sodium hydroxide, potassium hydroxide) are substances that are found in household products, such as Drano.

    a. Severe burns of the skin, mucous membranes, and eyes can occur on contact.

    b. They tend to be more severe injuries than seen with acid caustic ingestion.

    c. Immediate and extensive irrigation of affected areas is recommended.

    d. Oral ingestion requires dilution with water or milk.

    e. Steroid therapy for a 3-week course has been used when esophageal burns occur.

7. Benzodiazepine overdose (see Chapter 3 VI C 4 b)

8. Narcotics overdose (see Chapter 3 IX E 5)

III. MANAGEMENT OF POISONING

A. General principles

1. The exposure of the patient to the toxic substance should be avoided or reduced.

    a. The individual should be removed from the contaminated air if the toxic substance is airborne.

    b. The individual's clothing should be removed immediately if the clothing is soaked in the poison.

    c. When the poison has been ingested, vomiting should be induced or gastric lavage should be used except when that is contraindicated, as in the case of caustic poisons or a comatose patient.

2. Supportive therapy should be given to maintain basic respiratory and cardiovascular function.

3. Telephone management, especially the pediatric population, comprises the majority of this population's treatment. Most children under the age of 5 years accidentally ingest the poison.

4. Although few poisons have specific antidotes, the most common substance that is effective and generally available in a household is **milk**.

    a. Milk is amphoteric, and both acids and bases are compatible.

    b. Both the calcium and protein can serve as chelators.

    c. Milk coats the stomach, thereby protecting it and delaying absorption.

B. Induction of vomiting

1. Syrup of ipecac is the preferred emetic for inducing vomiting.

    a. It is best administered with a glass of warm water because this produces a diluting effect and solubilizes the stomach contents.

    b. Syrup of ipecac (or any emetic) must be used with particular caution when central nervous system (CNS) integrity is compromised because of the risk of aspiration pneumonia.

2. Salt water and **using a finger to promote emesis** are both dangerous.

3. Contraindications to induced emesis include:

    a. Caustic poisons, such as lye

    b. Petroleum distillates, such as lighter fluid or gasoline

    c. A comatose patient

    d. A patient in whom convulsions may be imminent, as with ingestion of a large dose of aspirin

4. **Alternatives to emesis.** The major alternatives to emesis include the following:
   a. **Gastric lavage** is especially useful in treating poisoning by aromatic substances, such as perfume, or when some contraindication for emesis exists.
   b. **Activated charcoal** adsorbs the poison or toxin and delays gastrointestinal absorption. It is especially helpful in the treatment of poisoning from aromatic and alkaloid compounds.
   c. **Cathartics** are used to hasten the removal of a toxic substance and are useful for ingestion of hydrocarbons and enteric-coated tablets. **Sodium sulfate** is a frequently used cathartic.
   d. Dialysis is most effective if the poison has a small volume of distribution and has low protein binding. Peritoneal dialysis and hemodialysis have limited use in the treatment of intoxication with chemicals.
   e. Pharmacologic antagonism can be effective with compounds that act at specific receptors (pharmacologic antagonism), but stimulation of physiologic mechanisms may be deleterious (physiologic antagonism); for example, CNS stimulants used in respiratory depression can cause convulsions.

STUDY QUESTIONS

Directions: Each of the numbered items or incomplete statements in this section is followed by answers or by completions of the statement. Select the **one** lettered answer or completion that is **best** in each case.

1. All of the following statements about toxicology are true EXCEPT

(A) certain heavy metals can be considered hazardous poisons

(B) chronic exposure to a toxic substance is likely to produce the same symptoms as acute exposure

(C) antidotes of poisons can act by preventing absorption of the poison

(D) antidotes of poisons can act by antagonizing the actions of poisons

(E) activated charcoal is a management alternative to syrup of ipecac

2. The therapeutic efficacy of sodium nitrite in the treatment of patients with cyanide poisoning is based upon

(A) the formation of methemoglobin

(B) an increase in oxidative phosphorylation

(C) an increase in coronary arterial blood flow

(D) a decrease in intracranial pressure

(E) relaxation of the nonvascular smooth muscle

3. Mercury is toxic because it

(A) complexes with hemoglobin to form methemoglobin

(B) inhibits hemoglobin synthesis, producing anemia

(C) binds to ferric ions of the cytochrome a–a_3 complex

(D) inhibits anaerobic glycolysis

(E) binds to sulfhydryl groups

4. All of the following statements about arsenic poisoning are true EXCEPT

(A) arsenic is used in household plant-spray pesticides

(B) the trivalent form is toxic and binds to sulfhydryl groups

(C) the antidote is dimercaprol

(D) a characteristic basophilic stippling of red blood cells often occurs

(E) tolerance to chronic arsenic poisoning can develop

5. Which of the following statements about lead poisoning is true?

(A) Lead poisoning is the least common cause of heavy metal poisoning

(B) Acute lead poisoning is more common than chronic exposure

(C) The most common route of absorption is through the skin

(D) Footdrop is the most common sign of lead poisoning

(E) A black "lead line" can occur on the gums

6. A comatose patient is brought to the emergency room after taking an overdose of secobarbital. Proper therapy would include all of the following EXCEPT

(A) ventilatory support

(B) frequent monitoring of blood pressure

(C) placement of an intravenous catheter

(D) an emetic agent

(E) monitoring urinary volume

1-B	4-D
2-A	5-E
3-E	6-D

7. A 2-year-old toddler accidentally ingests Drano. All of the following statements are true EXCEPT

(A) alkalies tend to cause more severe injury than acid ingestion
(B) extensive irrigation is indicated
(C) milk as a dilutant is contraindicated
(D) steroid therapy may be effective in the presence of esophageal burns
(E) patients may have respiratory distress

Directions: Each item below contains four suggested answers of which **one or more** is correct. Choose the answer

A   if **1, 2, and 3** are correct
B   if **1 and 3** are correct
C   if **2 and 4** are correct
D   if **4** is correct
E   if **1, 2, 3, and 4** are correct

8. Examples of inert gases that might be considered simple asphyxiants include

(1) nitrogen (N_2)
(2) carbon dioxide (CO_2)
(3) methane (CH_4)
(4) sulfur dioxide (SO_2)

9. True statements concerning the systemic toxicant cyanide include which of the following?

(1) It is a slow-acting poison
(2) It interferes with the cytochrome oxidase system
(3) It does not affect the odor of the breath
(4) It is treated by preventing or reversing the cyanide–ferric ion binding complex

10. Inducing emesis is contraindicated when a child has just swallowed which of the following substances?

(1) Drain cleaner
(2) Lighter fluid
(3) Gasoline
(4) Rubbing alcohol

ANSWERS AND EXPLANATIONS

1. The answer is B *[I C; II B; III B 4 b]*
Acute exposure to a toxic substance is likely to produce different symptoms than are seen with chronic exposure to lower concentrations. Antidotes act by both preventing the absorption and antagonizing the actions of poisons. Certain heavy metals can be dangerous poisons. Activated charcoal is a useful alternative to inducing vomiting with syrup of ipecac when a person has ingested a poison. It adsorbs the poison and delays gastrointestinal absorption.

2. The answer is A *[II A 3 a (3)]*
The inhalation of amyl nitrite and the intravenous administration of sodium nitrite cause the oxidation of hemoglobin to methemoglobin. Methemoglobin competes with cytochrome oxidase for the cyanide ion, allowing the cytochrome oxidase to function in normal oxidative metabolism.

3. The answer is E *[II B 1, 2 c (1) (c)]*
Mercury, like arsenic, binds to sulfhydryl groups on proteins, frequently inactivating those proteins that are enzymes or producing structural damage. Interaction with the ferric ions of the cytochrome oxidase system is the principal mechanism of cyanide damage. Hemoglobin synthesis is disrupted by lead, which causes a microcytic hypochromic anemia. A number of substances can cause methemoglobinemia (e.g., nitrites, nitrates, chlorates, quinones), but mercury is not one of them.

4. The answer is D *[II B 2 a, b (2) (f)]*
Lead arsenate is often used as a household plant-spray pesticide. The trivalent form of arsenic (As^{3-}) is toxic and binds to sulfhydryl groups. Dimercaprol can be used as an antidote because it contains sulfhydryl groups, which compete with sulfhydryl moieties on proteins for arsenic. Tolerance to chronic arsenic poisoning can develop (e.g., in agricultural workers). Basophilic stippling of red blood cells is seen with lead poisoning, not with arsenic poisoning.

5. The answer is E *[II B 2 b (1), (2)]*
Lead poisoning is the most common heavy metal poisoning. Chronic exposure is much more common than acute poisoning. The gastrointestinal and respiratory tracts are the most common routes of absorption. Wristdrop is seen more frequently than footdrop. The black "lead line" often seen on the gums can be missing in a person who practices good dental hygiene.

6. The answer is D *[II C 2]*
Treatment for an overdose of secobarbital, a barbiturate, would focus on maintaining basic life functions, including placement of an intravenous catheter and ventilatory support if indicated. Maintenance of cardiopulmonary stability is of prime importance, and alkalinization of the urine and promotion of diuresis is often beneficial. There are no specific antagonists for barbiturates, and generalized CNS stimulants such as amphetamines are not indicated. Hemodialysis is the most effective means of treating a severe barbiturate overdose. If the patient were conscious, emesis would indeed be indicated, but it should not be used in a comatose patient.

7. The answer is C *[III A 4]*
Milk and water are effective dilutants and can be used as part of an extensive irrigation process in a patient who ingests Drano. Alkalies tend to cause more severe injury than acid ingestion, and steroid therapy may help with esophageal burns. Patients may present with or develop respiratory distress.

8. The answer is A (1, 2, 3) *[II A 1, 2]*
Nitrogen, carbon dioxide, and methane are all examples of simple asphyxiants, which are usually inert gases that cause hypoxia by decreasing the oxygen available to the lungs. Sulfur dioxide can produce asphyxia by irritating the respiratory tract and can be corrosive to the lungs.

9. The answer is C (2, 4) *[II A 3 a]*
Hydrocyanic acid (cyanide) is one of the most rapidly acting poisons. Cyanide anions complex with ferric ions of the cytochrome oxidase system. With systemic toxicity, the patient's breath has a characteristic odor of oil of bitter almond. A combination of inhaled amyl nitrite and intravenous sodium nitrite is used to prevent or reverse the cyanide–ferric ion binding.

10. The answer is A (1, 2, 3) *[III B 3]*
Emesis would be indicated after ingestion of rubbing alcohol. Usually, vomiting should be induced promptly when anyone has swallowed a poison. However, emesis is contraindicated when the poison is a caustic, such as drain cleaner or dishwasher detergent, or a petroleum distillate, such as lighter fluid, gasoline, or kerosene. A caustic can do as much damage coming up as it did going down; it is better to dilute it with water or milk than to make the patient vomit. Petroleum distillates are much more hazardous to the respiratory tract than to the gastrointestinal tract, and emesis is contraindicated because of the risk of aspiration. Instead, milk is given, to dilute the ingested substance and protect the stomach. Emesis is also contraindicated when the patient is comatose or when convulsions are present or imminent.

Comprehensive
Exam

Introduction

One of the least attractive aspects of pursuing an education is the necessity of being examined on what has been learned. Instructors do not like to prepare tests, and students do not like to take them.

However, students are required to take many examinations during their learning careers, and little if any time is spent acquainting them with the positive aspects of tests and with systematic and successful methods for approaching them. Students perceive tests as punitive and sometimes feel that they are merely opportunities for the instructor to discover what the student has forgotten or has never learned. Students need to view tests as opportunities to display their knowledge and to use them as tools for developing prescriptions for further study and learning.

A brief history and discussion of the National Board of Medical Examiners (NBME) examinations [now the United States Medical Licensing Examination (USMLE)] are presented in this introduction, along with ideas concerning psychological preparation for the examinations. Also presented are general considerations and test-taking tips as well as how practice exams can be used as educational tools. (The literature provided by the various examination boards contains detailed information concerning the construction and scoring of specific exams.)

Before the various NBME exams were developed, each state attempted to license physicians through its own procedures. Differences between the quality and testing procedures of the various state examinations resulted in the refusal of some states to recognize the licensure of physicians licensed in other states. This made it difficult for physicians to move freely from one state to another and produced an uneven quality of medical care in the United States.

To remedy this situation, the various state medical boards decided they would be better served if an outside agency prepared standard exams to be given in all states, allowing each state to meet its own needs and have a common standard by which to judge the educational preparation of individuals applying for licensure.

One misconception concerning these outside agencies is that they are licensing authorities. This is not the case; they are examination boards only. The individual states retain the power to grant and revoke licenses. The examination boards are charged with designing and scoring valid and reliable tests. They are primarily concerned with providing the states with feedback on how examinees have performed and with making suggestions about the interpretation and usefulness of scores. The states use this information as partial fulfillment of qualifications upon which they grant licenses.

Students should remember that these exams are administered nationwide and, although the general medical information is similar, educational methodologies and faculty areas of expertise differ from institution to institution. It is unrealistic to expect that students will know all the

The author of this introduction, Michael J. O'Donnell, holds the positions of Assistant Professor of Psychiatry and Director of Biomedical Communications at the University of New Mexico School of Medicine, Albuquerque, New Mexico.

material presented in the exams; they may face questions on the exams in areas that were only superficially covered in their classes. The testing authorities recognize this situation, and their scoring procedures take it into account.

The Exams

The first exam was given in 1916. It was a combination of written, oral, and laboratory tests, and it was administered over a 5-day period. Admission to the exam required proof of completion of medical education and 1 year of internship

In 1922, the examination was changed to a new format and was divided into three parts. Part I, a 3-day essay exam, was given in the basic sciences after 2 years of medical school. Part II, a 2-day exam, was administered shortly before or after graduation, and Part III was taken at the end of the first postgraduate year. To pass both Part I and Part II, a score equalling 75% of the total points available was required.

In 1954, after a 3-year extensive study, the NBME adopted the multiple-choice format. To pass, a statistically computed score of 75 was required, which allowed comparison of test results from year to year. In 1971, this method was changed to one that held the mean constant at a computed score of 500, with a predetermined deviation from the mean to ascertain a passing or failing score. The 1971 changes permitted more sophisticated analysis of test results and allowed schools to compare among individual students within their respective institutions as well as among students nationwide. Feedback to students regarding performance included the reporting of pass or failure along with scores in each of the areas tested.

During the 1980s, the ever-changing field of medicine made it necessary for the NBME to examine once again its evaluation strategies. It was found necessary to develop questions in multidisciplinary areas such as gerontology, health promotion, immunology, and cell and molecular biology. In addition, it was decided that questions should test higher cognitive levels and reasoning skills.

To meet the new goals, many changes have been made in both the form and content of the examination. Changes include reduction in the number of questions to approximately 800 on Step 1 and Step 2 of the USMLE to allow students more time on each question, with total testing time reduced on Step 1 from 13 to 12 hours and on Step 2 from 12.5 to 12 hours. The basic science disciplines are no longer allotted the same number of questions, which permits flexible weighing of the exam areas. Reporting of scores to schools include total scores for individuals and group mean scores for separate discipline areas. Only pass/fail designations and total scores are reported to examinees. There is no longer a provision for the reporting of individual subscores to either the examinees or medical schools. Finally, the question format used in the new exams is predominately multiple-choice, best answer.

The New Format

New question formats, designed specifically for Step 1, are constructed in an effort to test the student's grasp of the sciences basic to medicine in an integrated fashion. The questions are designed to be interdisciplinary. Many of these questions are presented as a vignette, or case study, followed by a series of multiple-choice, best-answer questions.

The scoring of this exam also is altered. Whereas, in the past, the exams were scored on a normal curve, the new exam has a predetermined standard, which must be met in order to pass. The exam no longer concentrates on the trivial; therefore, it has been concluded that there is a common base of information that all medical students should know in order to pass. It is anticipated that a major shift in the pass/fail rate for the nation is unlikely. In the past, the average student could only expect to feel comfortable with half the test and eventually would complete approximately 67% of the questions correctly, to achieve a mean score of 500. Although with the standard setting method it is likely that the mean score will change and become higher, it is unlikely that the pass/fail rates will differ significantly from those in the past. During the first testing in 1991, there was not differential weighing of the questions. However, in the future, the NBME will be researching methods of weighing questions based on both the time it takes to answer questions vis à vis their difficulty and the perceived importance of the information. In addition, the NBME is attempting to design a method of delivering feedback to the student that will have considerable importance in discovering weaknesses and pinpointing areas for further study in the event that a retake is necessary.

Materials Needed for Test Preparation

In preparation for a test, many students collect far too much study material only to find that they simply do not have the time to go through all of it. They are defeated before they begin because either they cannot get through all the material, leaving areas unstudied, or they race through the material so quickly that they cannot benefit from the activity.

It is generally more efficient for the student to use materials already at hand; that is, class notes, one good outline to cover or strengthen areas not locally stressed and for quick review of the whole topic, and one good text as a reference for looking up complex material needing further explanation.

Also, many students attempt to memorize far too much information, rather than learning and understanding less material and then relying on that learned information to determine the answers to questions at the time of the examination. Relying too heavily on memorized material causes anxiety, and the more anxious students become during a test, the less learned knowledge they are likely to use.

Positive Attitude

A positive attitude and a realistic approach are essential to successful test taking. If concentration is placed on the negative aspects of tests or on the potential for failure, anxiety increases and performance decreases. A negative attitude generally develops if the student concentrates on "I must pass" rather than on "I can pass." "What if I fail?" becomes the major factor motivating the student to **run from failure rather than toward success**. This results from placing too much emphasis on scores rather than understanding that scores have only slight relevance to future professional performance.

The score received is only one aspect of test performance. Test performance also indicates the student's ability to use information during evaluation procedures and reveals how this ability might be used in the future. For example, when a patient enters the physician's office with a problem, the physician begins by asking questions, searching for clues, and seeking diagnostic information. Hypotheses are then developed, which will include several potential causes for the problem. Weighing the probabilities, the physician will begin to discard those hypotheses with the least likelihood of being correct. Good differential diagnosis involves the ability to deal with uncertainty, to reduce potential causes to the smallest number, and to use all learned information in arriving at a conclusion.

This same thought process can and should be used in testing situations. It might be termed **paper-and-pencil differential diagnosis**. In each question with five alternatives, of which one is correct, there are four alternatives that are incorrect. If deductive reasoning is used, as in solving a clinical problem, the choices can be viewed as having possibilities of being correct. The elimination of wrong choices increases the odds that a student will be able to recognize the correct choice. Even if the correct choice does not become evident, the probability of guessing correctly increases. Just as differential diagnosis in a clinical setting can result in a correct diagnosis, eliminating incorrect choices on a test can result in choosing the correct answer.

Answering questions based on what is incorrect is difficult for many students since they have had nearly 20 years experience taking tests with the implied assertion that knowledge can be displayed only by knowing what is correct. It must be remembered, however, that students can display knowledge by knowing something is wrong, just as they can display it by knowing something is right. **Students should begin to think in the present as they expect themselves to think in the future.**

Paper-and-Pencil Differential Diagnosis

The technique used to arrive at the answer to the following question is an example of the paper-and-pencil differential diagnosis approach.

> A recently diagnosed case of hypothyroidism in a 45-year-old man may result in which of the following conditions?

(A) Thyrotoxicosis
(B) Cretinism
(C) Myxedema
(D) Graves' disease
(E) Hashimoto's thyroiditis

It is presumed that all of the choices presented in the question are plausible and partially correct. If the student begins by breaking the question into parts and trying to discover what the question is attempting to measure, it will be possible to answer the question correctly by using more than memorized charts concerning thyroid problems.

- The question may be testing if the student knows the difference between "hypo" and "hyper" conditions.
- The answer choices may include thyroid problems that are not "hypothyroid" problems.
- It is possible that one or more of the choices are "hypo" but are not "thyroid" problems, that they are some other endocrine problems.
- "Recently diagnosed in a 45-year-old man" indicates that the correct answer is not a congenital childhood problem.
- "May result in" as opposed to "resulting from" suggests that the choices might include a problem that **causes** hypothyroidism rather than **results from** hypothyroidism, as stated.

By applying this kind of reasoning, the student can see that choice **A**, thyroid toxicosis, which is a disorder resulting from an overactive thyroid gland ("hyper") must be eliminated. Another piece of knowledge, that is, Graves' disease is thyroid toxicosis, eliminates choice **D**. Choice **B**, cretinism, is indeed hypothyroidism, but it is a childhood disorder. Therefore, **B** is eliminated. Choice **E** is an inflammation of the thyroid gland—here the clue is the suffix "itis." The reasoning is that thyroiditis, being an inflammation, may **cause** a thyroid problem, perhaps even a hypothyroid problem, but there is no reason for the reverse to be true. Myxedema, choice **C**, is the only choice left and the obvious correct answer.

Preparing for Board Examinations

1. **Study for yourself.** Although some of the material may seem irrelevant, the more you learn now, the less you will have to learn later. Also, do not let the fear of the test rob you of an important part of your education. If you study to learn, the task is less distasteful than studying solely to pass a test.

2. **Review all areas.** You should not be selective by studying perceived weak areas and ignoring perceived strong areas. This is probably the last time you will have the time and the motivation to review **all** of the basic sciences.

3. **Attempt to understand, not just memorize, the material.** Ask yourself: To whom does the material apply? When does it apply? Where does it apply? How does it apply? Understanding the connections among these points allows for longer retention and aids in those situations when guessing strategies may be needed.

4. **Try to anticipate questions that might appear on the test.** Ask yourself how you might construct a question on a specific topic.

5. **Give yourself a couple days of rest before the test.** Studying up to the last moment will increase your anxiety and cause potential confusion.

Taking Board Examinations

1. In the case of the USMLE, be sure to **pace yourself** to use time optimally. Each booklet is designed to take 2 hours. You should check to be sure that you are halfway through the booklet at the end of the first hour. You should use all your allotted time; if you finish too early, you probably did so by moving too quickly through the test.

2. **Read each question and all the alternatives carefully** before you begin to make decisions. Remember the questions contain clues, as do the answer choices. As a physician, you would not make a clinical decision without a complete examination of all the data; the same holds true for answering test questions.

3. **Read the directions for each question set carefully.** You would be amazed at how many students make mistakes in tests simply because they have not paid close attention to the directions.

4. It is not advisable to leave blanks with the intention of coming back to answer the questions later. Because of the way board examinations are constructed, you probably will not pick up any new information that will help you when you come back, and the chances of getting numerically off on your answer sheet are greater than your chances of benefiting by skipping around. If you feel that you must come back to a question, mark the best choice and place a note in the margin. Generally speaking, it is best not to change answers once you have made a decision, unless you have learned new information. Your intuitive reaction and first response are correct more often than changes made out of frustration or anxiety. **Never turn in an answer sheet with blanks.** Scores are based on the number that you get correct; you are not penalized with incorrect choices.

5. **Do not try to answer the questions on a stimulus–response basis.** It generally will not work. Use all of your learned knowledge.

6. **Do not let anxiety destroy your confidence.** If you have prepared conscientiously, you know enough to pass. Use all that you have learned.

7. **Do not try to determine how well you are doing as you proceed.** You will not be able to make an objective assessment, and your anxiety will increase.

8. **Do not expect a feeling of mastery** or anything close to what you are accustomed. Remember, this is a nationally administered exam, not a mastery test.

9. **Do not become frustrated or angry** about what appear to be bad or difficult questions. You simply do not know the answers; you cannot know everything.

Specific Test-Taking Strategies

Read the entire question carefully, regardless of format. Test questions have multiple parts. Concentrate on picking out the pertinent key words that might help you begin to problem solve. Words such as "always," "all," "never," "mostly," "primarily," and so forth play significant roles. In all types of questions, distractors with terms such as "always" or "never" most often are incorrect. Adjectives and adverbs can completely change the meaning of questions—pay close attention to them. Also, medical prefixes and suffixes (e.g., "hypo-," "hyper-," "-ec-tomy," "-itis") are sometimes at the root of the question. The knowledge and application of everyday English grammar often is the key to dissecting questions.

Multiple-Choice Questions

Read the question and the choices carefully to become familiar with the data as given. Remember, in multiple-choice questions there is one correct answer and there are four distractors, or incorrect answers. (Distractors are plausible and possibly correct or they would not be called distractors.) They are generally correct for part of the question but not for the entire question. Dissecting the question into parts aids in discerning these distractors.

If the correct answer is not immediately evident, begin eliminating the distractors. (Many students feel that they must always start at option A and make a decision before they move to B, thus forcing decisions they are not ready to make.) Your first decisions should be made on those choices you feel the most confident about.

Compare the choices to each part of the question. **To be wrong,** a choice needs to be incorrect for only part of the question. **To be correct,** it must be **totally** correct. If you believe a choice is partially incorrect, tentatively eliminate that choice. Make notes next to the choices regarding tentative decisions. One method is to place a minus sign next to the choices you are certain are incorrect and a plus sign next to those that potentially are correct. Finally, place a zero next to any choice you do not understand or need to come back to for further inspection. Do not feel that you must make final decisions until you have examined all choices carefully.

When you have eliminated as many choices as you can, decide which of those that are left has the highest probability of being correct. Remember to use paper-and-pencil differential diagnosis. Above all, be honest with yourself. If you do not know the answer, eliminate as many choices as possible and choose reasonably.

Vignette-Based Questions

Vignette-based questions are nothing more than normal multiple-choice questions that use the same case, or grouped information, for setting the problem. The NBME has been researching question types that would test the student's grasp of the integrated medical basic sciences in a more cognitively complex fashion than can be accomplished with traditional testing formats. These questions allow the testing of information that is more medically relevant than memorized terminology.

It is important to realize that several questions, although grouped together and referring to one situation or vignette, are independent questions; that is, they are able to stand alone. Your inability to answer one question in a group should have no bearing on your ability to answer subsequent questions.

These are multiple-choice questions, and just as is done with the single best answer questions, you should use the paper-and-pencil differential diagnosis, as was described earlier.

Single Best Answer—Matching Sets

Single best answer—matching sets consist of a list of words or statements followed by several numbered items or statements. Be sure to pay attention to whether the choices can be used more than once, only once, or not at all. Consider each choice individually and carefully. Begin with those with which you are the most familiar. It is important always to break the statements and words into parts, as with all other question formats. **If a choice is only partially correct, then it is incorrect.**

Guessing

Nothing takes the place of a firm knowledge base, but with little information to work with, even after playing paper-and-pencil differential diagnosis, you may find it necessary to guess the correct answer. A few simple rules can help increase your guessing accuracy. Always guess consistently if you have no idea what is correct; that is, after eliminating all that you can, make the choice that agrees with your intuition or choose the option closest to the top of the list that has not been eliminated as a potential answer.

When guessing at questions that have choices in numerical form, you will often find the choices listed in an ascending or descending order. It is generally not wise to guess the first or last alternative, since these are usually extreme values and are most likely incorrect.

Using the USMLE to Learn

All too often, students do not take full advantage of practice exams. There is a tendency to complete the exam, score it, look up the correct answers to those questions missed, and then forget the entire thing.

In fact, great educational benefits can be derived if students would spend more time using practice tests as learning tools. As mentioned earlier, incorrect choices in test questions are plausible and partially correct or they would not fulfill their purpose as distractors. This means that it is just as beneficial to look up the incorrect choices as the correct choices to discover specifically why they are incorrect. In this way, it is possible to learn better test-taking skills as the subtlety of question construction is uncovered.

Additionally, it is advisable to go back and attempt to restructure each question to see if all the choices can be made correct by modifying the question. By doing this, four times as much will be learned. By all means, look up the right answer and explanation. Then, focus on each of the other choices and ask yourself under what conditions they might be correct? For example, the entire thrust of the sample question concerning hypothyroidism could be altered by changing the first few words to read:

> "Hyperthyroidism recently discovered in . . . ."
> "Hypothyroidism prenatally occurring in . . . ."
> "Hypothyroidism resulting from . . . ."

This question can be used to learn and understand thyroid problems in general, not only to memorize answers to specific questions.

In the Comprehensive Exam that follows, every effort has been made to simulate the types of questions and the degree of question difficulty in the USMLE Step 1. While taking this exam, the student should attempt to create the testing conditions that might be experienced during actual testing situations.

Summary

Ideally, examinations are designed to determine how much information students have learned and how that information is used in the successful completion of the examination. Students will be successful if these suggestions are followed:

- Develop a positive attitude and maintain that attitude.
- Be realistic in determining the amount of material you attempt to master and in the score you hope to obtain.
- Read the directions for each type of question and the questions themselves closely and follow the directions carefully.
- Guess intelligently and consistently when guessing strategies must be used.

- Bring the paper-and-pencil differential diagnosis approach to each question in the examination.
- Use the test as an opportunity to display your knowledge and as a tool for developing prescriptions for further study and learning.

The USMLE is not easy. It may be almost impossible for those who have unrealistic expectations or for those who allow misinformation concerning the exam to produce anxiety out of proportion to the task at hand. It is manageable if it is approached with a positive attitude and with consistent use of all the information the student has learned.

Michael J. O'Donnell

STUDY QUESTIONS

Directions: Each of the numbered items or incomplete statements in this section is followed by answers or by completions of the statement. Select the **one** lettered answer or completion that is **best** in each case.

1. All of the following statements about therapeutic iron preparations are true EXCEPT that

(A) ferrous sulfate is the drug of first choice for iron-deficiency anemia
(B) ferrous sulfate contains about 20% elemental iron
(C) adverse effects of ferrous sulfate are often inversely related to the amount of soluble iron in the upper gastrointestinal tract
(D) iron dextran is useful in treating patients with malabsorption syndromes
(E) reticuloendothelial cells phagocytize iron dextran

2. The principles of drug interactions are correctly described by all of the following statements EXCEPT

(A) an interaction occurs whenever the pharmacologic action of a drug is altered by a second substance
(B) clinically important changes that result from interactions are often seen with agents having a low therapeutic index
(C) clinically important changes that result from interactions are often seen with agents having a poorly defined therapeutic endpoint
(D) interactions can often be avoided by using a different drug having the desired pharmacologic effect
(E) no drug interactions result from the use of the H$_2$-receptor antagonist cimetidine

3. A hypertensive crisis might be seen with which of the drug classes listed below?

(A) Tricyclic antidepressants
(B) Barbiturates
(C) Narcotic analgesics
(D) Monoamine oxidase inhibitors
(E) Phenothiazines

4. All of the following statements regarding salicylate preparations are true EXCEPT

(A) sodium salicylate cause less gastric irritation than aspirin
(B) acetyl salicylic acid may cause thrombosis in predisposed individuals
(C) buffered aspirin has a slightly enhanced absorption rate
(D) diflunisal is more potent than aspirin when used in the treatment of osteoarthritis
(E) 5-aminosalicylic acid has poor oral absorption

5. True statements about cimetidine include which of the following?

(A) It is a competitive H$_2$-receptor antagonist
(B) It is useful for the treatment of duodenal ulcers
(C) It is used in the tretment of Zollinger-Ellison syndrome
(D) It causes somnolence
(E) It reduces blood flow in the liver

Questions 6–9

A 29-year-old black man presents to the clinic for a routine examination. His family history is significant for cardiovascular disease, including a father who died of a myocardial infarction at 49 years of age and a grandfather who is presently 70 years old and has severe congestive heart failure. Physical examination is unremarkable except that the patient is 20 pounds heavier than ideal body weight, and his blood pressure is 160/100. Repeat blood pressure evaluation confirms this reading.

6. First line therapy for this patient should be

(A) initiation of captopril therapy
(B) initiation of propranolol therapy
(C) initiation of verapamil therapy
(D) dietary restriction
(E) initiation of hydralazine therapy

1-C	4-B
2-E	5-D
3-D	6-D

7. The recommended therapy made little difference. Which therapy should be tried next?

(A) Reserpine
(B) Dietary restriction
(C) Methyldopa
(D) Thiazide diuretic
(E) Diltiazem

8. Two months later, the patient's blood pressure is 156/98. The physician discontinues previous therapy and initiates therapy with a selective β-blocker, such as

(A) atenolol
(B) propranolol
(C) nadolol
(D) timolol
(E) labetalol

9. One month later, the patient's blood pressure is 140/86. However, the patient reports persistent dizziness. The physician stops the current therapy and initiates therapy that was initially well tolerated but ultimately caused bronchospasm and cough. An agent capable of producing these effects is

(A) methyldopa
(B) captopril
(C) diltiazem
(D) reserpine
(E) propranolol

(end of group question)

10. All of the following statements regarding central dopamine receptors are true EXCEPT

(A) D_1 receptor activation inhibits the adenylate cyclase system
(B) D_2 receptors are inhibitory in some brain tissue
(C) neuroleptic side effects are thought to be mediated through D_2 receptors in the pituitary
(D) D_3 receptors are principally found in the limbic system
(E) D_3 receptors are associated with emotional and cognitive behavior

11. A 67-year-old man is found to have tachypnea, pitting edema, and audible S_3 and S_4 heart sounds. A chest x-ray supports the diagnosis of congestive heart failure. Which of the following is an appropriate diuretic?

(A) Mannitol
(B) Hydrochlorothiazide
(C) Bumetanide
(D) Triamterene
(E) Spironolactone

12. A 55-year-old patient with mild type II diabetes lives half of the time in hotels because his job involves traveling. He has trouble maintaining a suitable diet with restaurant meals and cannot take insulin easily because of sterilization problems. All of the following agents could be tried in this patient EXCEPT

(A) acetohexamide
(B) chlorpropamide
(C) glyburide
(D) sulfanilamide
(E) tolbutamide

13. Which of the following drugs, if given concomitantly with warfarin, would require an increase in warfarin dosage?

(A) Aspirin
(B) Barbiturates
(C) Disulfiram
(D) Phenylbutazone
(E) Trimethoprim-sulfamethoxazole

14. Pharmacologic effects of the classic antihistamines (H_1-receptor antagonists) include all of the following EXCEPT

(A) sedation with low doses
(B) convulsions with high doses
(C) useful for the treatment of motion sickness
(D) inhibition of gastric acid secretion
(E) an antipruritic effect

7-D   10-A   13-B
8-A   11-C   14-D
9-B   12-D

15. Oral contraceptives containing an estrogen and norethindrone act mainly by which of the following mechanisms?

(A) Speeding up the growth of ovarian follicles
(B) Increasing the secretion of follicle-stimulating hormone
(C) Hastening the release of luteinizing hormone
(D) Suppressing ovulation
(E) Thickening the consistency of the cervical mucus

16. Which antineoplastic drug acts during a specific phase of the cell cycle?

(A) Methotrexate
(B) 5-Fluorouracil
(C) Mechlorethamine
(D) Cyclophosphamide
(E) Melphalan

17. A young woman presents with candidal vaginitis. Her past medical history reveals that she has just completed a 10-day course of antibiotic therapy for streptococcal pharyngitis. Antibiotics capable of producing this untoward effect include all of the following EXCEPT

(A) amoxicillin
(B) ampicillin
(C) cefaclor
(D) cephalexin
(E) erythromycin

18. Drugs that are likely to aggravate bronchial asthma include all of the following EXCEPT

(A) morphine
(B) tubocurarine
(C) propranolol
(D) amphetamine
(E) meperidine

19. Correct statements concerning vitamin B_{12} deficiency include all of the following EXCEPT

(A) it can be caused by intrinsic factor deficiency
(B) dietary vitamin B_{12} deficiency is uncommon
(C) pernicious anemia requires parenteral vitamin B_{12} therapy
(D) vitamin B_{12} will reverse the neurologic changes of pernicious anemia

20. Disadvantages of alimentary administration include all of the following EXCEPT

(A) the rate of absorption is variable
(B) irritation of the mucosal surfaces can occur
(C) the compliance of the patient is not ensured
(D) it is the least safe route of administration
(E) hepatic metabolism may occur before the drug reaches its site of action

21. Tamoxifen induces the most favorable response in which of the following forms of cancer?

(A) Estrogen receptor-rich breast cancer
(B) Testicular cancer
(C) Ovarian cancer
(D) Cervical cancer
(E) Kaposi's sarcoma

22. Substances that act as inhibitors of the mixed-function oxygenase system include all of the following EXCEPT

(A) carbon monoxide
(B) cimetidine
(C) carbon tetrachloride
(D) organophosphorous insecticides
(E) phenobarbital

23. In patients with congestive heart failure, digitalis glycosides are used because they produce a positive inotropic effect that can best be defined as an increase in

(A) the force of myocardial contraction
(B) cardiac filling pressure
(C) the heart rate
(D) venous pressure
(E) cardiac conduction velocity

24. A patient complaining of abnormal movements is found to have a parkinsonian tremor and tardive dyskinesia. Chronic use of which of the following drugs would cause these symptoms?

(A) Flurazepam
(B) Codeine
(C) Chloral hydrate
(D) Triflupromazine
(E) Carbamazepine

15-D	18-D	21-A	24-D
16-A	19-D	22-E	
17-E	20-D	23-A	

25. Characteristics of aspirin include all of the following EXCEPT

(A) its analgesic, antipyretic, and anti-inflammatory actions are due to inhibition of prostaglandin synthesis
(B) toxic doses are capable of producing respiratory and metabolic acidosis
(C) it can increase mean bleeding time
(D) excretion can be increased by alkalinizing urine
(E) low doses increase urate excretion

26. Which of the following agents is a selective B_1-adrenergic antagonist that is also available as a topical formulation for the treatment of glaucoma?

(A) Betaxolol
(B) Carteolol
(C) Labetalol
(D) Nadolol
(E) Timolol

27. All of the following drugs are correctly matched with a form of cancer that they are used to treat EXCEPT

(A) busulfan—colon cancer
(B) cisplatin—testicular cancer
(C) cyclophosphamide—Hodgkin's disease
(D) 5-fluorouracil—breast cancer
(E) methotrexate—lymphoblastic leukemia

28. Synonyms for sympathetic antagonists include all of the following EXCEPT

(A) adrenergic blocking agents
(B) antiadrenergic agents
(C) sympatholytics
(D) cholinomimetics

29. Aspirin, phenylbutazone, and sulfamethoxazole have all of the following characteristics in common EXCEPT

(A) they are all highly protein bound
(B) they can all cause agranulocytosis
(C) they all interact with warfarin
(D) they can all affect platelet function
(E) they all cause hypersensitivity reactions

30. A 3-month-old infant is brought to the emergency room with seizures of the tonic–clonic type. His mother reports that these seizures have been occurring for the past 50 minutes. The treatment of choice is

(A) a benzodiazepine
(B) a barbiturate
(C) phenytoin
(D) carbamazepine
(E) valproate

31. All of the following statements about the therapeutic index (TI) are true EXCEPT

(A) it is used to evaluate the safety of a drug
(B) a low TI indicates that the drug is dangerous to use therapeutically
(C) a high TI indicates that the ED_{50} far exceeds the LD_{50}
(D) aspirin has a high TI
(E) the TI may be a less useful indicator than the standard margin of safety

32. A patient who is being treated for hypertension, recurrent ventricular tachycardia, and congestive heart failure presents with anorexia, nausea, and color vision changes. Discontinuation of which of the following agents will most likely improve these adverse effects?

(A) Disopyramide
(B) Procainamide
(C) Clonidine
(D) Digoxin
(E) Enalapril

33. Characteristics of ergot alkaloids include all of the following EXCEPT

(A) they stimulate smooth muscle
(B) they are agonists at tryptamine receptors
(C) they show central nervous system stimulating effects
(D) they can produce vasoconstriction
(E) they can be blocked by propranolol

25-E	28-D	31-C
26-A	29-B	32-D
27-A	30-B	33-E

34. A 47-year-old man suffers from chronic anemia secondary to chronic renal failure; thus treatment with erythropoietin is indicated. All of the following statements about erythropoietin are true EXCEPT

(A) erythropoietin administration could decrease the need for transfusion
(B) erythropoietin would also be excellent to correct acute severe anemia
(C) erythropoietin works by stimulating the proliferation of immature erythroid progenitor cells
(D) erythropoietin cannot be administered orally
(E) erythropoietin's pharmacokinetics are not affected by dialysis

35. A patient who recently had prostate surgery develops a urinary tract infection. *Pseudomonas aeruginosa* is cultured. Suitable therapy would include all of the following agents EXCEPT

(A) amoxicillin and clavulanate
(B) aztreonam
(C) ceftazidime
(D) ciprofloxacin
(E) tobramycin

36. All of the following statements about procaine are true EXCEPT that

(A) it is nonaddictive
(B) it is nontoxic in the normal dose range
(C) it has a short duration of action
(D) it is active topically
(E) it is metabolized in the blood

37. Metoclopramide can be used to treat all of the following conditions EXCEPT

(A) diabetic gastroparesis
(B) chemotherapy-induced vomiting
(C) gastroesophageal reflux disease
(D) peptic ulcer disease
(E) radiation-induced vomiting

Questions 38 and 39

A 10-year-old boy is admitted to the hospital with an initial diagnosis of acute lymphoblastic leukemia. His liver, spleen, and lymph nodes are extensively infiltrated.

38. Which of the following drug combinations would be most appropriate for inducing remission?

(A) Prednisone and vincristine
(B) Cyclophosphamide and methotrexate
(C) Cyclophosphamide and vinblastine
(D) 6-Mercaptopurine and methotrexate
(E) Cytarabine and 5-fluorouracil

39. The patient is given allopurinol to reduce the complications of his cancer chemotherapy. The rationale underlying the allopurinol therapy is that

(A) allopurinol increases the renal clearance of uric acid
(B) the most effective therapeutic regimens interfere with purine biosynthesis
(C) rapid lympholysis produces large quantities of uric acid
(D) lower doses of the remission-inducing drugs can be given
(E) allopurinol inhibits the metabolism of pyrimidine analogs

(end of group question)

40. A postmenopausal woman presents with a breast carcinoma that is rich in estrogen receptors. The drug most likely to be administered is

(A) bleomycin
(B) vinblastine
(C) mitomycin
(D) dacarbazine
(E) tamoxifen

41. Diisopropyl fluorophosphate increases all of the following effects EXCEPT

(A) lacrimation
(B) bronchodilation
(C) salivation
(D) muscle twitching
(E) muscle weakness

34-B	37-D	40-E
35-A	38-A	41-B
36-D	39-C	

42. A patient with arthritis presents with a sore throat, fever, and dependent edema. The patient had been in good health previously. A complete blood count reveals a white cell count of 500 (normal = 5000–8000). A drug capable of causing this effect is

(A) aspirin
(B) indomethacin
(C) sulindac
(D) phenylbutazone
(E) diclofenac

43. Monoamine oxidase inhibitors can be used concurrently with all of the following agents EXCEPT

(A) α-adrenergic blocking agents
(B) aspirin
(C) sulfonamide antibiotics
(D) tricyclic antidepressants
(E) flurazepam

44. Isoniazid is the most widely used agent in the treatment of tuberculosis. True statements regarding this agent include all of the following EXCEPT

(A) it is used in conjunction with other agents in the treatment of tuberculosis
(B) its metabolism is partly under genetic control
(C) it is ineffective against many atypical mycobacteria
(D) it can be administered as a prophylactic agent to children or young adults who have converted from a tuberculin-negative to tuberculin-positive skin test
(E) fast acetylators have a higher concentration of free isoniazid

45. Therapeutic uses for propranolol include all of the following EXCEPT

(A) atrial fibrillation
(B) atrial flutter
(C) paroxysmal atrial tachycardia
(D) ventricular arrhythmias
(E) low-output congestive heart failure

46. Characteristics of adrenergic receptors include all of the following EXCEPT

(A) nonselective β-receptor blocking agents are not yet available
(B) β_1-adrenergic receptors predominate in cardiac tissue
(C) β_1-adrenergic receptors are found in smooth muscle
(D) α_2-adrenergic receptors mediate presynaptic feedback inhibition
(E) α_1-adrenergic receptors are found at postsynaptic effector sites

47. All of the following anesthetic drugs and descriptions are correctly matched EXCEPT

(A) lidocaine—an ester but metabolized in the liver
(B) mepivacaine—an amide metabolized in the liver
(C) procaine—a short-acting local anesthetic that lacks topical activity
(D) tetracaine—a good spinal anesthetic
(E) bupivacaine—in certain situations a duration of action that can exceed 24 hours

48. The response to a dose of an oral anticoagulant is often changed by concomitant administration of other drugs, which affect the dose–response by different mechanisms. True statements about such drugs and their mechanisms include all of the following EXCEPT

(A) phenylbutazone impairs platelet aggregation
(B) phenobarbital induces the drug microsomal metabolizing system
(C) acetylsalicylic acid impairs platelet aggregation
(D) glutethimide inhibits the drug microsomal metabolizing system
(E) cimetidine inhibits the drug microsomal metabolizing system

---

42-D   45-E   48-D
43-D   46-A
44-E   47-A

49. Agents that produce neuromuscular blockade act by inhibiting which of the following events?

(A) Synthesis of acetylcholine from acetyl coenzyme A and choline
(B) Release of acetylcholine from the prejunctional membrane
(C) Packaging of acetylcholine into synaptic vesicles
(D) Interaction of acetylcholine with cholinergic receptors
(E) Re-uptake of acetylcholine into the nerve ending

50. Which cancer chemotherapeutic agent could be used for a patient with rheumatoid arthritis who did not respond to nonsteroidal anti-inflammatory agents?

(A) Cyclophosphamide
(B) Pentostatin
(C) Cytarabine
(D) Methotrexate
(E) Doxorubicin

51. Which of the following antibiotics should be administered to a patient whose renal function is severely compromised?

(A) Erythromycin
(B) Tobramycin
(C) Piperacillin
(D) Cefazolin
(E) Norfloxacin

52. Terfenadine and astemizole differ by which important property when compared to classical antihistamines?

(A) They are ineffective for the treatment of seasonal rhinitis
(B) They produce less sedation
(C) They are available for topical use
(D) They have greater adverse anticholinergic effects
(E) They have very short half-lives

53. Which of the following statements best characterizes potentiation?

(A) Potentiation occurs if a drug lacking an effect of its own increases the effect of a second, active drug
(B) Potentiation occurs if two drugs with the same effect, when given together, produce an effect that is equal in magnitude to the sum of the effects when the drugs are given individually
(C) Potentiation occurs if two drugs with the same effect, when given together, produce an effect that is greater in magnitude than the sum of the effects when the drugs are given individually
(D) Potentiation occurs if two drugs with the same effect, when given together, produce an effect that is equal in magnitude to the effect of each drug given alone
(E) None of the above statements correctly characterizes potentiation

54. The use of "replacement" hormones or their antagonists can be of medical benefit. Which benefit is incorrectly matched to the hormone?

(A) Estrogen—relieves atrophic vaginitis after menopause
(B) Progestins—can be used in the treatment of prostate carcinoma
(C) Clomiphene—a nonsteroidal partial antagonist, induces ovulation
(D) Human menopausal gonadotropin is useful in women who do not respond to clomiphene
(E) Androgens—replacement therapy in women with hyperpituitarism

55. Enalopril is an antihypertensive agent that acts by competitive inhibition of angiotensin converting enzyme. Properties of enalopril include all of the following EXCEPT

(A) it reduces total peripheral resistance and mean arterial pressure
(B) it is used alone and in combination therapy
(C) by inhibiting angiotensin II production, it decreases renin secretion
(D) its blood pressure–lowering effects appear to be additive with thiazide diuretics
(E) it has a longer duration of action than captopril

49-D   52-B   55-C
50-D   53-A
51-A   54-E

56. An 18-year-old woman presents with urgency, frequency, and burning urination. She is afebrile. Urinalysis reveals the presence of red blood cells. Appropriate therapy after urine culture would include which of the following agents?

(A) Aztreonam
(B) Carbenicillin
(C) Gentamicin
(D) Trimethoprim-sulfamethoxazole

57. A patient with renal failure is to undergo abdominal surgery. Which competitive neuromuscular blocking agent could be used in this patient as an adjunct to the surgery?

(A) Pipercuronium
(B) Gallamine
(C) Atracurium
(D) Succinylcholine
(E) Decamethonium

58. The following pairs consist of a chelating agent (i.e., an agent used to treat heavy metal poisoning) and a heavy metal. Which pair is correctly matched?

(A) Dimercaprol—iron
(B) Calcium disodium EDTA—arsenic
(C) Penicillamine—copper
(D) Deferoxamine—lead

59. Pharmacologic doses of glucocorticoids can result in all of the following effects EXCEPT

(A) stimulation of leukocyte migration
(B) stabilization of lysosomal membranes
(C) reduced activity of fibroblasts
(D) reversal of a histamine-stimulated increase in capillary permeability
(E) inhibited antibody synthesis

60. A patient with progressive rheumatoid arthritis is no longer benefiting from the administration of nonsteroidal anti-inflammatory agents, and auranofin is prescribed. All of the following statements about auranofin are true EXCEPT

(A) it may be somewhat less effective than injectable gold for the treatment of rheumatoid arthritis
(B) it is more likely to cause renal or mucocutaneous toxicity than injectable gold
(C) a high incidence of diarrhea is associated with its use
(D) eosinophilia and proteinuria often occur with its use
(E) cutaneous reactions are often seen

61. Allopurinol is most likely to potentiate the pharmacologic action of

(A) 5-fluorouracil
(B) bleomycin
(C) 6-mercaptopurine
(D) doxorubicin
(E) methotrexate

62. A 57-year-old farmer of Swedish descent presents with several hard, gray lesions on his nose. After suitable diagnostic studies, a topical preparation is prescribed, which is most likely to contain

(A) cisplatin
(B) mercaptopurine
(C) vincristine
(D) 5-fluorouracil
(E) mitotane

63. The diuretic of choice for a patient receiving the nephrotoxic antitumor agent cisplatin is

(A) ethacrynic acid
(B) mercaptomerin
(C) acetazolamide
(D) chlorothiazide
(E) mannitol

56-D   59-A   62-D
57-C   60-B   63-E
58-C   61-C

64. Adverse effects of cardiac glycosides include all of the following EXCEPT

(A) they have a low margin of safety
(B) intoxication is often precipitated by the depletion of Na^+
(C) they can cause vision changes
(D) decreased renal function can predispose to toxicity
(E) they can cause ventricular tachycardia

65. A teenager overdoses on heroin. In the emergency room, the patient's blood pressure is 100/60, but his respiratory rate is 4/min, and he is comatose. Which of the following would be most important to this patient's management?

(A) Syrup of ipecac
(B) Direct respiratory stimulant
(C) Pharmacologic antagonist (e.g., naltrexone)
(D) Use of a cathartic
(E) Gastric lavage

66. A 62-year-old patient who is known to have glaucoma is scheduled for a cholecystectomy. Which neuromuscular blocking agent is contraindicated?

(A) Tubocurarine
(B) Pancuronium
(C) Succinylcholine
(D) Gallamine
(E) Metocurine

67. A patient being treated for endogenous depression also has an obsessive–compulsive disorder. The psychiatrist treats the patient with an agent that is a selective inhibitor of serotonin reuptake in the central nervous system. This agent is most apt to be

(A) bupropion
(B) fluoxetine
(C) tranylcypromine
(D) amitriptyline
(E) deprenyl

68. A diabetic patient presents with cough, hemoptysis, and a single shaking chill. His temperature is 101° F, and a chest x-ray demonstrates lobar pneumonia. Gram staining reveals gram-positive diplococci. Correct therapy would be to administer

(A) gentamicin
(B) penicillin G
(C) carbenicillin and gentamicin
(D) ampicillin
(E) ciprofloxacin

69. Each of the following antiarrhythmic agents is correctly matched with an appropriate adverse effect EXCEPT

(A) quinidine—cinchonism
(B) procainamide—hypotension with intravenous administration
(C) lidocaine—systemic lupus erythematosus–like syndrome
(D) disopyramide—untoward anticholinergic effects
(E) flecainide—excessive mortality and nonfatal cardiac arrest

70. A 67-year-old man with acute pulmonary coccidioidomycosis. Proper therapy includes

(A) high doses of penicillin G
(B) griseofulvin
(C) flucytosine
(D) amphotericin B
(E) pentamidine

71. A teenaged girl presents with a pruritic dermatitis on her earlobes. The cause is found to be a recently purchased set of earrings. She should be advised to avoid jewelry containing which of the following metals?

(A) Gold
(B) Nickel
(C) Platinum
(D) Silver
(E) Zinc

64-B	67-B	70-D
65-C	68-B	71-B
66-C	69-C	

72. Which of the following agents used to treat gout could actually increase the frequency of acute gouty attacks during initial therapy?

(A) Sulfinpyrazone
(B) Allopurinol
(C) Colchicine
(D) Probenecid
(E) Indomethacin

73. Fluconazole is emerging as an important systemic antifungal agent. Reasons for this include all of the following EXCEPT

(A) when administered orally, it is highly bioavailable
(B) its mechanism of action is unique in that it does not block the synthesis of ergosterol
(C) it is active against acquired immune deficiency syndrome–related *Cryptococcus neoformans*
(D) it penetrates the blood–brain barrier
(E) it is less toxic than amphotericin B

74. All of the following points should be kept in mind when considering long-term corticosteroid therapy EXCEPT

(A) abrupt withdrawal may cause signs of adrenal insufficiency
(B) therapy may precipitate peptic ulcers
(C) patients may become intolerant to stressful situations for as long as 1 year after therapy is stopped
(D) therapy may lead to increased infections
(E) hypoglycemia is an adverse effect

75. Quinidine can produce all of the following effects on the heart EXCEPT

(A) a reduction in the maximal rate of rise ($\dot{V}_{max}$) of depolarization
(B) an increase in the effective refractory period
(C) a decrease in automaticity
(D) an increase in inotropic action
(E) a decrease in conduction velocity

76. The thrombolytic agent streptokinase has all of the following properties EXCEPT

(A) it is obtained from group C β-hemolytic streptococci
(B) it can produce significant hypertension, especially on reperfusion
(C) it has been used to treat acute pulmonary embolism
(D) it stimulates the conversion of endogenous plasminogen to plasmin
(E) it can produce gastrointestinal bleeding in 5%–10% of patients

77. A patient with severe hypertension is being treated with an agent that stimulates presynaptic α_2 receptors in the vasomotor center of the brain. The patient might be taking

(A) guanethidine
(B) reserpine
(C) clonidine
(D) prazosin
(E) minoxidil

78. Pairs of compounds with opposing effects on blood glucose concentrations include all of the following EXCEPT

(A) tolbutamide and diazoxide
(B) insulin and cortisol
(C) insulin and glucagon
(D) glucagon and isoproterenol
(E) glucagon and propranolol

79. A 67-year-old man is started on warfarin sodium therapy for the prophylactic treatment of venous thrombosis. The patient asks for full disclosure of possible adverse effects. All of the following drugs or adverse effects are correctly matched with causes or results EXCEPT

(A) major bleeding—2% of patients treated
(B) warfarin necrosis—occurs 3–10 days after initiation of therapy
(C) purple toe syndrome—caused by venous emboli
(D) cimetidine—increases anticoagulant action
(E) phenobarbital—decreases anticoagulant action

72-B	75-D	78-D
73-B	76-B	79-C
74-E	77-C	

80. The pharmacologic actions of scopolamine most closely resemble those of

(A) hexamethonium
(B) atropine
(C) succinylcholine
(D) acetylcholine
(E) curare

Directions: Each group of items in this section consists of lettered options followed by a set of numbered items. For each item, select the **one** lettered option that is most closely associated with it. Each lettered option may be selected once, more than once, or not at all.

Questions 81–85

For each clinical condition, select the drug that is most likely to be used in its management.

(A) Carmustine
(B) Cyclophosphamide
(C) Dacarbazine
(D) Methotrexate
(E) Mitotane

81. Adrenal carcinoma

82. Brain tumor

83. Malignant melanoma

84. Psoriasis

85. Renal transplants

Questions 86–89

Disease-modifying antirheumatic agents can be used in conjunction with a nonsteroidal anti-inflammatory drug regimen to treat rheumatoid arthritis. For each description that follows, select the drug that it best describes.

(A) Aurothioglucose
(B) Hydroxychloroquine
(C) Cyclophosphamide
(D) Penicillamine
(E) Azathioprine

86. Immunosuppressive drug that rarely causes severe toxicity with the dosage used for rheumatoid arthritis

87. In high doses, can be effective in patients with refractory rheumatoid arthritis but is highly toxic and teratogenic

88. Can produce irreversible retinal damage as a result of ocular deposition

89. Chrysotherapy that has fewer cutaneous adverse effects than gold thiomalate

80-B	83-C	86-E	89-A
81-E	84-D	87-D	
82-A	85-B	88-B	

Questions 90–94

Barbiturates can be involved in drug interactions with many other drugs. For each drug listed below, select the mechanism that is the most likely cause of an interaction with a barbiturate.

(A) Incompatibility in vitro
(B) Induction of microsomal enzymes
(C) Inhibition of nonmicrosomal enzymes
(D) Enhancement of pharmacologic effects
(E) Interference with renal excretion

90. Warfarin

91. Dextran

92. Tranylcypromine

93. Digitoxin

94. Phenothiazines

Questions 95–98

Match each of the following autacoid antagonists to the enzyme that it inhibits.

(A) Cyclooxygenase
(B) Peptidyl dipeptidase
(C) Phospholipase A_2
(D) Thromboxane synthetase
(E) Cystathionine synthetase

95. Captopril

96. Hydralazine

97. Ibuprofen

98. Prednisolone

Questions 99–102

For each of the following descriptions of drug actions, select the agent with which it is most likely to be associated.

(A) Phenylephrine
(B) Amphetamine
(C) Diisopropyl fluorophosphate
(D) Neostigmine
(E) Methacholine

99. Purely muscarinic in its action

100. Irreversible cholinesterase inhibitor

101. Closely resembles norepinephrine in its cardiovascular actions

102. Enzyme inhibitor as well as receptor agonist

Questions 103–105

Match each statement about drug action with the drug that is most likely to be associated with it.

(A) Cyclophosphamide
(B) 5-Fluorouracil
(C) Cytarabine
(D) Vincristine
(E) Mitomycin

103. In addition to being a natural product, this drug is an alkylating agent because it is reduced intracellularly and alkylates DNA.

104. This drug inhibits DNA polymerase and can be incorporated into DNA and RNA.

105. This drug is a phase-specific agent, producing metaphase arrest.

90-B	93-B	96-D	99-E	102-D	105-D
91-A	94-D	97-A	100-C	103-E	
92-C	95-B	98-C	101-A	104-C	

Questions 106–110

For each diuretic agent that follows, select its major mechanism of action.

(A) Inhibits carbonic anhydrase
(B) Inhibits electrolyte reabsorption in the ascending limb of the loop of Henle
(C) Competitively antagonizes aldosterone
(D) Binds to sulfhydryl enzymes
(E) Inhibits active Na^+ secretion, decreasing K^+ excretion in the distal nephron

106. Ethacrynic acid

107. Spironolactone

108. Chlorothiazide

109. Acetazolamide

110. Triamterene

Questions 111–114

Match each description that follows with the anti-infective agent most likely to be associated with it.

(A) Clindamycin
(B) Gentamicin
(C) Nafcillin
(D) Tetracycline
(E) Rifampin

111. This agent is very effective in the treatment of *Chlamydia* infections.

112. This agent is often administered along with isoniazid and ethambutol.

113. This agent is the drug of choice for *Bacteroides fragilis* infection.

114. This agent is poorly absorbed orally because it is polycationic.

Questions 115–117

Match the correct propionic acid derivative with the statement that best describes it.

(A) Ibuprofen
(B) Naproxen
(C) Fenoprofen
(D) Ketoprofen
(E) Flubiprofen

115. A more effective analgesic than aspirin, it is available "over the counter" in low doses.

116. When treated concurrently with methotrexate, the patient can develop life-threatening hepatotoxicity.

117. It is available in ophthalmic dosage form for the treatment of postoperative meiosis.

106-B	109-A	112-E	115-A
107-C	110-E	113-A	116-D
108-B	111-D	114-B	117-E

ANSWERS AND EXPLANATIONS

1. The answer is C *[Ch 7 I C, D]*
Ferrous sulfate, which contains 20% elemental iron, is the drug of first choice for iron-deficiency anemia. The adverse effects seen with ferrous sulfate are directly, not inversely, related to the amount of soluble iron in the upper gastrointestinal tract. Iron dextran, which is parenterally administered, is useful in patients with malabsorption syndromes. The iron is split off from the sugar molecule of iron dextran by phagocytization in the reticuloendothelial cells.

2. The answer is E *[Ch 8 IV A 2 a; Ch 13 I A, B]*
Interactions occur whenever the pharmacologic action of a drug is altered by a second substance. They often can be avoided by using a different drug having the desired pharmacologic effect. Clinically important changes that result from drug interactions often are seen with agents that have either a low therapeutic index or a poorly defined therapeutic endpoint. Cimetidine is safe, but it inhibits the activity of the cytochrome P-450 system, thereby slowing the metabolism of many drugs that are substrates for hepatic mixed-function oxidases.

3. The answer is D *[Ch 3 VII B 2 d (2) (b)]*
Tricyclic antidepressants, barbiturates, narcotic analgesics, and phenothiazines can be associated with hypotension, not hypertension. Monoamine oxidase inhibitors can interact with sympathomimetic amines, especially indirectly acting ones (e.g., amphetamine, tyramine), and with certain foods (e.g., cheese, beer), which have a high tyramine content. Catecholamines are released from nerve terminals, producing the hypertensive crisis.

4. The answer is B *[Ch 9 II A 3 h (2) 5, a–e]*
Acetyl salicylic acid prolongs bleeding time. It can acetylate and inactivate the platelet cyclooxygenase system when administered in appropriate doses. All of the other statements in the question are true.

5. The answer is D *[Ch 8 V A 2 a]*
Cimetidine is the prototype H_2-receptor antagonist. It is used in the treatment of duodenal ulcers and hypersecretory states such as the Zollinger-Ellison syndrome. The H_2 blockers are not sedating and would not cause somnolence, in contrast to H_1 blockers. Because cimetidine reduces liver blood flow, it can markedly decrease the hepatic clearance of drugs whose metabolism is dependent on liver blood flow.

6–9. The answers are: 6-D *[Ch 5 IV A 1, 2]*, **7-D** *[Ch 5 IV A 2, B 1]*, **8-A** *[Ch 5 IV C 3 a]*, **9-B** *[Ch 5 IV 1 1 g (6), (7)]*
Because the patient described in the question did not have severe hypertension and the physical examination was unremarkable, dietary restriction was indicated. However, the patient was told to return for a checkup in 1 month.

After 1 month, no perceptible difference was seen in the blood pressure reading. First-line therapy for black hypertensive men should include thiazide diuretics. In general, black individuals respond better to volume loss as opposed to β-blockers, but this is a generalization.

After 2 months of thiazide diuretics, the patient was switched to atenolol. In low doses, the only cardioselective β blocker listed is atenolol. All of the other agents are nonselective.

One month later, the blood pressure is 140/86; however, the patient reports feeling dizzy. The physician stops the atenolol and initiates captopril, which was initially well tolerated but ultimately caused cough and bronchospasm. Captopril is a competitive inhibitor of peptidyl dipeptidase, an angiotensin-converting enzyme, which is finding increased use for the treatment of mild to moderate hypertension.

10. The answer is A *[Ch 2 II C 3]*
All of the statements in the question are true except that the central D_1 receptor is excitatory and directly activates the adenylate cyclase system.

11. The answer is C *[Ch 6 VII C 3]*
A rapid-acting, potent "loop" diuretic is needed in a patient presenting with acute congestive heart failure. Bumetanide is such a diuretic. Neither mannitol, hydrochlorothiazide, triamterene, nor spironolactone would give the immediate diuretic response that is needed.

12. The answer is D *[Ch 10 V B, C; Ch 12 II A]*
The patient in the question is a candidate for therapy with an oral hypoglycemic agent. These drugs, the sulfonylureas, are used to treat non–insulin-dependent (type II) diabetes in patients who cannot be treated by dietary control or insulin therapy. Sulfanilamide is one of the sulfonamides, which are antimicrobial agents. The sulfonylureas were developed in the 1940s after the discovery that some sulfonamide drugs had a hypoglycemic effect. Today's antimicrobial sulfonamides are not likely to cause hypoglycemia, but they may increase the hypoglycemic effects of the sulfonylureas.

13. The answer is B *[Ch 7 IV B 3; Table 7-1]*
Warfarin, a coumarin-derived anticoagulant, acts by interfering with the vitamin K–dependent synthesis of active coagulation factors II, VII, IX, and X. Disulfiram, aspirin, trimethoprim-sulfamethoxazole, and phenylbutazone increase the response to warfarin and other oral anticoagulants, and thus, their use would probably require a reduction in warfarin dosage. Disulfiram affects warfarin activity by prolonging the half-life of levowarfarin, and this effect increases hypoprothrombinemia. Aspirin and phenylbutazone both impair platelet aggregation. Barbiturates and glutethimide have the reverse effects on anticoagulation. These drugs reduce the response to warfarin and, thus, would probably require an increase in warfarin dosage, because they induce the hepatic enzyme system that increases drug metabolism.

14. The answer is D *[Ch 8 V A 1 d, e, g]*
All of the pharmacologic effects listed in the question, with the exception of inhibition of gastric acid secretion, are associated with the classic antihistamines (H_1-receptor antagonists). They are used prophylactically for motion sickness and for vestibular disturbances, such as Meniere's disease. Overdosage can lead to convulsions, while low (therapeutic) doses cause sedation. The principal pharmacologic effect of the H_2-receptor antagonists, not the H_1-receptor antagonists, is to inhibit histamine-stimulated gastric acid secretion.

15. The answer is D *[Ch 10 III D 2 a (1) (c)]*
Oral contraceptives that combine an estrogen and a progestin act by blocking the surge of luteinizing hormone (LH) and folllicle-stimulating hormone (FSH) that normally occurs in the middle of the menstrual cycle. In this way, they suppress ovulation and ovarian follicle growth. The "minipill," which contains progestin alone, acts by thickening the consistency of the cervical mucus, forming a barrier to the entry of sperm.

16. The answer is A *[Ch 11 I C 3; II B 2 c; III B 1 d, D 1 b (5)]*
Methotrexate acts during the DNA synthetic phase of the cell cycle. Although 5-fluorouracil is proliferation-dependent, it is phase-nonspecific, perhaps due to its RNA actions. Alkylating agents, such as mechlorethamine, cyclophosphamide, or melphalan, are not phase-specific.

17. The answer is E *[Ch 12 I C; II B 2 f (5), i (2) (d), F 7 a]*
All of the antibiotics listed in the question with the exception of erythromycin (i.e., amoxicillin, ampicillin, cefaclor, cephalexin) are broad-spectrum agents and, therefore, can produce fungal superinfections. Local application of an appropriate antifungal agent is often sufficient therapy for the treatment of a fungal vaginitis.

18. The answer is D *[Ch 2 II G; III B 1 d (3); VIII D 3; Ch 3 VIII A; IX B 1 b, 4, C 1 d]*
Morphine, merperidine, and tubocurarine are capable of releasing histamine and, thus, aggravate bronchial asthma. Since propranolol is a nonselective β-adrenergic blocker, it too can aggravate bronchial asthma. Amphetamine, being a sympathomimetic agent, does not aggravate bronchial asthma.

19. The answer is D *[Ch 7 II C 2, 4]*
Vitamin B_{12} is so prevalent in foodstuffs from animal sources that a dietary deficiency of the vitamin is very uncommon. The usual cause of vitamin B_{12} deficiency is a lack of intrinsic factor, as occurs in pernicious anemia and following gastrectomy. In such cases, parenteral vitamin B_{12} therapy is given, because oral B_{12} alone will not be absorbed, and oral combinations of vitamin B_{12} plus intrinsic factor are too unreliable. Antibodies to intrinsic factor can develop, preventing absorption of the vitamin; also, patients can eventually become refractory to oral intrinsic factor. Because the neurologic damage that results from vitamin B_{12} deficiency is **not** reversible, prompt, adequate therapy with parenteral vitamin B_{12} is important, to prevent further neurologic damage from occurring.

20. The answer is D *[Ch 1 II B 1 a (3)]*
Drugs that are orally administered will have variable rates of absorption. Compliance is not ensured, and irritation of the mucosal surfaces can occur with some drugs (e.g., nonsteroidal anti-inflammatory drugs). The oral route of administration is considered to be a relatively safe route. First-pass metabolism results when hepatic metabolism occurs before the drug reaches its site of action.

21. The answer is A *[Ch 11 V B 2, 4]*
Tamoxifen, an antiestrogen, shows a favorable response rate in both estrogen receptor-rich and estrogen receptor-poor breast carcinoma, but a more favorable response occurs in the receptor-rich variant. Tamoxifen is not indicated for the treatment of testicular cancer, ovarian cancer, cervical cancer, and Kaposi's sarcoma.

22. The answer is E *[Ch 13 II D 5 b]*
Inhibitors of the mixed-function oxygenase system include carbon monoxide, ozone, cimetidine, carbon tetrachloride, and organophosphorus insecticides. Inhibition of the microsomal enzymes causes the metabolism of certain drugs to be reduced, resulting in higher systemic levels of the drug. Thus, poisoning by any of these toxic substances might cause an increased drug effect as well as the effects of the poison itself. Phenobarbital is capable of inducing the hepatic microsomal drug-metabolizing enzyme system.

23. The answer is A *[Ch 5 I B 3 a, b]*
The most important property of the cardiac glycosides is to increase the force of myocardial contraction (positive inotropic effect). In patients with congestive heart failure, this leads to an increase in cardiac output, a decrease in cardiac filling pressures, and decreases in heart size and venous and capillary pressures. Digitalis also tends to slow the heart rate in patients with congestive heart failure; this negative chronotropic effect is the result of a decrease in sympathetic activity brought about by increased cardiac output. Digitalis also decreases conduction velocity through the atrioventricular (A-V) node; this effect is unrelated to the positive inotropic effect.

24. The answer is D *[Ch 3 V A 3, B 3, 5 a]*
The presenting symptoms of this patient are compatible with chronic use of a phenothiazine, such as triflupromazine. Patients who develop such extrapyramidal side effects often display rigidity and tremor at rest as well as sucking and smacking of the lips. Flurazepam, codeine, chloral hydrate, and carbamazepine do not produce extrapyramidal side effects.

25. The answer is E *[Ch 9 I A 1; II A 3 a–d, h, i, 6 d]*
Aspirin has analgesic, antipyretic, and anti-inflammatory actions, all of which are mediated by an inhibition of prostaglandin synthesis. Aspirin can increase mean bleeding time, and toxic doses can produce respiratory and metabolic acidosis. Excretion is increased by alkalinizing the urine. Low doses of aspirin decreases urate excretion and could produce a gout attack in predisposed patients.

26. The answer is A *[Ch 2 III B 9]*
Betaxolol is a selective β_1-adrenergic antagonist, which is available as a topical formulation for the treatment of glaucoma. Nadolol and carteolol are nonselective β blockers. Carteolol also possesses intrinsic sympathomimetic activity. Labetalol is a nonselective β blocker with selective α_1-blocking activity. Timolol is used topically for the treatment of glaucoma but is a nonselective β blocker.

27. The answer is A *[Ch 11 II B 4 c, D 4; III B 4 a, D i e (1); VI D 4 b]*
Busulfan, an alkyl sulfonate alkylating agent, is a myelosuppressive drug and is used to treat chronic granulocytic leukemia. Cisplatin has a mechanism of action similar to that of the alkylating agents. It is one of the most effective agents against solid tumors. Cyclophosphamide, a nitrogen mustard, is also an alkylating agent and is used to treat a variety of cancers; it is also useful as an immunosuppressant for organ transplantation. 5-Fluorouracil and methotrexate are both antimetabolites and are used to treat a number of solid tumors. 5-Fluorouracil is also used topically for certain premalignant and malignant skin cancers. Methotrexate is also used in the therapy of acute lymphoblastic leukemia in children and in the treatment of psoriasis.

28. The answer is D *[Ch 2 III]*
Synonyms abound for drugs acting on the autonomic nervous sytem. Drugs that mimic the actions of the sympathetic nervous system are called sympathomimetics or adrenergic agents. Drugs with the opposite effect are known as sympathetic antagonists, sympatholytics, adrenergic blocking agents, and antiadrenergic agents, while subsets of this class are called α blockers and β blockers. Drugs that mimic the actions of the parasympathetic nervous system and the effects of acetylcholine are called parasympathetic, parasympathomimetic, cholinomimetic, or cholinergic agents. Drugs that mimic atropine are known as antimuscarinic agents. To complicate the terminology further, the catecholamines are not cholinergic but adrenergic, so termed because epinephrine was originally called adrenalin and norepinephrine was originally called noradrenalin.

29. The answer is B *[Ch 7 II A; J; Table 7-1; Ch 9 II B 6 a, c, C 3; IV E 3, 5, 6; Ch 12 II A 7 c]*
Aspirin does not affect the leukocyte count, whereas phenylbutazone and sulfonamides can cause agranulocytosis. Aspirin, phenylbutazone, and sulfamethoxazole all are highly protein bound, affect platelet function, and interact with warfarin. They are all capable of producing hypersensitivity reactions.

30. The answer is B *[Ch 3 III A 1, 2, C 1, E, F 1 a, 2 a]*
Barbiturates are the drugs of choice for infantile tonic–clonic seizures. It should be noted, however, that they are no longer the treatment of choice for the prophylactic control of generalized seizure states. The various benzodiazepines differ in the types of seizures that they control. Diazepam, given intravenously, is the drug of choice for status epilepticus in adults, but not in children. Phenytoin and carbamazepine are also used for tonic–clonic seizures, but neither of these agents would be the treatment of choice in the situation described. Valproate is more useful for absence seizures, although it is also used for grand mal seizures.

31. The answer is C *[Ch 1 III D 6]*
The therapeutic index (TI) is a measure that is used in evaluating the safety and usefulness of a drug. The formula for the TI is:

$$TI = \frac{LD_{50}}{ED_{50}}$$

where LD_{50} is the minimum dose that is **lethal** for 50% of the population, and ED_{50} is the minimum dose that is **effective** for 50% of the population. Therapeutically, the standard margin of safety has been considered more useful because the numerator is more restrictive. The standard margin of safety $[(LD_1/ED_{99}) - 1 \times 100]$ shows how much the dose that is effective for 99% of the population must be increased to be toxic for 1% of the population.

32. The answer is D *[Ch 5 I B 6 e]*
The patient described in the question presents with symptoms that are consistent with the symptoms of digoxin toxicity (i.e., anorexia, nausea, color vision changes). When the serum digoxin level rises above 2 ng/ml, therapy with the glycoside should be discontinued until the level falls below this concentration.

33. The answer is E *[Ch 2 III A 4]*
Ergot alkaloids are tryptaminergic and dopaminergic agonists; in addition, they interact at α-adrenergic receptors. Their chemical structure resembles lysergic acid diethylamide, and thus, central nervous system stimulation can occur. They also directly stimulate smooth muscle. Ergot alkaloids are weak α blockers and partial α agonists; they would not be blocked by propranolol, which is a nonselective β blocker.

34. The answer is B *[Ch 7 III A 2, B 1, 3, C 1–3]*
Erythropoietin is not intended for patients needing immediate correction of severe anemia. By stimulating erythroid progenitor cells, it elevates or maintains red blood cell levels, decreasing the need for transfusions. It must be administered parenterally because peptidases inactivate it in the gastrointestinal tract. Erythropoietin's pharmacokinetics is not affected by dialysis.

35. The answer is A *[Ch 12 II B 2 f (7), 3 i (3) (b), 5 d, C 5 d, G 5 c, d]*
Ceftazidime, a third-generation cephalosporin, has greater activity against *Pseudomonas aeruginosa* than other third-generation cephalosporins. Tobramycin is an aminoglycoside with excellent activity against *P. aeruginosa*. Both agents are administered parenterally. Aztreonam is also administered parenterally and is effective against gram-negative pathogens but has poor activity against gram-positive cocci and anaerobic bacteria. Amoxicillin and clavulanate have no activity against *P. aeruginosa*. Ciprofloxacin is highly active against bacteria that cause enteritis and against staphylococci. It is somewhat less active against *P. aeruginosa* but is indicated for both complicated and uncomplicated urinary tract infections.

36. The answer is D *[Ch 4 II C 2]*
Procaine is nonaddictive and causes minimal systemic toxicity and no local irritation. It is rapidly metabolized and has a short duration of action. It is not active topically.

37. The answer is D *[Ch 2 IV F, G]*
Metoclopramide, a parasympathetic (cholinergic) agonist, has proved useful for the treatment of delayed gastric emptying (gastroparesis) due to diabetes, for gastroesophageal reflux disease, and as an antiemetic in vomiting induced by certain types of radiation and cancer chemotherapy. Because it is a parasympathetic drug, it could exacerbate peptic ulcer disease.

38 and 39. The answers are: 38-A *[Ch 11 IV C 5 b (5)]*, **39-C** *[Ch 9 IV A 3 a, E 2]*
Vincristine is far superior to vinblastine in the treatment of lymphocytic leukemia. When combined with prednisone, it is the treatment of choice for inducing remission in acute lymphoblastic leukemia in children.
    Rapid lympholysis produces large quantities of uric acid via nucleic acid release and catabolism. The xanthine oxidase inhibitor allopurinol is given because it inhibits uric acid formation and, thus, is effective in preventing acute gouty arthritis attacks during antineoplastic therapy. Because allopurinol is an inhibitor of xanthine oxidase, it increases the renal excretion of xanthine and hypoxanthine. Since allopurinol is an analog of hypoxanthine, it inhibits the metabolism of purines, not pyrimidines.

40. The answer is E *[Ch 11 V B 2, 4]*
Tamoxifen is a nonsteroidal antiestrogen that competes with estrogen for the cytoplasmic estrogen receptor. Tumors with many estrogen receptors are frequently dependent on estrogen for cell proliferation. Thus, tamoxifen blocks the growth of such tumors. Bleomycin, mitomycin, and vinblastine are natural products that have little activity against breast carcinomas. Decarbazine is a triazene alkylating agent that is effective against melanomas but is not effective against breast carcinomas.

41. The answer is B *[Ch 2 V E 1 a, 2]*
Diisopropyl fluorophosphate is an irreversible cholinesterase inhibitor, which increases acetylcholine levels. Increased lacrimation, salivation, muscle twitching and weakness are cholinergic (cholinomimetic) effects; increased bronchodilation is not.

42. The answer is D *[Ch 9 II A 3 h, C 7, D 6, J 7 a, b, K 5]*
Phenylbutazone, by directly affecting the renal tubules, can cause significant salt and water retention, leading to edema. Phenylbutazone can also cause agranulocytosis or aplastic anemia. Although indomethacin also can cause blood dyscrasias, its salt-retaining properties are much less significant than those occurring with phenylbutazone. The properties of sulindac are similar to those of indomethacin. Aspirin would not affect the leukocyte count or cause edema. Gastrointestinal symptoms and elevated hepatic transaminases are the most frequent adverse effects associated with diclofenac use.

43. The answer is D *[Ch 3 VII B 3 g (3)]*
Of the agents listed in the question, monoamine oxidase (MAO) inhibitors should not be used with tricyclic antidepressants: Their interaction has produced hyperpyrexia, hypertension, convulsions, and coma. The underlying mechanism is unknown; however, MAO inhibitors interfere with various drug-metabolizing enzymes and can, therefore, interact with a number of drugs. Most important is the potential for inducing hypertensive crises with certain amines or their precursors, including those present in some foods.

44. The answer is E *[Ch 12 IV B 3 b, c, 4 b]*
Isoniazid is the most widely used agent in the treatment of tuberculosis. To prevent the development of mycobacterial resistance, isoniazid is used in conjunction with rifampin or other agents in the treatment of active disease. It can be used alone as prophylaxis in persons who have converted from tuberculin-negative to tuberculin-positive and also in close contacts of patients who have newly diagnosed active disease. Isoniazid is not effective against atypical mycobacteria. Its metabolism depends in part on genetically determined acetyl transferase activity. Patients who are fast acetylators will have lower concentrations of unchanged or free isoniazid.

45. The answer is E *[Ch 5 II E 1 d; Table 5-5]*
Propranolol is used to control supraventricular tachyarrhythmias, including atrial fibrillation, atrial flutter, and paroxysmal supraventricular tachycardia. It is useful in ventricular arrhythmias that are due to enhanced adrenergic stimulation (e.g., from emotional stress). It is also sometimes used to abolish digitalis-induced ventricular arrhythmias, but it can cause conduction problems, resulting in A-V dissociation. Propranolol administration can exacerbate congestive heart failure, asthma, and chronic obstructive pulmonary disease.

46. The answer is A *[Ch 2 I D 2]*
All of the statements regarding receptors are true except that nonselective β-receptor blocking agents, such as propranolol and timolol, are currently available. Those drugs that act principally on β_1 receptors produce cardiac effects, while those acting on β_2 receptors produce minimal cardiac effects but possess significant smooth muscle (e.g., bronchiolar) relaxant activity. Alpha$_1$ receptors are found at postsynaptic effector sites, while α_2 receptors mediate presynaptic feedback inhibition.

47. The answer is A *[Ch 4 II C 2–4, 8, 9]*
Lidocaine is an amide and, like mepivacaine, is metabolized in the liver. Procaine is rapidly metabolized by pseudocholinesterase and is short-acting. It has no topical activity and is given parenterally. Tetracaine is the most frequently used spinal anesthetic agent. Bupivacaine is an amide local anesthetic, is more potent and has a longer duration of action than mepivacaine, and can last more than 24 hours in some situations.

48. The answer is D *[Ch 7 IV B; Table 7-1]*
Both phenylbutazone and aspirin affect platelet aggregation. These two drugs **increase** the response to oral anticoagulants, which can cause severe hemorrhage. Phenylbutazone, in addition, can displace warfarin from albumin, which increases the warfarin blood level. Glutethimide, like phenobarbital and other barbiturates, induces the drug microsomal metabolizing system. This **decreases** the response to oral anticoagulants, so that higher doses are required to produce the desired anticoagulant effect. Cimetidine inhibits the drug microsomal metabolizing system, increasing blood levels of oral anticoagulants.

49. The answer is D *[Ch 2 VIII A]*
Both competitive and noncompetitive neuromuscular blocking agents interact with cholinergic receptors to produce neuromuscular blockade. Competitive agents, such as tubocurarine, act at the skeletal muscle cholinergic receptor in a reversible fashion. Succinylcholine, however, acts at this site in a more complex manner, and metabolism is required for the termination of its action.

50. The answer is D *[Ch 11 III B 4 d]*
Methotrexate is considered by some rheumatologists to be "first-line" therapy for the treatment of rheumatoid arthritis. The drug has also been used in the treatment of psoriasis. Methotrexate is used in combination with a number of agents for a variety of cancers.

51. The answer is A *[Ch 12 II B 2 e (3) (b), 3 i (1) (b), C 3 b (3), F 3 a (2), G 4 d]*
In a patient with renal disease, any antibiotic that is renally excreted should be administered with caution. Erythromycin is concentrated in the liver and is excreted primarily in bile and feces and, thus, may be useful in the treatment of infections in renally compromised patients. Tobramycin, piperacilin, cefazolin, and norfloxacin are principally excreted via the kidney.

52. The answer is B *[Ch 8 V A f (2), (3)]*
Both terfenadine and astemizole lack significant central nervous system sedating effects. Both agents are effective for seasonal rhinitis, and both agents are administered orally. Astemizole has a half-life of 9 days. Because astemizole is extremely long-acting, adverse effects may be a problem. Terfenadine lacks significant adverse anticholinergic effects.

53. The answer is A *[Ch 1 III D 5 c]*
Potentiation occurs if a drug lacking an effect of its own increases the effect of a second, active drug. If two drugs with the same effect, when given together, produce an effect that is equal in magnitude to the sum of the effects when the drugs are given individually, the effects of the two drugs are additive. If two drugs with the same effect, when given together, produce an effect that is greater in magnitude than the sum of the effects when the drugs are given individually, synergism has occurred. If two drugs with the same effect, when given together, produce an effect that is less than the combined effect of the two drugs individually, antagonism has occurred.

54. The answer is E *[Ch 10 III D 4 c (1), (3), d (1), 5 a, b (2) (b), 7 c]*
Estrogen therapy is given to women with failure of ovarian development (dysgenesis) that may result in dwarfism due to hypopituitarism. In this situation, estrogen, given in combination with an androgen for a growth spurt, can emulate endogenous release. All of the other medical benefits are correctly matched with replacement hormones or their antagonists.

55. The answer is C *[Ch 5 IV I 1 b–d, f (1) (b); Ch 8 V C 2 c]*
Enalopril decreases the secretion of aldosterone, not renin, by inhibiting the production of angiotensin II. In addition, vasoconstrictor properties associated with angiotensin II are inhibited. Enalopril is a specific competitive inhibitor of peptidyl dipeptidase (angiotensin-converting enzyme), the enzyme that converts angiotensin I to angiotensin II. Enalopril is more potent and has a longer duration of action than captopril.

56. The answer is D *[Ch 12 II A 5 a (1)]*
The major indication for the use of sulfa drugs such as trimethoprim-sulfamethoxazole is the treatment of acute uncomplicated urinary tract infections. Carbenicilin and gentamicin represent broad-spectrum therapy, which is unnecessary for the treatment of an uncomplicated cystitis. Aztreonam, a monobactam, is often substituted for parenteral aminoglycoside therapy and would not be used for the treatment of uncomplicated cystitis.

57. The answer is C *[Ch 2 VIII B 4 d, C 2, 3]*
Succinylcholine and decamethonium are depolarizing, not competitive, agents. The competitive blocking agents gallamine and pipercuronium are excreted via the kidney and, therefore, would be contraindicated in patients with renal failure. Atracurium, on the other hand, can be used in patients with renal failure since it does not rely on the kidney for excretion but is largely dependent on a nonenzymatic process known as Hoffmann elimination.

58. The answer is C *[Ch 14 II B 3 a–d]*
Dimercaprol is useful in the treatment of mercury poisoning, as well as in poisoning by arsenic, antimony, gold, and lead. Penicillamine is an orally effective treatment for copper and lead poisoning. Calcium disodium EDTA ($CaNa_2EDTA$) is useful in the treatment of lead, iron, copper, and zinc poisoning, but not in arsenic poisoning. Deferoxamine exhibits a high affinity for the ferric ion and is used in iron poisoning.

59. The answer is A *[Ch 10 III G 3 d (2)]*
Leukocyte migration is suppressed, not stimulated, by glucocorticoids. This effect is thought to be one component of the overall anti-inflammatory effect of corticosteroids. Pharmacologic doses of glucocorticoids can result in stabilization of lysosomal membranes, reduced activity of fibroblasts, reversal of a histamine-stimulated increase in capillary permeability, and inhibited antibody synthesis—all of the other effects listed in the question.

60. The answer is B *[Ch 9 III B 5 c (4), 6 e]*
Auranofin is a recently approved analog of gold thioglucose that can be administered orally. Although it may be less effective than injectable gold for the treatment of arthritis, it is less toxic than injectable gold. There is a high incidence of diarrhea, but this is often self-limiting and rarely requires discontinuation of therapy. Cutaneous reactions, mucosal lesions, eosinophilia, and proteinuria are other common side effects.

61. The answer is C *[Ch 11 III C 1 g (4)]*
Attempts to inhibit the degradation of 6-mercaptopurine (and thus enhance its effects) led to the development of the xanthine oxidase inhibitor, allopurinol. Allopurinal blocks not only the metabolism of 6-mercaptopurine but also the formation of uric acid from hypoxanthine and xanthine. Therefore, allopurinol can inhibit the hyperuricemia and hyperuricosuria that occurs with 6-mercaptopurine therapy. Because allopurinol prevents the inactivation of 6-mercaptopurine, the dose of 6-mercaptopurine must be reduced when a patient is also given allopurinol.

62. The answer is D *[Ch 11 III D 1 e (4)]*
The patient described in the question has actinic keratoses—premalignant skin lesions that develop most often in fair-skinned persons who are chronically exposed to sunlight. 5-Fluorouracil, an antimetabolite type of antineoplastic agent, has proved very successful in treating actinic keratoses, although the lesions are apt to recur. The other drugs listed in the question are also antineoplastic agents, but they are used parenterally, and not for this form of cancer.

63. The answer is E *[Ch 6 VIII C 4; Ch 11 VI D 5; Ch 13 II E 3]*
The antitumor agent cisplatin causes severe nephrotoxicity if it is given without concomitant hydration or a diuretic. The osmotic diuretic mannitol is most commonly employed to reduce this side effect. Mannitol is also useful prophylactically to reduce the risk of acute renal failure in conditions such as cardiovascular operations and severe trauma. Ethacrynic acid, mercaptomerin, acetazolamide, and chlorothiazide are not as effective as mannitol in these situations.

64. The answer is B *[Ch 5 I B 6 a–e]*
Digitalis glycosides have a low margin of safety. In most patients, the lethal dose is likely to be only 5–10 times the minimal effective dose. Intoxication can be precipitated by depletion of K^+, not Na^+. The hypokalemia is often the result of diuretic therapy but can also be the result of protracted vomiting or diarrhea. Other signs of toxicity include abnormal color perception and, more importantly, ventricular tachycardia.

65. The answer is C *[Ch 3 IX E 6; Ch 14 III B]*
Syrup of ipecac should not be used if central nervous system integrity is compromised. A physiologic antagonist (direct respiratory stimulant) is not useful and could induce convulsions. A pharmacologic antagonist (e.g., naltrexone) is the drug of choice. Gastric lavage is not indicated, while use of a cathartic is best reserved for hydrocarbons and enteric-coated tablets.

66. The answer is C *[Ch 2 VIII A 1, D 2 c]*
Because succinylcholine can depolarize cholinergic skeletal muscle receptors, it affects the extraocular muscles and, therefore, can cause an increase in intraocular pressure. This effect is contraindicated in glaucoma.

67. The answer is B *[Ch 3 VII B 5 b]*
Fluoxetine selectively inhibits serotonin reuptake in the central nervous system and produces little effect on central norepinephrine or dopamine function. It is used to treat endogenous depression and obsessive–compulsive disorder. Bupropion weakly blocks dopamine reuptake. Tranylcypromine and deprenyl work by inhibiting monoamine oxidase. Amitriptyline inactivates the reuptake of amines after release from the presynaptic neuron.

68. The answer is B *[Ch 12 II B 2 f (1) (a) (i), (5), (6), C 5 c, 6 b (1), G 5 d]*
The diabetic patient described in the question most likely has pneumococcal pneumonia for which the drug of first choice would be penicillin G. Gentamicin is not active against pneumococcal pneumonia, while carbenicillin and ampicillin, although effective, are not the drugs of first choice. Ciprofloxacin has only modest activity against many streptococci.

69. The answer is C *[Ch 5 II B 1 f (3), 2 f (4) (c), (5), 3 d (2), C 1 f, D 2]*
All of the listed adverse effects are paired correctly with their respective therapeutic agents except that a syndrome resembling systemic lupus erythematosus can occur with procainamide, not lidocaine. This syndrome is reversible on discontinuation of therapy but can develop in as many as 30% of patients taking procainamide for long periods of time.

70. The answer is D *[Ch 12 III B 5 c (2)]*
Amphotericin B is effective in the treatment of acute pulmonary coccidioidomycosis. The other agents listed would be ineffective. Griseofulvin is used for mycotic diseases of the skin, hair, and nails. Flucytosine is used for systemic infections caused by *Candida albicans* or *Cryptococcus meningitidis*. Penicillin G has no antifungal activity. Pentamidine is most useful for the prophylaxis and treatment of *Pneumocystis carinii* pneumonia. It has no antifungal activity.

71. The answer is B *[Ch 14 II B 2 d (3)]*
Nickel is sensitizing and can cause a pruritic dermatitis. Nickel is often used in inexpensive jewelry and as components of wearing apparel, such as the buckles on bra or slip straps. Of all the metals listed in the question, nickel is the most likely to cause a contact dermatitis.

72. The answer is B *[Ch 9 IV E 4 b]*
Acute attacks of gout occur more frequently during initial therapy with allopurinol. This effect may be explained by the active dissolution of microcrystalline deposits of sodium urate (tophi) in subcutaneous tissue, which results in brief episodes of hyperuricemia and crystal deposition in joints. Simultaneous administration of colchicine decreases the frequency of these attacks.

73. The answer is B *[Ch 12 III F 2–4, 7]*
Fluconazole is highly bioavailable. It penetrates the blood–brain barrier and is active against *Cryptococcus neoformans*. It is less toxic than amphotericin B and flucytosine, but its mechanism of action is similar to most antifungal agents. It inhibits cytochrome P-450–dependent enzymes, blocking the synthesis of ergosterol.

74. The answer is E *[Ch 10 III G 3 i]*
Because corticosteroids alter the mucosal defense mechanisms, peptic ulceration can result from prolonged therapy. The immunosuppressive effects of corticosteroids increase susceptibility to infection. Sudden withdrawal of corticosteroids can result in signs of adrenal insufficiency. The patient may have to be protected during stressful situations for 1 year or more after withdrawal. Hyperglycemia can result from prolonged therapy.

75. The answer is D *[Ch 5 II B 1 c, f]*
Quinidine reduces the maximal rate of rise ($\dot{V}_{max}$) of depolarization during phase 0. It increases the effective refractory period but decreases automaticity and conduction velocity in ventricular tissue. Quinidine depresses myocardial contractility, and caution must, therefore, be used if quinidine is administered to patients with any degree of congestive heart failure.

76. The answer is B *[Ch 7 IV C 2 a]*
Streptokinase on intravenous administration reduces blood pressure, total peripheral resistance, and cardiac afterload, which can result in hypotension. All of the other statements about this thrombolytic agent are correct. Streptokinase is a protein without known enzymatic activity that is obtained from group C β-hemolytic streptococci. Its interaction with a proactivator of plasminogen results in a proteolytic activity that converts plasminogen to plasmin, which is then capable of hydrolyzing fibrin clots. This property is the basis for the use of streptokinase in treating acute pulmonary embolism. Gastrointestinal bleeding occurs in 5%–10% of patients.

77. The answer is C *[Ch 5 IV G 1]*
Clonidine, by stimulating presynaptic α_2 receptors in the vasomotor center of the brain, decreases sympathetic outflow to the peripheral vessels. Both guanethidine and reserpine are agents that block postganglionic adrenergic neurons. Prazosin is a selective postsynaptic α_1-adrenergic receptor blocker. Minoxidil directly relaxes anteriolar smooth muscle.

78. The answer is D *[Ch 2 II B 2 g; Ch 5 IV E 4 b (1); Ch 10 III G 3; IV E, I 1 c; V]*
The oral hypoglycemic agent tolbutamide decreases blood glucose concentrations, while the antihypertensive agent diazoxide increases them. Insulin decreases blood glucose concentrations, while cortisol, glucagon, and isoproterenol all increase blood glucose concentrations. Propranolol decreases blood sugar.

79. The answer is C *[Ch 7 IV B 6 a–c; Table 7-1]*
All of the drugs or adverse effects are correctly matched with the causes or results listed except the purple toe syndrome, which is caused by cholesterol emboli from athermatous plaques, following bleeding into the plaque. It can occur 3–8 weeks after starting warfarin therapy.

80. The answer is B *[Ch 2 VI B]*
Scopolamine is a competitive muscarinic blocker and, therefore, most closely resembles atropine in its mechanism of action. It is more potent than atropine in decreasing bronchial, salivary, and sweat gland secretions, in its sedative effect, and in producing mydriasis and cycloplegia. It is less potent than atropine in its effects on the heart, bronchial muscle, and intestines.

81–85. The answers are: 81-E *[Ch 11 VI C 4]*, **82-A** *[Ch 11 II C 3 c]*, **83-C** *[Ch 11 II E 4]*, **84-D** *[Ch 11 III B 4 b]*, **85-B** *[Ch 11 II B 4 c (2)]*
Mitotane is a derivative of the insecticide DDT that shows selective activity against cells of the adrenal cortex, both normal and neoplastic. It is, therefore, used in the management of inoperable adrenal carcinoma.
    Carmustine, a nitrosourea, is lipid-soluble and crosses the blood–brain barrier. Thus, it is useful in treating brain tumors.
    Dacarbazine, an alkylating agent, is one of the most useful drugs for malignant melanoma.
    Methotrexate, a folic acid analog, can be given orally or parenterally. It has proved useful for the treatment of severe psoriasis, a nonmalignant condition characterized by overproliferation of epidermal cells.
    Cyclophosphamide is a nitrogen mustard that can be given orally as well as parenterally. Because of its potent immunosuppressant properties, it is used to control rejection of transplanted organs.

86–89. The answers are: 86-E *[Ch 9 III C 1 a (1)]*, **87-D** *[Ch 9 III C 3 a]*, **88-B** *[Ch 9 III C 4 b]*, **89-A** *[Ch 9 III B 5 a]*
Disease-modifying antirheumatic drugs (DMARDs) are used in conjunction with nonsteroidal anti-inflammatory drugs (NSAIDs) to modify immunologic response.
    Azathioprine and cyclophosphamide have been used to treat refractory rheumatoid arthritis. Azathioprine rarely causes severe toxicity with the dosage used for rheumatoid arthritis. Cyclophosphamide because of its severe adverse effects is reserved for life-threatening rheumatoid vasculitis. Penicillamine is highly toxic, though effective in high doses in patients with refractory rheumatoid arthritis.
    The antimalarial drug hydroxychloroquine can produce irreversible retinal damage. Thus, an ophthalmic examination prior to therapy and every 3 months after is recommended.
    Cutaneous reactions, including exfoliative dermatitis and lesions of the mucous membrane are often observed with gold thiomalate but rarely with aurothioglucose.

90–94. The answers are: 90-B *[Ch 3 II A 5 g; Table 7-1]*, **91-A** *[Ch 13 II B 1 a]*, **92-C** *[Ch 13 II D 4 a]*, **93-B** *[Ch 13 II D 5]*, **94-D** *[Ch 3 V B 3 b (9)]*
Most drug interactions involving the barbiturates result from induction of hepatic microsomal enzymes by the barbiturate; this causes accelerated metabolism of the other drug (e.g., warfarin, digitoxin, corticosteroids, and β blockers, to name only a few). However, other mechanisms can also be involved. Thus, a barbiturate plus another central nervous system depressant (e.g., a phenothiazine, ethanol, or an antihistamine) can cause marked depression. Tranylcypromine is an inhibitor of monoamine oxidase, a nonmicrosomal enzyme, and this can retard the metabolism of a barbiturate. Dextran solutions are incompatible with various drugs, including barbiturates. Barbiturates can also interfere with the absorption of some drugs (e.g., dicumarol, griseofulvin), and some barbiturates compete with other drugs (e.g., aspirin) for plasma protein binding sites.

95–98. The answers are: 95-B *[Ch 8 V C 2]*, **96-D** *[Ch 8 IV C 3 a]*, **97-A** *[Ch 9 II G 3 d (4)]*, **98-C** *[Ch 8 V D 1 a, 2]*
Captopril belongs to the class of drugs known as angiotensin-converting enzyme (ACE) inhibitors because they inhibit peptidyl dipeptidase, the ACE that normally converts angiotensin I to angiotensin II. The autacoid angiotensin II is a potent vasoconstrictor that raises blood pressure, and thus, ACE inhibitors are used clinically to treat hypertension.

Hydralazine inhibits thromboxane synthetase, the enzyme involved in the formation of thromboxanes from prostaglandin H. Thromboxane A_2 is, like angiotensin II, a potent vasoconstrictor, and hydralazine is used clinically as an antihypertensive vasodilator.

Ibuprofen is a nonsteroidal anti-inflammatory drug (NSAID). These agents act by inhibiting cyclooxygenase, and thus, they inhibit the synthesis of both prostaglandins and thromboxanes. Several prostaglandins serve as mediators of the inflammatory response. Some NSAIDs inhibit 15-lipoxygenase as well as cyclooxygenase, and aspirin, by inhibiting platelet cyclooxygenase, also interrupts the thromboxane synthetase pathway.

Prednisolone and other glucocorticoids inhibit phospholipase in a number of tissues, thereby blocking all eicosanoid formation in these tissues. Thus, glucocorticoids block the synthesis of prostaglandins, leukotrienes, and thromboxanes, which probably explains their potent anti-inflammatory effects. Moreover, since leukotrienes play a role in hypersensitivity reactions, their suppression may explain the efficacy of glucocorticoids in allergic disorders.

99–102. The answers are: 99-E *[Ch 2 IV B 1 b]*, **100-C** *[Ch 2 V E 1 a]*, **101-A** *[Ch 2 II E 1]*, **102-D** *[Ch 2 V B]*
Methacholine, because of the addition of the β-methyl group, is purely muscarinic in action. Diisopropyl fluorophosphate is an irreversible organophosphate cholinesterase inhibitor. Phenylephrine, though less potent, resembles norepinephrine in its cardiovascular effects. Neostigmine, besides being a reversible cholinesterase inhibitor, also stimulates nicotinic receptors.

103–105. The answers are: 103-E *[Ch 11 IV B 4 b]*, **104-C** *[Ch 11 III D 2 b]*, **105-D** *[Ch 11 IV C 2 b]*
Mitomycin is both a natural product and an alkylating agent. Isolated from a *Streptomyces* species, mitomycin C is reduced by a reduced nicotinamide adenine dinucleotide phosphate (NADPH)–dependent reductase and alkylates DNA.

Cytarabine inhibits DNA polymerase and, thus, kills cells in S phase. Cytarabine nucleotides can be incorporated into DNA and RNA, but the significance of this is not known.

Vincristine, a natural product, is an M-phase–specific agent, blocking proliferating cells as they enter metaphase.

106–110. The answers are: 106-B *[Ch 6 VII A]*, **107-C** *[Ch 6 IX B 1 a]*, **108-B** *[Ch 6 VI A 1, 2]*, **109-A** *[Ch 6 IV A 1]*, **110-E** *[Ch 6 IX A 1 a]*
Ethacrynic acid inhibits electrolyte reabsorption in the ascending limb of the loop of Henle, producing an increased urinary excretion of Na^+, Cl^-, and K^+.

Spironolactone is a competitive antagonist of the mineralocorticoid aldosterone. It competes for the aldosterone receptor site in the distal convoluted tubule. It interferes with the aldosterone-mediated Na^+–K^+ exchange, increasing Na^+ loss at the distal tubular site while decreasing K^+ loss.

Chlorothiazide inhibits Cl^- reabsorption in the ascending limb of the loop of Henle in addition to inhibiting Cl^- reabsorption in other areas of the nephron. The thiazides also can inhibit carbonic anhydrase, but this is not the major mechanism of action.

Acetazolamide is a carbonic anhydrase inhibitor. It inhibits this enzyme at both the proximal and distal convoluted tubule. Carbon dioxide reabsorption from the glomerular filtrate is suppressed, and HCO_3^- excretion is increased. Due to a decrease in the reabsorption of Na^+ in exchange for H^+, the Na^+–K^+ exchange in the distal convoluted tubule increases. The result is an alkaline urine.

Triamterene inhibits active Na^+ reabsorption and, thus, increases the excretion of Na^+ and Cl^-. There is a net change in the electrogenic force across tubular membranes, which reduces the net driving force for K^+ secretion, resulting in the decreased excretion of K^+. The major site of action is the distal nephron.

111–114. The answers are: 111-D *[Ch 12 II D 5 b]*, **112-E** *[Ch 12 IV C 5 a]*, **113-A** *[Ch 12 II F 3 b, 4 b]*, **114-B** *[Ch 12 II C 3 a, 6 b, 8]*
Tetracyclines (e.g., demeclocycline) are effective in the treatment of *Chlamydia* infections. Agents such as demeclocycline can produce a severe phototoxic skin reaction.

Rifampin, which is used in combination with isoniazid and ethambutol for the treatment of tuberculosis, may cause urine, sweat, tears, and contact lenses to have a harmless orange color.

Clindamycin is the drug of first choice for *Bacteroides fragilis* infections. It can produce pseudomembranous colitis as an untoward effect.

The aminoglycosides (e.g., gentamicin) are polycations, which accounts for their pharmacokinetic properties, including poor oral absorption. These agents have a predilection for causing both ototoxicity and nephrotoxicity.

115–117. The answers are: 115-A *[Ch 9 II G 3 b]*, **116-D** *[Ch 9 II G 6 b (3)]*, **117-E** *[Ch 9 II G 7 b (2)]*
Ibuprofen is equal to aspirin in its anti-inflammatory effect but is a more effective analgesic than aspirin or acetaminophen. Ketoprofen exhibits a profile similar to ibuprofen, but if used concurrently with methotrexate, the patient can develop life-threatening methotrexate hepatotoxicity.

Flubiprofen is the only nonsteroidal anti-inflammatory drug approved for ophthalmic use. It decreases meiosis without affecting intraocular pressure.

Index